THE CLINICAL INTERVIEW USING DSM-IV-TR

Volume 1: Fundamentals

THE CLINICAL INTERVIEW USING DSM-IV-TR

Volume 1: Fundamentals

Ekkehard Othmer, M.D., Ph.D.
Sieglinde C. Othmer, Ph.D.

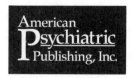

Washington, DC
London, England

Copyright © 2002 Ekkehard Othmer and Sieglinde C. Othmer
ALL RIGHTS RESERVED

Manufactured in the United States of America on acid-free paper
06   05   04   03   02   5   4   3   2   1
First Edition

American Psychiatric Publishing, Inc.
1400 K Street, N.W.
Washington, DC   20005
www.appi.org

Library of Congress Cataloging-in-Publication Data
Othmer, Ekkehard.
    The clinical interview using DSM-IV-TR   /   Ekkehard Othmer, Sieglinde
C. Othmer.— 1st ed.
        p.   cm.
    Includes bibliographical references and index.
    Contents: v. 1. Fundamentals — v. 2. The difficult patient.
    Vol. 1: ISBN 1-58562-050-5 (alk. paper; hardcover) — ISBN 1-58562-051-3
(alk. paper; softcover)
    1. Interviewing in psychiatry. 2. Mental illness—Diagnosis. 3. Diagnostic and
statistical manual of mental disorders. I. Title: DSM-IV-TR. II. Othmer, Sieglinde C.
III. Diagnostic and statistical manual of mental disorders. 4th ed., text revision.
IV. Title.
    [DNLM: 1. Interview, Psychological. 2. Mental Disorders—diagnosis.
3. Psychiatric Status Rating Scales.   WM 141 O87cb 2002]
RC480.7.O744 2002
616.89′075—dc21

                                                                                    2001041373

British Library Cataloguing in Publication Data
A CIP record is available from the British Library.

To our children

Konstantin,
Johann Philipp,
Julia Christie

CONTENTS

CHAPTER 3
STRATEGIES TO GET INFORMATION: TECHNIQUES . . . 45

CHAPTER 4
THREE METHODS TO ASSESS MENTAL STATUS 101

CHAPTER 5
TESTING. 169

LIST OF FIGURES

LIST OF TABLES

ABOUT THE AUTHORS

(Who are married to each other)

Ekkehard Othmer, M.D., Ph.D., is Adjunct Professor of Psychiatry at the University of Kansas Medical Center and Medical Director of Picture Hills Psychiatric Center in Kansas City. He is a Diplomate of the American Board of Psychiatry and Neurology and one of its examiners. He is a fellow of the American Psychiatric Association and a member of the Society of Biological Psychiatry. He was a member of the psychiatric hospital surveyor panel of the Health Care Financing Administration (HCFA) of the Department of Health and Human Services, Baltimore, Maryland. Dr. Othmer graduated from the Department of Psychology (Ph.D.) and the Medical School (M.D.) of the University of Hamburg and trained in psychoanalysis at the Psychoanalytical Institute in Hamburg, Germany. He completed his residency in psychiatry at Renard Hospital, Washington University Medical School in St. Louis, Missouri.

Sieglinde C. Othmer, Ph.D., studied Romance languages at the Sorbonne in Paris, France, and history at the Social Sciences Department of the University of Hamburg, Germany. She earned her doctorate in the social sciences at the University of Hamburg. Her thesis on the expansion of human rights in Europe in the prerevolution era was selected for publication as a book by the Berlin Historical Commission at the Friedrich-Meinecke Institut of the Free University of Berlin, Germany. She completed a postdoctoral fellowship in genetics at Renard Hospital, Department of Psychiatry at Washington University, St. Louis, Missouri. As Research Assistant Professor, she conducted investigational drug studies at the University of Kansas Medical School, Department of Psychiatry, Kansas City, Kansas.

Foreword to the Second Edition

This edition of *The Clinical Interview Using DSM-IV, Volume 1: Fundamentals* arrives at just the right moment, with the publication of DSM-IV. DSM-IV provides text and criteria for currently recognized psychiatric disorders; this book provides interviewing techniques to determine, assess, and implement these criteria. The Othmers illustrate how to approach patients in a way that illuminates the diagnostic criteria and points the way toward treatment. With case examples drawn directly from their clinical work, the Othmers lead clinicians through the steps that will help them to include or exclude appropriate DSM-IV categories in their differential diagnoses, and engage the patient to help in this process.

This text will benefit even the experienced clinician, but it is most critical reading for young psychiatrists, clinical psychologists, social workers, and other mental health professionals. It shows students the full complexity of the interview process. By the time the reader encounters the final chapters—detailed interviews showing the interviewer's process of diagnostic inclusion and exclusion—the reader has a highly developed understanding of the four components advocated by the Othmers: rapport, techniques to gather information, mental status assessment, and diagnostic decision making.

This book helps teach DSM-IV in a way that usefully illustrates the diagnostic criteria. It sets the standard for clinical, diagnostic interviewing. Superb teachers and clinicians, the Othmers have established the classic book on how to conduct an interview.

Allen J. Frances, M.D.
Chairperson, Task Force on DSM-IV

Foreword to the First Edition

I read this book with keen interest. Not only because it has DSM-III-R in its title (I had the privilege of being in a leadership role in the development of both DSM-III and DSM-III-R) but also because I have a special interest in teaching clinical interviewing. For almost 10 years, I have been teaching a course, on the initial psychiatric interview, to the first-year residents at the New York State Psychiatric Institute. In the course a variety of patients are interviewed, each by both a resident and by me. (The resident and I alternate conducting the first interview, and sometimes one or both interviews are videotaped prior to the class.) In the discussions that follow the interview we attempt to dissect each interview to see what worked, what didn't work, and what alternative strategies either the resident or I could have used that would have made the interview more effective.

The course has always been well received as the students recognize the value of having the opportunity to observe and critically evaluate their own and my own interviewing (as well as the interviewing of other senior staff members who help teach the course). However, I have always recognized that with the limited time available (the course is only about fourteen 2-hour sessions), and with the vagaries of patient selection, countless problems encountered in clinical interviewing are never discussed. For that reason I always wished that I could recommend a suitable text that would systematically and comprehensively present the principles of clinical interviewing.

What would be the basic approach of such a text? It would recognize that the clinical interview of a psychiatric patient should have three main goals: to make a tentative psychiatric diagnosis according to DSM-III (and more recently, DSM-III-R); to understand how the patient experiences his difficulties and inner world; and, if possible, to understand what events in the patient's life might have contributed to the current difficulties. Not only are these three goals not incompatible, but they should supplement and complement each other. I am much more confident about a DSM-III-R diagnosis of a major depressive episode if, in addition to information about symptoms included in the diagnostic criteria, I also have information from my interview that the patient experiences his world as empty, his difficulties as overwhelming and his future as bleak, and that the onset of the current difficulties followed an event that was a blow to his self-esteem or reactivated a long-standing inner conflict.

There have been many books (and even more chapters in psychiatric texts) that focus on teaching clinical interviewing. However, none have seemed to me to be successful in the difficult task of integrating these three goals of the clinical interview in a book that is comprehensive, full of examples of clinical interviews (some very good, and some, for illustrative purposes, very, very bad), and fun to read. That is why, as I started to read this book I had two thoughts. The first was that this is the kind of book that I have always wished I could recommend to the residents in my interviewing course. The second was that I wished I had written such a book myself!

Robert L. Spitzer, M.D.

PREFACE TO THE DSM-IV-TR EDITION

We welcome the opportunity to update our two interview books to make their content compatible with DSM-IV-TR. We hope the update will aid the reader in becoming current with the consensus judgment of the experts consulted for DSM-IV-TR.

Our update did not change the structure of the books or the interviews; we applied the changes in DSM-IV-TR to the comments on the interviews. Some case vignettes concerning assessment of patients with homicidal tendencies have been added.

Ekkehard Othmer, M.D., Ph.D.
Sieglinde C. Othmer, Ph.D.
Kansas City, Missouri
August 2001

Preface to the Second Edition

Our readers and reviewers all urged us to keep our same basic approach in the second edition of *The Clinical Interview Using DSM-IV*. Nothing has changed in our emphasis on empathy for the patient and the four-prong approach to interviewing. We once again stress the simultaneous establishing of rapport, the application of effective interviewing techniques, the assessment of the essentials of the mental status, and the pursuit of an efficient diagnostic decision process. But there have been some major changes.

First, and most importantly, we have changed the official nomenclature. This edition has been adapted to the DSM-IV.

Second, we have divided our description of the mental status examination into two chapters: the first covers observation, conversation, and exploration and the second the subject of testing. In the chapter on testing, we offer a roster of tests responding to the DSM-IV emphasis on the assessment of cognitive functions. Furthermore, the Health Care Financing Administration (HCFA) guidelines require the routine evaluation of at least three cognitive areas for all inpatients: orientation, memory, and intelligence. The expanded testing of cognitive functions improves accuracy of diagnosis and the quality of patient care, especially in regard to our growing geriatric population. We thus offer a step-by-step guide that shows how to conduct tests, with whom, and what can be determined diagnostically from the results.

Third, the previous edition contained seven phases of interviewing. We have reduced the number of phases to five, thus simplifying the procedure and, we hope, enhancing your understanding of the stages in the interview process.

Fourth, with major changes in our health care system currently under way, it has become imperative for all mental health professionals to keep clear, accessible records. In Chapter 7, we offer an example of a write-up of a psychiatric evaluation, one that will satisfy most third-party payors' expectations. We take you through this write-up step by step and show you how it can be adapted to your own procedural and insurance needs.

And, finally, recent findings in mental health research and clinical work have been included.

We wrote this book to assemble the basic tools of psychiatric and psychological interviewing. The undertaking is most successful if we collaborate with you. We thank all health professionals who shared their views of our first edition; we've tried to incorporate their comments in this revision. We trust that this second edition will encourage additional comments and invite you once again to give us your suggestions and insights. We truly enjoy this feedback.

ACKNOWLEDGMENTS

We thank some corresponding readers of the first edition for their insightful comments: Mariano Alemany, Ph.D.; Barbara A. Bebensee, Ed.D.; Philip Coons, M.D.; Jennifer McIntyre; Louis A. Pagliaro, Pharm.D., Ph.D.; John Praylor; Philinda Smith Hutchings, Ph.D.; and Melvin S. Wise, M.D.

We thank Jane Carver and the staff at Dykes Library, University of Kansas Medical Center, Kansas City, for their capable detective work and help with the literature search.

We thank Kitty Moore, our superb editor, for her assistance with the second edition. It was her professionalism, punctuality, and humor that pulled us through. We thank Despina Papazoglou Gimbel for her gracious attention to the details of the production process.

We thank American Psychiatric Publishing and New York University Press for again collaborating on the DSM-IV-TR edition.

We are especially grateful that American Psychiatric Publishing pursued the translation of our work into Greek, Italian, Portuguese, and Spanish. Such acceptance by foreign publishers confirms that the DSM-IV-based approach is of interest beyond U.S. borders.

We thank Mr. James R. Wyrsch and Mr. W. Brian Gaddy, attorneys with Wyrsch, Hobbs, Mirakian & Lee, P.C., in Kansas City, Missouri, for reviewing the law regarding the proposed strategies applied in the cases described under assessment of homicidal tendencies.

We thank Claire Reinburg, Editorial Director at American Psychiatric Publishing, Inc., for her encouragement to make this volume compatible with DSM-IV-TR.

CHAPTER ONE

PROLOGUE: FRAMEWORK

1. **Insight- and Symptom-Oriented Interviewing**
2. **The Four Components**
3. **The Multiphasic Approach**
4. **Disorder-Specific Interviewing**

SUMMARY

Chapter 1 provides the framework and rationale of descriptive psycho-diagnostic interviewing. It compares the psychodynamic, insight-oriented interview with the descriptive, symptom-oriented interview and shows their integration.

The interview takes place in four dimensions and therefore has four components: rapport, technique, mental status, and diagnosing. This interviewing process usually progresses through five phases. When the patient's pathology interferes with this process, the interviewer has to modify the strategy of his or her approach.

▲ ▲ ▲ ▲ ▲

Insanity, even in its mildest forms, involves the greatest suffering that the physicians have to meet.

Emil Kraepelin
Lectures on Clinical Psychiatry, 2nd ed., 1906

▼ ▼ ▼ ▼ ▼

The ability to conduct a comprehensive clinical interview is the critical first step in the assessment and treatment of patients. To develop or refine an effective, flexible, and fluid interview style, the mental health professional needs to know the basic principles underlying the interview process. In this first chapter, we will explore the rationale of descriptive, diagnostic interviewing and give you the foundation for conducting a successful interview.

1. INSIGHT- AND SYMPTOM-ORIENTED INTERVIEWING

There are two interview styles used by mental health professionals: *insight-oriented (psychodynamic)* and *symptom-oriented (descriptive)*. The symptom-oriented approach is much more compatible with the descriptive approach required by DSM-IV-TR (American Psychiatric Association 2000). Both approaches have advantages and can be integrated to develop an interview style that will elicit information from the patient on many different levels. Let us compare in detail both styles, focusing on their respective underlying concepts of illness, goal, and method of interviewing.

Insight-oriented interviewing originates from the concept that deep-seated, often infantile conflicts become chronic pathogens of the mind that interfere with the patient's actions, distort his perceptions, and lead to symptoms, maladjusted behavior, and suffering.[*]

Insight-oriented interviewing attempts to uncover these unconscious conflicts and bring them to the patient's awareness, with the expectation that he may resolve them. The patient often resists this unraveling by using what have been termed "unconscious defense mechanisms."

The methods employed by the insight-oriented interviewer are as follows: he interprets the patient's free associations and dreams; he detects his anxieties; he confronts him with his interpersonal behavior toward the therapist and others; and he identifies defenses and analyzes the patient's resistance to the discussion of his conflicts. He pursues such an interview with the dual purpose of diagnosis and therapy.

Symptom-oriented interviewing originates from the concept that psychiatric disorders manifest themselves in a characteristic set of signs, symp-

---

[*] Sigmund Freud (1856–1939) developed both the psychodynamic theory of psychiatric illness and the methods of insight-oriented interviewing (Freud 1952–1955). Over the last 100 years, other investigators have elaborated on this concept and established its place in psychiatry (for example, Adler 1964; Berne 1964; Dubois 1913; Erikson 1969; Horney 1939; Jaspers 1962; Jung 1971; Klein 1952; Masserman 1955; Menninger 1958; Meyer 1957; Rado 1956; Reich 1949; Rogers 1951; Sullivan 1954; Wolberg 1967).

toms, and behaviors; a predictable course; a somewhat specific treatment response; and often a familial occurrence (American Psychiatric Association 2000). As twin and adoption studies show, heredity as well as learning may contribute to this observed familial occurrence (Goodwin and Guze 1989).

We do not know all the etiological factors that contribute to the manifestation of these disorders. Investigators have identified some biological and psychological components, but these findings are insufficient to classify these disorders by etiology. Therefore, classification is based on clinical criteria rather than underlying (assumed) pathology (Ludwig and Othmer 1977; Akiskal and Webb 1978).

The goal of symptom-oriented interviewing is to classify the patient's complaints and dysfunctions according to defined diagnostic categories (by criteria in DSM-IV-TR). Such a diagnosis helps to predict the future course (prognosis) and to select empirically the most effective treatment—but may not allow conclusions about its causes.

The method of the symptom-oriented interviewer is to observe the patient's behavior and to motivate her to describe her problems in detail. The interviewer translates his perception into symptoms and signs for a descriptive diagnosis (DSM-IV-TR Axis I and Axis II disorders). He includes the evaluation of the patient's adjustment and coping skills, her personal way of dealing with her disorder, and an assessment of the patient's medical condition and psychosocial and environmental problems.

Manifestations of the same disorder vary from patient to patient, as do coping mechanisms and treatment responses. Furthermore, the comorbidity of clinical and personality disorders, and the impact of general medical conditions, life stressors, and interpersonal conflicts complicate psychosocial adjustment and prognosis. To acknowledge these factors, the symptom-oriented interviewer incorporates mental retardation and personality disorders (Axis II), general medical conditions (Axis III), psychosocial and environmental problems (Axis IV), global assessment of functioning (Axis V), and defensive functioning (proposed Axis VI) in a multiaxial diagnosis.

Goals and methods of this descriptive type of interview have been pursued over the last 3,000 years by physicians of all medical specialties. In psychiatry, this tradition is exemplified in the work of Emil Kraepelin (1856–1926), and of his contemporaries, followers, and critics (Kleist 1928; Leonhard 1979). Several recent books approach psychiatric interviewing from such a descriptive point of view (Leon 1989; Hersen and Turner 1985; MacKinnon and Yudofsky 1986; Shea 1988; Simms 1988; Morrison 1993).

In summary, the insight- and symptom-oriented interviews serve different goals in psychiatry and psychology. The insight-oriented interview with an interpretative approach *explains* signs, symptoms, and behaviors. The symptom-oriented interview with a descriptive approach *classifies* signs and symptoms into disorder categories.

Both approaches are compatible and can be used effectively in conjunction with one another. Mental health professionals seem to agree that they can best understand the patient's personality, conflicts, and problems of living by a psychodynamic approach, but that major psychiatric and personality disorders are best assessed by the descriptive method. A synthesis of interpretation and description can bridge the different points of departure.

An interviewer may use both types of interviewing in a two-step fashion. He assumes that a patient may have both major psychiatric and personality disorders and unconscious conflicts. He may diagnose major psychiatric and personality disorders according to DSM-IV-TR Axes I and II by means of a symptom-oriented interview. If, after treatment, interpersonal conflicts persist or surface, he may switch to an insight-oriented interview as a second step, thus complementing his symptom-oriented interview.

Indeed, you can often observe an interaction between interpersonal conflicts and psychiatric disorders. Psychiatric disorders may revive and magnify existing, or evoke new, interpersonal conflicts, while preexisting conflicts may trigger the outbreak or aggravate the course of psychiatric disorders.

In 1916, E. Bleuler was the first prominent psychiatrist to integrate the two approaches (Bleuler 1972). Many psychiatrists followed this integrative approach under the label of eclectic psychiatry. A clearly separated, two-step approach assures appropriately tailoring the interview to the patient's needs.

Using Both Methods

The following case report illustrates the two-step method, with description first and interpretation second.

> Georgia is a 36-year-old, white single female who has been in treatment for the last 6 years. Diagnostically, she fulfills DSM-IV-TR criteria for major depressive disorder, delusional disorder, and obsessive-compulsive disorder. A worsening of her mood disorder intensified both obsessive-compulsive symptoms and persecutory ideas, but a remission of the depression was not associated with a remission of either the obsessive-compulsive or the delusional disorders. She was single. She was functioning at work but was socially isolated. Her symptoms did not respond to clomipramine (Anafranil) but improved with a combination of amitriptyline (Elavil) and thiothixene hydrochloride (Navane). Since her persecutory ideas had diminished, her dose of Navane was slowly tapered to lower the risk of tardive dys-

kinesia and to respond to the patient's complaint that she felt less alert and lively on Navane. She had recently lost her job because her company transferred to another city.

She found a new job with a mail-order business where she had to correct purchase orders on a computer screen that had the errors highlighted. She loved this type of work and was very proficient and fast in her corrections. Within the first few weeks she managed to make up to 8,000 corrections a day.

Serendipitously, she detected that some of the frames had more than one area highlighted. She realized that she had outperformed her colleagues by working on the false assumption of only one error per frame. She was devastated. She calculated that she literally had messed up thousands of orders, that she possibly had caused irreparable harm to her company—all due to her wish to be the best.

For a few days she concealed the error and continued her routine. She finally felt she could not take it any more and stayed home from work without notifying her employer. Her supervisor called her, she admitted her mistake, and was grateful that the supervisor did not make a major point out of her failure. Georgia worked for 2 days, each day looking forward to her job. On the third day, she took some pizzas to work for everybody to express her gratitude.

That afternoon, one of her colleagues walked up to her and said: "Don't you have to cool off your fingers?" and repeated this remark on another occasion. Georgia was shocked. She started to ruminate about this remark. Then she noticed that the number of purchase orders that she had to pick up from a front window was only a tenth of the usual amount, forcing her to interrupt her work frequently, to leave her terminal, walk to the window, and pick up a new set of orders. On her way there, she could not help but notice that all the other 30 employees in the room typed very slowly, nearly like in a rhythm, tap-tap-tap, and there was no chitchat at all, just tap-tap-tap.

Immediately, she understood what was going on. The small amount of purchase orders were placed there to distract her from her work, so that she had to notice the slow typing, giving her the message: "You messed up, we have to do your work, slow down so that you don't mess up again." She realized letting her come back to work was an evil plot to punish her for her failure. Every tap was a condemnation, revenge for what she had done.

She returned to her work station in tears. They had gotten her good. And she deserved it. It was so mean and cruel, yet so clever. If anybody knew how to torture her, they did.

The next day, she did not report to work and was fired.

Here is how the interviewer uses a two-step approach with this patient.

Step 1: The phenomenological part in Georgia's evaluation is straightforward. She had persecutory delusions in the past. At times, they were associated with vegetative symptoms of depression and dysphoric mood, never with hallucinations. Since the neuroleptic was discontinued when she became unemployed, she relapsed and the persecutory delusions returned. Georgia's clinical picture again fulfilled criteria for delusional disorder (DSM-IV-TR 297.1). Treatment with Navane was reinstated.

Step 2: We chose a psychodynamic, interpretative intervention when Georgia made an appointment and reported her problem. Here is a segment of this portion of the interview.

1. I: You went through quite an ordeal.
   P: Isn't it awful? I don't understand how human beings can do that to one another.
2. I: I agree. It is a merciless torture.
   P: I don't understand it. They all seemed so nice, and I really liked my supervisor. He let me come back and he was not down on me at all. I don't understand why he did this to me.
3. I: But it was not him who has done it; it was not them.
   P: [excited, panicky] But Dr. O., what do you mean? I just told you what they did to me. How can you say it was not them?
4. I: Because it was you . . . You did it yourself. You thought you deserved that punishment for the big crime you committed. And when the punishment did not come, you brought it on yourself.
   P: [more excited] But Dr. O., you don't believe me—you were my last hope, you are my only friend—and you don't believe me . . .
5. I: I believe everything you told me. Most of your observations were right. What I have problems with is your interpretations, what you think it all means.
   P: [with slightly lower, less pressed voice] But how do you explain what the fellow said about my hot fingers, and that they all typed so slowly?
6. I: I don't know. But let me ask you a few questions. Since you worked there, how many new people started in that month?
   P: Six out of thirty.
7. I: You see, in a job like yours there is a high turnover. How do you think a supervisor would get everybody together to type slowly just to punish you? How do you think he'll get that kind of cooperation? They all would think, "If they do it to Georgia, they'll do it to me too." [uses Georgia's own persecutory tendencies to break through her delusional beliefs]
   P: I thought about that on the way home that night, but then I thought no, no—it was all too real.
8. I: Yes, it is real. You have no way of telling that it isn't. And you are right. You made a mistake, and the supervisor made a mistake of not catching your mistake, and I made a mistake of stopping the Navane that would have helped you to tell the difference between what is going on on the outside and on your inside. So we all made mistakes. Let's try to correct what we can. I'll give you a new prescription. In a few weeks those things won't happen to you anymore.

P: [shakes her head] Dr. O., I can't believe that you think I'm that paranoid.

9. I: I know you can't. And I don't expect you to believe what I told you. You may even think I'm in with them too.

P: Yes, that crossed my mind. I thought they had talked to you.

10. I: Yes, that happens. You can't think any differently.

P: [less intense] They really did it.

11. I: Do you want to call the supervisor right now?

P: But Dr. O., they would never admit it.

12. I: Would they not just talk to you about your mistake, rather than punishing you like this?

P: Hmm . . . I would think . . .

13. I: Is there anything that would convince you?

P: Yeah . . . if they pay me. Of course, they will not pay me for what I did.

14. I: If they pay you, that will tell you that it might have been you who did the torturing . . . No matter what, here is a prescription and I want you to start with your medicine now.

Comment: The patient called her company to find out whether there was a check for her, which there was. She apologized to the supervisor. At the next visit with the interviewer, 1 week later and back on the neuroleptic:

P: It is terrible how paranoid I am. It still feels real.

I: It will be over soon when the medicine works fully—and we will not stop it again. I apologize for my mistake. It cost you your job.

This case demonstrates the two-step approach. Step 1: Georgia had long-standing symptoms qualifying her for a diagnosis of delusional disorder (DSM-IV-TR), a diagnosis that may predict return of symptoms when the neuroleptic is stopped.

Step 2: This case also shows that Georgia has a strong punitive super-ego that will punish her when she fails, intentionally or not. A psycho-dynamic interpretation can explain the content of her delusion to her; however, it cannot remove her tendency to form delusions around stressful or everyday events when not taking neuroleptics.

Do not misconstrue this example to mean that the content of every delu-sion should or can be interpreted, or that the way this case was handled should be considered as a model. The interpretation as presented was intended to give the patient some relief and to motivate her to take medicine again. More-over, this type of aggressive interpretation should not be attempted in a first-time interview with a patient whom the therapist does not know.

This book describes a systematic approach to phenomenological inter-viewing in psychiatry (step 1). However, our approach is not pure, because it includes a descriptive approach to transference patterns in Chapter 2 (Rapport) and defense mechanisms in Chapter 3 (Techniques), and, in Chapters 4 and 5 (Mental Status and Testing), to the interface with psychodynamic interviewing (Vaillant 1986).

2. THE FOUR COMPONENTS

An emphasis on phenomenology requires a fresh look at the interviewing techniques to match the diagnostically driven interviewing goal if one follows DSM-IV-TR: assessment of signs and symptoms in a psychodiagnostic interview.

A useful comparison to this technique is the way in which twentieth-century artists began to portray the human face and figure. Pablo Picasso's 1957 portrait of Sylvette, which hangs in the Chicago Art Institute (Gedo 1980), shows this innovation. Picasso portrayed the woman from all sides: the front, the side, and the back, all simultaneously. He gives a "total" picture, a "stereo view" for a comprehensive representation of the persona.

A psychodiagnostic interview requires a similar approach. You see a patient in four dimensions: in her rapport with you, in her response to your interviewing techniques (to get all the data you need and to keep the interview flowing), in her mental status, and in the signs and symptoms of her disorder(s) as they unfold during the interviewing process. You have to keep track of these four components throughout the interview. Both the insight- and the symptom-oriented interviews adopt a similar four-pronged approach.

Rapport: Rapport refers to how the interviewer and her patient relate. Establishing rapport is equally important for the reporter who in an interview chases the four W's—what-where-when-why—and for the corporate executive who wants to market his product and has to recognize the customer's needs.

Both types of psychodiagnostic interviewing emphasize the importance of establishing, monitoring, and maintaining rapport. The insight-oriented interview conceptualizes rapport in terms of *transference and countertransference patterns,* thus looking for repetitions of previous infantile relationships in the interview situation. The descriptive approach describes rapport as *patient-interviewer interaction* that progresses from understanding to trust.

Technique: This refers to the methods used by interviewers to establish rapport and to obtain information. Interviewers take pride in their technique.

For instance, Barbara Walters, the television host, wrote a book called *How to Talk to Anybody About Anything*. Techniques range from open-ended questions to confrontation, and from interpretation to interrogation.

Both insight-oriented and descriptive interviewing emphasize technique, but draw on different methods. The insight-oriented interview uses techniques that uncover unconscious conflicts, such as free association, confrontation, and interpretation, while the descriptive interview stresses techniques that are geared toward the assessment of symptoms, signs, behaviors, and psychological dysfunctions.

Mental Status: This refers to the patient's general state of mind while you talk to him. Is he clear or fuzzy in his answers, quick-witted or slow in remembering, pleasant or angry, open or suspicious and concealing, reality-oriented or full of strange and bizarre ideas? This is the same for the insight- or symptom-oriented interviewer. She monitors psychological and psychosocial functioning during the interview and recognizes its importance. The descriptive interviewer describes and focuses on dimensions of functions such as psychomotor behavior, speech and thinking, affect, mood, thought content, memory, orientation, insight, and judgment, while the insight-oriented interviewer goes beyond the description of these functional disturbances and identifies underlying defense mechanisms and conflicts.

Diagnosing: The more the interviewer learns about the patient's strengths, weaknesses, and suffering, the better able she is to render an appropriate and accurate diagnosis. The more experienced she is and the more she knows about the disorder, stressors, and coping skills, the better she can assess them.

Both types of interview pursue diagnosis, but they follow different routes. The insight-oriented interview identifies conflicts and unconsciously directed behavior patterns for a psychodynamic formulation, while the symptom-oriented interview strives to collect a set of symptoms and signs that fit diagnostic criteria of categorical disorders.

Chapters 2 through 6 describe separately the four components of the symptom-oriented, descriptive, psychodiagnostic interview. This dissecting approach to interviewing is similar to the medical school approach to the human body: the same organ system is repeatedly described under the aspects of anatomy, histology, physiology, and biochemistry. Obviously, anatomy, histology, physiology, and biochemistry of the organs do not exist independently of each other. On the contrary, they are highly interrelated, and different aspects of the same organ system are examined to better study, teach, research, and understand the body and its organs and treat its disorders. Similarly interconnected are rapport, assessment techniques, mental status examination, and diagnosing, but for heuristic purposes they will be separately treated.

Interviewing a patient can be compared to two people assembling a puzzle where the patient has the pieces and the interviewer the image of the completed design.

1. Both must be willing to do it together—rapport.
2. The interviewer must know how to get the right pieces from the patient—he asks for them, and assembles small sections—assessment techniques.
3. The interviewer has to inspect and move all pieces in front of him continuously—mental status.
4. The interviewer constantly compares what he has put together with the design, to see which pieces are still missing—diagnosis.

3.   THE MULTIPHASIC APPROACH

All interviewing takes place as a process in time. Most books on interviewing, both psychodynamic and descriptive, divide the interview into three phases: an opening, a middle, and an end (MacKinnon and Michels 1971). These phases differ in their respective goals.

In the *opening phase* the interviewer warms up the patient, establishes rapport, and prepares the patient for the main task of the interview.

In the *middle phase* he performs the bulk of the work; therefore it takes the longest time. Some subdivide this phase further to emphasize the shift of interviewing goals. So do we. Obviously, such divisions are arbitrary but of heuristic value.

In the *end phase* the interviewer prepares the patient for the closure. He avoids highly emotional topics, summarizes for the patient what has been learned, and provides an outlook for the future.

We have further refined the stages of the interview to enable the clinician to better understand the process. We have five phases, as follows.

1. Warm-up and screening of the problem
2. Follow-up of preliminary impressions
3. Psychiatric history
4. Diagnosis and feedback
5. Prognosis and treatment contract.

The five phases and their integration with the four components of the interview (see Figure 1–1) are described in Chapter 6 and illustrated by edited, taped interviews in Chapters 7 and 8.

In your own interviews you will often deviate from such an order of phases because you follow the patient's leads and jump back and forth among phases. Yet it is critical to know the logical sequence of phases; most interviews do follow this pattern of unfolding. In addition, if the interview goes awry, an understanding of these distinct phases offers places to which the interviewer can return to regain his bearings.

4. DISORDER-SPECIFIC INTERVIEWING

If a patient is difficult, the skilled interviewer changes her strategies. How else can she get through to the patient or client? What about those who don't understand that you want to help them or who won't talk? Whether you dig for conflicts or collect symptoms, the patient's shyness, withdrawal, or hostility may get in your way. Thus, the patient's pathology may obstruct a standard approach that you use with the cooperative patient (Chapter 7). You have to adjust your interviewing strategies to the patient's behavior typical for his illness. Chapters 8 through 10 describe how to do that for some clinical and personality disorders. You may also refer to our book *The Clinical Interview Using DSM-IV-TR, Volume 2: The Difficult Patient* (Othmer and Othmer 2002), which provides specific techniques and approaches for working with these individuals.

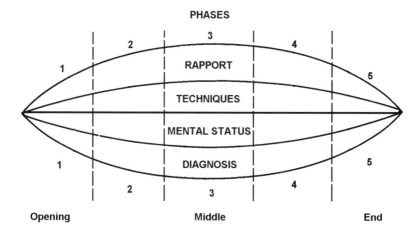

Figure 1–1. The five phases of the standard interview.

In the chapters that follow, we first show you the general strategies of interviewing, and then their modification for selected disorders. You may use two measuring sticks to judge the quality of your interviewing technique: short- and long-term outcome.

In the short term, see whether the patient gets involved in the interviewing process and provides useful and spontaneous information. If so, your approach is obviously productive. In the long term, if your patient returns after the initial interview, cooperates with your treatment, and improves in his functioning, your approach was obviously effective.

CHAPTER TWO

STRATEGIES FOR RAPPORT

1. **Put the Patient and Yourself at Ease**
   Recognize Signs
   Respond to Signs
2. **Find the Suffering—Show Compassion**
   Assess the Suffering
   Respond With Empathy
3. **Assess Insight—Become an Ally**
   Levels of Insight
   Split Off the Sick Part of the Patient
   Set Therapeutic Goals
4. **Show Expertise**
   Put the Illness Into Perspective
   Show Knowledge
   Deal With Doubt
   Instill Hope
5. **Establish Leadership**
6. **Balance the Roles**
   The Roles of the Interviewer
      The Empathic Listener
      The Expert
      The Authority
   The Roles of the Patient
      Carrier of an Illness
      The Sufferer
      The "VIP"
   Role Interaction
      Dependence on the Interviewer's Leadership

SUMMARY

The first component of the interview, achieving rapport, is divided into six strategies: 1) putting the patient and yourself at ease, 2) finding the pain and expressing compassion, 3) evaluating the patient's insight and becoming an ally, 4) showing expertise to the patient, 5) establishing leadership as a therapist, and 6) balancing the roles in the therapeutic setting.

▲▲▲▲▲

30 . . . A certain man went down from Jerusalem to Jericho, and fell among thieves, which stripped him of his raiment, and wounded him, and departed, leaving him half dead.
31 And by chance there came down a certain priest that way: and when he saw him, he passed by on the other side.
32 And likewise a Levite, when he was at the place, came and looked on him, and passed by on the other side.
33 But a certain Samaritan, as he journeyed, came where he was: and when he saw him, he had *compassion* on him,
34 And went to him, and bound up his wounds, pouring in oil and wine, and set him on his own beast, and brought him to an inn, and took care of him.
35 And on the morrow when he departed, he took out two pence, and gave them to the host, and said unto him, Take care of him; and whatsoever thou spendest more, when I come again, I will repay thee . . .
37 . . . And then said Jesus . . . , Go, and do thou likewise.

—The Holy Bible, King James Version,
Luke 10:30–37

▼▼▼▼▼

1. PUT THE PATIENT AND YOURSELF AT EASE

The first-time psychiatric patient is often skeptical, apprehensive, and anxious. He overcame the stigma of seeing a mental health professional, but the taboo about psychiatric or psychological problems lingers and troubles him. He is unsure of the people who take care of such matters; he does not know what to expect. He rarely verbalizes what plagues him before the visit:

"Will she listen to me?"
"Will she really understand what I'm telling her?"
"Will she care for me?"
"Will she respect or ridicule me?"
"Will she be able to help me?"
"Can I trust her enough to follow her advice?"

It is your role to convey that you sense these doubts, that you are on his side, respecting him and his concerns and trying to help him—then he will hear an internal all-clear signal and you can carefully initiate rapport with him. But if his fears and hopes are ignored, reservation and frustration may prevail.

How do you put yourself at ease? The patient will immediately sense your own anxiety or lack of control. Remember, the patient is another human being and generally wants very much to be understood. Beginning the interview with an interlude of easy conversation will help to settle both you and the patient and get past any initial awkwardness. Your first goal is simply to get a sense of the patient, and initiate rapport, not to arrive at an immediate diagnosis. Let yourself ease into the interview and get your bearings if you feel anxious or nervous.

When the patient arrives, it is often best to put him at ease by requesting basic information (see also Chapter 4, section 2: Conversation). First, you introduce yourself and ask him for his name and its proper pronunciation. Find out whether he prefers to be addressed by his first or last name. Some therapists recommend always using the last name to show respect. They maintain that since the patient usually addresses you with your last name (often with a Dr. in front of it), you should do the same. For many patients this is awkward, creates distance, and aggravates anxiety. True, some patients feel compelled to offer you a first name, when they actually prefer a last name. There is no quick way to find that out for sure. By asking the patient, you show you don't make decisions for him but that you take his wishes into account. The numerous interview vignettes that will follow use either first or last names, according to the patient's wishes. With patients who seem dependent, very anxious, or psychotic you may skip that question.

With most patients, you will want to engage in small talk. You might ask how he found out about you, and how he found his way to your office.

Hemingway probably put it best—know a man's dialect. Failing that, try to get him to talk of his area of geographical origin, where he was raised, and any common knowledge you might have of places or occupations familiar and comfortable to him, thus establishing common ground.

During this interlude, you can note whether he indeed settles down as you expect him to do, or whether he becomes more tense. Some patients with an anxiety disorder, for instance, may want to get to the point, that is, their problems; some obsessive patients may figure that they waste time, that is, money, by beating around the bush.

How do you know what to do when? By reading the patient's signs—his nonverbal behavior, voice, and mode of expression.

Recognize Signs

The moment you meet a new patient, his mental state may be expressed by signs. A sign is the nonverbal language of the face, body, and voice that is often hard to control. It tells you the patient's feelings without words. You can deal with such signs here and now to put the patient at ease and to re-assure him that he did the right thing to come and see you. Initiate rapport by reading these signs. They are of different nature:

1. territorial (locomotor)
2. behavioral (psychomotor)
3. emotional (expressive)
4. verbal (voice and mode of expression)

When the patient enters your office, notice how he moves into the new territory. If he is timid, he avoids coming close to you. He shies away from shaking hands. He takes a seat by the door. Your desk becomes a barrier, physical and emotional.

In contrast, the intrusive patient gets too close to you. She may expose you to her breath, spit, loud voice, or the touch of her hands.

Her psychomotor behavior fits her locomotor behavior. The timid pa-tient looks down in her lap, avoiding eye contact. The intrusive patient may fiddle with your pencils, rearrange the furniture, turn on your computer, or put her feet on your desk.

Emotional signs surface in the patient's posture, gestures, facial expression, eye contact, and tone of voice. He may walk in with erect posture, chin up, full of energy, or stooped and slowed down. He may smile or look tense, avoiding your eyes. His voice may be quivering or barking. There may be tears.

A patient gives verbal signs about his mental state by the choice of his words. Pick up his vocabulary, especially his metaphors. This will help to reflect back to him your understanding of his unique problems. It will also help you get inside the patient's way of thinking and experiencing his world.

The patient may represent his problems in a visual, kinesthetic, auditory, or more abstract way. Here are examples:

Visual:
   "There is no light at the end of the tunnel."
   "Everything looks bleak."
   "No silver lining."
   "Can't see the way out."

Kinesthetic:
   "I feel trapped."
   "I feel pushed to the wall."
   "I'm dead-headed."
   "Feels like I'm paralyzed."
   "I feel choked."
   "Everything is closing in."
   "It's like walking through quicksand."

Auditory:
   "There is a constant buzz in my head."
   "Everything sounds far away."
   "I feel like screaming."

Abstract:
   "Feeling depressed."
   "Unable to concentrate."
   "Confused thinking."
   "Less energy than usual."
   "No initiative."
   "Anxious."
   "Getting hypomanic."
   "Feeling guilty."

When a patient uses visual, kinesthetic, auditory, or abstract language, pick it up initially. If he says, for instance:

"There is no light at the end of the tunnel."

Ask him,

"Since when did things look so dark?"

Try to continue his metaphor (Cameron-Bandler 1978; Bandler and Grinder 1979).

All of these efforts add up to helping the patient feel comforted by your presence. Decoding his signs, helping him to express his state of mind, may be experienced with great relief by the patient. He feels understood, and you have accomplished your goal of establishing an initial sense of rapport.

Respond to Signs

The four types of signs—territorial, behavioral, emotional, and verbal—hit you at once. You get an immediate impression. Your patient may be tense, anxious, aggressive, overbearing, elated, depressed, or relaxed. There are different ways of responding to signs.

In the early stages of the interview, you may want to simply observe these signs. You may decide to give the patient space and time—to express himself more—and relax. But you *always* monitor his signs. They are part of his mental status and give you clues for the diagnosis.

In some instances, you may want to alert him to his signs. If you draw his attention to them and discuss their meaning, you may use them as a lead into diagnosing.

In many cases it is best to respond in kind, with or without reflecting on them. This response is often the most effective. For example, you can respond territorially to territorial signs. If your patient avoids you, remain standing, move slowly toward him. Show him you are concerned about his well-being and make inviting gestures. With an anxious patient who has come accompanied by a family member, you might invite the escort to join. If a patient is intrusive, you can reestablish distance. Your response to intrusion of your personal space can determine whether you stay in control. Make a gesture that stops his advance and follow up verbally.

> "Why don't you sit down over there? That way we can talk more comfortably."

While not every interview situation requires strict delineation of boundary lines, their absence can create serious problems, as the following example indicates.

> Dr. L. is a 40-year-old, small-framed psychiatrist who looks younger than his age. Although well trained in his field, he has a timid interpersonal style. He lets patients stand close to him, and put their hands on his shoulders. He responds by cowering, wincing, and backing off. By his nonverbal signs, he

shows his patients that they put him in an uncomfortable position and that they can invade his personal space. The resulting disrespect is detrimental for rapport with some patients. Other patients, who share a similar sense of interpersonal boundaries, may respond very well to this approach and find this nonconfrontational style comforting.

With emotional signs you can respond by shaking your head, or raising your eyebrows; smiling or looking away; raising or lowering your voice.

Hopkinson et al. (1981) found no significant correlation between the rate of a listener's nonverbal response such as head nodding and the amount of emotional expression by interviewed mothers. However, Heller et al. (1966) and Siegman and Pope (1972) contradict this point. No expression or strong emotional expression by the interviewer may inhibit, while a moderate expression may facilitate emotional response. Picking up an emotional sign or talking about it, confronting the patient with it, and exploring its origin appears effective for an emotional response. In a 30-minute session, interviewers who picked up their clients' emotions elicited three or more spontaneous self-disclosures in eight out of nine cases. Interviewers who ignored their patients' emotional signals elicited 3 spontaneous self-disclosures in only 6 out of 27 cases.

An example will illustrate how a response to an emotional (and not to a verbal) sign deepened rapport.

Novice: What can I do for you?
    P: I'm so angry and mad, I had 2 bad years. What these people did to me in North Carolina! [looks away, bites his lip, and clenches his fist] They stripped me of the right to see my children. I'm angry and depressed about that.

The patient gives two types of signs, an emotional one (looks away, bites his lip, clenches his fist) and a verbal one (I'm angry and depressed). The novice responds to the *word* "depressed."

Novice: You say you are depressed. Did it affect your sleep?
    P: Yeah [the patient whips his crossed-over leg].
Novice: What about your appetite?
    P: What about it?
Novice: Was it affected?
    P: Nope [looks away].

The supervisor interrupts. He hones in on the suspiciousness and anger that was expressed by body language:

I: [raises his hand, moves forward on his chair] Excuse me, you said people have stripped you of the right to see your children.

P: Yes, that's right, they really did me in.

I: [raises his eyebrows]

P: The judge and the lawyer down in that little whoretown . . . I'm sure you know judges and lawyers in such a place must be crooked. All they deal with is prostitutes, illegal drugs, bribery, it's all a big scam.

I: Hmm . . . [shakes his head in disapproval].

P: At my divorce, these people listened only to my wife. I could not go down there, because I was sick, and my wife paid them off. So they gave me a bad deal.

I: How can we help?

P: I'm so mad, I'm afraid somebody will get hurt if I don't get any help.

The supervisor addressed what the patient had expressed by his body language rather than by words. These signs led him to the patient's persecutory ideas, the core pathology.

As we suggested earlier, you can respond with a metaphor to metaphorical language. Initially use the patient's terms instead of psychological or psychiatric terminology. For instance, when he talks about his "spells," use that word. This gives him the feeling that you understand him. Then ask him to describe what he means by "spell" to help you understand what he is talking about (see Chapter 4, section 3: Exploration). (With some patients from Hispanic cultures, "spells" will have a particular religious connotation and should be considered in light of the cultural meaning.)

Later, if indicated, you may introduce technical terms such as seizure, panic attack, cataplectic attack, hypnagogic hallucination, restless leg syndrome, or hyperventilation episode to assure him that you have the expertise to understand his problems.

The following interview section, recorded in a rural outpatient mental health center, shows how a novice missed connecting with his patient's use of language.

Mr. Huber, a 58-year-old farmer dressed in blue overalls, leans back in his chair with legs spread apart. His face is weather-beaten, with wrinkles around the eyes from squinting.

P: I don't know what's going on, I'm not with it anymore!

Novice: How would you compare your present level of mental functioning with the level you were at prior to the onset of your problems?

P: What do you mean?

Novice: I obviously mean how you can concentrate, memorize, and think now, in comparison to the time before you got sick.

P: You mean if I think different now?

Novice: Yes, that's part of it, but not just thinking, also memorizing and concentrating.

P: Well, I think a lot about losing my farm and why my son can't take it over.

Novice: That's not what I mean. I mean, is your thinking slower now, is it more of an effort to get your thoughts out?

P: You mean if I'm crazy or something?

The novice talks above the patient's head. He interviews him as if the patient were a psychology major. The supervisor continued the interview, and it went like this:

I: You said you are not really with it anymore.

P: That's right.

I: Can you give me an example?

P: Yes, I often stand and stare. Don't know what to do next.

I: How's that?

P: Well, I just can't remember what I wanted to do.

I: You mean it just does not come to you?

P: Yeah, that's it.

I: Does that mean that your thoughts just don't pop up in your mind as they used to?

P: Right. It's just all blank up there [points to his head].

In contrast to the novice, the supervisor tunes into his patient's language. The patient feels understood and responds more openly. The interviewer retrieves the information he seeks.

To recognize and respond to your patient's signs is difficult if you yourself are tense, anxious, or nervous. This will hinder your efforts to establish rapport. You cannot come up with appropriate questions, you may miss finer points of the mental status, or you may lose contact with the patient, because you focus your attention on yourself. The most powerful technique to help you overcome self-consciousness and insecurity is to shift the focus from yourself to your suffering patient. If you find you are tense, allow yourself to listen to your patient and avoid putting pressure on yourself to find the "right" question. Once you get back into the flow of the patient's experience you can return to a more directive interview style.

2. FIND THE SUFFERING—SHOW COMPASSION

After responding to the patient's signs and putting him at ease, search for the patient's suffering. "Give me a place to stand and I will move the earth,"

Archimedes allegedly said (c. 287–212 B.C.). This Greek mathematician and scientist illustrated to Hieron II, king of Syracuse in Sicily, that a very great weight could be moved by a very small force, provided you have a distant point from which to apply the leverage. In psychiatric interviewing, the point from which you can set the patient's emotions free is his suffering.

There are usually two aspects to the patient's problems: the facts and the associated emotions. The facts may be symptoms such as loss of appetite, early morning awakenings, shortness of breath, unexplained abdominal pain; they may be stressors such as the death of a child, marital problems, job loss, relocation, or recurrent adjustment problems. The emotions are the feelings that these facts stir up in the patient and make him suffer. He may hide this aspect because of fear of being embarrassed or ashamed. You will intensify rapport if you bring out not only the facts but also his suffering.

Assess the Suffering

To determine the ways in which the patient is suffering, you can try questions such as:

> "What is bothering you?"
> "What are you going through?"

When the patient describes his problems, often called the *chief complaint,* help him to put his distress into words:

> "How did that make you feel?"

indicating that you are interested in his emotions and want to know more about his anguish. In this early phase of the interview it is more important to allow him to ventilate his suffering than to list his symptoms. Giving the patient the opportunity to talk freely about his suffering and bringing the patient's affect to his awareness accomplishes two goals: 1) it allows you to judge his affect and mood, and to detect the underlying quality, such as depression, anxiety, or anger; 2) it shows the patient your interest in his feelings, which brings you closer to each other and deepens rapport.

Respond With Empathy

When the patient reveals his suffering, tell him that you understand. Show your empathy. Express your compassion. Research supports this clinical instinct. Out of 19 criteria used to choose a physician, 205 adults rated empathy as the second-most-important criterion ("seems interested in my particular problem") after expertise (Hill 1991). In this group, females especially appeared to appreciate a personal, empathic attitude. More than males, they valued that the physician is not "pushy or abrasive . . . treats me in a personal manner, and puts me at ease with small talk" (Hill 1991). Thus, empathy and compassion are highly rated facilitators of rapport.

A patient, for instance, tells you that she can hardly make ends meet on her salary since her husband returned to school, forcing them to take out a loan. The patient grows increasingly tense and angry as she speaks, clenching her fists, spitting out her words. Before focusing on the content of her talk, express empathy for her distress: "You sounded angry while you said that. You must be fed up with the situation to carry the burden alone." Try to be genuine, spontaneous, and accurate in your response to her affect:

"You must feel awful."
"You must feel harassed."
"I can see how that shook you up."
"That must have made you feel deserted."

As interviewer you should express empathy if you want the patient to entrust you with his suffering. Hopkinson et al. (1981) found that the novice uses empathetic statements in only 4% of all his questions and remarks. However, the quality, timing, and context of statements are at least as important as the number. As many as 51% of empathic statements by the interviewer elicited emotional responses in the patient. This figure rose to 62% when the interviewer expressed his own emotions before he made the empathic statement, as compared to 36% when he did not disclose his own emotions. This combined interaction is effective, yet rare. It was used in only 1.5% of all questions and remarks.

Some therapists experience difficulty in feeling empathy. Indeed, some difficult patients can tax even the most empathic interviewer. If you have chronic difficulty in feeling empathy, don't try to express it. Focused attention and appropriate questions convey your interest in the patient better than phony empathy. Patients get annoyed when they are confronted with mannerisms:

I: I heard you say you were apprehensive about coming here.
P: You heard right, damn it, that's what I said.

or

I: It sounds to me that you were pretty upset when you . . .
P: [sarcastically] Really? It sounds to you? . . . Doc, you are just playing thera-
     pist—I know that spiel—I have been to too many damn psychologists.

If you express empathy but the patient withdraws from you, check whether
you were genuine. Did you really understand his distress? Did you truly feel
empathic? Did you communicate your empathy in a language and manner
accessible to the patient?

  You can acquire an empathic, patient-centered, genuine interview style
such that it becomes second nature. One systematic way is to recapitulate
interviews with difficult patients. Jot down how the patient's attitudes toward you changed, and analyze what caused it. Did you use his vocabulary
when you formulated your questions? Were you clearly aware of how the
patient's problems affected him? Did you make an effort to explore these
feelings? Did you tune into his emotions when you expressed your empathy
and your understanding (Rogers 1951; Corsini 1984; Dobson 1988)? Were
you always aware of and responsive to the patient's attitudinal changes?

  If you want to improve your rapport with your patients, focus on your
ability to feel empathic and to communicate genuine concern.

3.   ASSESS INSIGHT—BECOME AN ALLY

Once you have expressed your empathy, begin to understand your patient's
own view of his problem, that is, his insight. This allows you not only to
share his emotional but also his cognitive attitude toward his problems.

  Why is this assessment necessary? Because you need to use the patient's insight in two ways: 1) When you interview him, you look at his
problem from *his* point of view; and 2) You use the distance between *his*
degree of insight and full insight as a measure for his reality testing. It will
be part of the therapeutic goal to correct any distortion and help him to gain
full insight.

  If you misjudge the patient's level of insight, rapport will deteriorate
rapidly. For example, if you treat the patient who feels controlled by a computer as delusional or crazy, he will feel insulted, because he feels his beliefs are true. Or if you assume a patient understands that he abuses
substances, you may quickly discover he loses interest in talking with you
further.

Levels of Insight

There are three levels of insight: full, partial, and no insight.

Full Insight

A patient who describes his psychiatric symptoms as a result of a disorder demonstrates full insight. For instance, a patient with panic attacks who recognizes them as part of her illness has full insight. Or a patient with phobic avoidance or obsessive-compulsive worries who considers this behavior as a symptom of a disorder has full insight. (Such patients were called "neurotic" in DSM-II [American Psychiatric Association 1968].)

Usually rapport develops with a patient who has full insight. She talks freely about her symptoms because she recognizes them as ego-dystonic, as part of an illness and not as part of her normal self. However, she may attempt to withhold embarrassing details such as suicide attempts, or violations of the law. You will typically find these patients in psychiatric outpatient settings, as clients of psychologists, or other mental health professionals.

Partial Insight

In contrast, psychotic patients with schizophrenia, bipolar illness, or major depression often lack the awareness of being sick; so do substance abusers who deny the impact of their illness on themselves and their environment. Since there is such disparity in insight, you have to gauge the patient's ability to understand that he is ill.

Partial insight is also seen in a patient who recognizes that there is something wrong but blames it on external circumstances, as the following example illustrates.

> Rose, a 32-year-old, white, single female who lives in an old neighborhood in an industrial city, learned to use psychiatric terminology for her problem without accepting it as a disorder. Her mother brought her to the emergency room.

P: I'm getting paranoid again.
I: What do you mean by that?
P: Well, I think that my neighbors are spying on me again.
I: Why do you call that paranoid?
P: My other doctor told me so.
I: So what do you think we should do about it?
P: I guess I need the Haldol shots again.
I: What does that medication do for you?

P: I'll be less bothered by my paranoia.
I: What do you think the neighbors are really doing to you?
P: One of them comes at night toward my house and listens at my bedroom window. Another one talked to the police to put a bug in my house.
I: Do you really think they are doing this?
P: Of course, what do you think? I'm really paranoid about it.

This patient understands her doctor considers her ill and in need of pharmacological treatment. In spite of her willingness to cooperate with his treatment and not report the neighbors to the police, her own beliefs are unshaken. Symptoms can be elicited from Rose as long as she is not inappropriately pressed to accept them as indicators of a mental illness. Rose knows that she is suffering and expects that medication will help her, even though she does not concede that the source of her suffering is an illness.

Your awareness of the patient's level of insight is important for rapport since it determines the phrasing of your questions throughout the interview. For instance, when you ask for family history, it would be a mistake to ask a patient with partial insight:

> "Does anybody else in your family suffer from beliefs like you, or show suspicious behavior?"

Rather, rephrase the question as if unrelated to the patient's problem; for instance:

> "Were there any medical illnesses in your family, or any psychiatric disorders?" or
> "Were some other members of your family also harassed by their neighbors?"

When you discuss treatment, emphasize initially that the medication will make the patient less sensitive to the neighbors' activities; not that it will relieve her delusional suspiciousness.

No Insight

A patient without insight demonstrates complete denial that he suffers from any illness, or even that he suffers at all. Characteristic features clue you in right away. He is accompanied by someone who urges him to be treated; his response to your opening question shows passive compliance, angry resistance, or muteness; he does not admit to psychosocial problems or a psychiatric disorder; and often he is noncommittal about his chief complaint.

"My wife sent me."
"I don't know why I'm here."

You will need to find a way to motivate the patient to be interviewed. The way to do this is to find out what leverage was used by the person who brought him in. This person can be a source to determine the patient's point of view regarding his behavior. For example, he may believe that the voices on the radio order him to commit acts; if you know this you can ask the patient directly about his experience of the voices.

> Richard is a 37-year-old African American who works at his father's farm; he suffers from recurrent delusions and hallucinations: "Spacemen are coming in at night; they are shooting darts, and I wake up with a splitting headache. Call the FBI, I want to file a complaint!"

The patient recognizes the spacemen as disturbing—but not as a symptom of an illness. To initiate rapport with such a patient, consider the spacemen as *his* reality and choose your words accordingly. Do not imitate this psychology student:

Student: Really? Have you had these hallucinations for a long time?
P: What do you mean? I don't know what you are talking about.
Student: I mean your hallucinations about the spacemen?
P: They aren't imagined, they are real—I get headaches from their shots. Would I get headaches if I imagined that?
Student: Well . . . sometimes our minds play tricks on us.
P: Maybe your mind plays tricks with you. I better go.

The supervisor interrupts.

I: Wait a minute.
P: [angry] Why? I don't want to talk to you either.
I: I see you get annoyed that we don't understand . . .
P: Yeah, you are like my brother. He says I'm crazy.
I: He probably hasn't seen spacemen and has a hard time understanding what's going on. Tell me how long have these spacemen been bothering you?
P: It started again 4 weeks ago.
I: Is there anything else going on?
P: Well, I have a splitting headache in the morning.
I: Do the spacemen bother you during the day?
P: No, not really.
I: Do they keep track of you in any way?
P: I don't know. They just seem to come at night.
I: Do they have any power over you?

P: No, they just bug me.

I: Can you hear them? Do they talk about you?

P: Well, once in a while at night I hear a whisper that comes from the air condi-
    tioner. They say, "See, there he is, see, there he is, and we will get him."

Some patients without insight refuse to be interviewed. If you can identify the patient's vantage point of his illness (which can sometimes be elicited from the persons who accompanied him to the hospital or your office),
you at least can approach the patient on his own terms. For instance, after
you have introduced yourself, you may say to the patient's escort who
brought him in:

     I: I'm glad that you accompanied Mr. Combs to my office. He told me that
        you thought he should see a psychiatrist. Mr. Combs doesn't really know
        why. Maybe you can help me.

Escort: Well, I've been George's neighbor for over 20 years. And during that time
        he got concerned about the mailman twice.

     I: What were his concerns?

Escort: Well, he felt that the mailman is not really the mailman but a spy who's
        been exchanged with our old mailman. So when I got that Fedex letter
        yesterday, George came over with a gun to protect me against the Fedex
        man.

     P: Oh, shut up, Tom, that's not what the doctor wants to know. He doesn't
        want to know about that spy that tries to sneak up on us. He wants to
        know why I'm here!

     I: Wait a minute, Mr. Combs! Maybe your neighbor has a point! It seems you
        were pretty upset about that mailman, if you felt you had to use your gun.
        Maybe I can give you something that will help to regain your cool. Maybe
        we should get you out of that situation for a few days so that you can feel
        safe and sort things out.

     P: You think that guy is that dangerous?

     I: Well, *you* must think he is, if you feel you need a gun to protect yourself.
        I really respect your feelings and your anxiety, and I'll do my best to help
        you to feel safe again.

     P: You're the first one who takes me seriously. Even Tom thinks I'm nuts.

Talk to the patient repeatedly from his point of view and express empathy for what he is going through. Like the above example, he may often
open up when he feels you understand him and want to help him.

Split Off the Sick Part of the Patient

After you have learned what the patient considers as her disturbance, appeal to the healthy observer in her, and offer your help against the trouble.

Communicate to her that you are on her side in the battle against her pain. Thus, you create a split between healthy observer and perceived perturbation.

To a patient with full insight you can explain the nature of her disorder. Review treatment options and their implementation. Full insight does not mean that the patient fully grasps the nature of her illness or the implications of potential treatment possibilities. You should not expect that the phobic patient, for example, will be able to arrest her behavior just because she understands it! In addition, the interviewer should be cautious and recognize distortions due to the illness. A depressed patient, for instance, may describe his depressive symptoms in a seemingly distant objective manner, but this cool presentation may belie his bleak view about the course of his illness. Is his past riddled by guilt feelings? Does he expect he can ever feel good again? Does he underestimate himself? Recognize where the disorder warps his perception.

In a patient with partial insight the healthy observer within the patient is harder to define. For instance, Rose truly believes that her neighbors are spying on her. You have to accept her delusions as *her* reality. Therefore, base the phrasing of your questions on her perception and you will have tapped into the part of her that wants help with feeling bothered by her neighbors' spying.

With Richard and with Mr. Combs, neither of whom has insight, the disturbance is the alleged encroachment on them by the spacemen or the mailman, respectively. They feel harassed and fearful about these persecutors. There may be no healthy observer, but there is a part of Richard and Mr. Combs that is scared, concerned, and aware that they are suffering. This is the part you need to appeal to with your suggestions of treatment. Express to these patients how terrible it must feel to be harassed. Offer them the hospital as security and medication as protection, so that the intruders will no longer upset them.

Set Therapeutic Goals

Define two goals, commensurate with the patient's insight: a goal that you discuss with him, and a therapeutic one based on the nature of his illness that you keep to yourself like a trade secret.

In a patient with full insight both goals are one and the same. For instance, you and the depressed patient may view his symptoms as expressions of a treatable illness. State this goal and offer your help.

There are two goals for a patient with partial insight. For Rose, the overt goal is to overcome her neighbors' hostility; your therapeutic goal is to eradicate the delusional thinking. The patient is barred from this insight and would be hostile or unresponsive to your goal.

For patients with partial insight, one goal of treatment is to try to bring them to full insight and prevent relapse. For Rose, with treatment she will recognize the delusional nature of her beliefs. Then the treatment of the delusion itself becomes the overt goal. After remission, the prevention of a relapse becomes a new overt goal. At this time, the overt and therapeutic goals have merged.

As the delusion melts away, the patient may start to challenge you and ask:

"Do you think my neighbors are really against me, or do you think I'm crazy?"

In reply, ask her what she thinks, and tell her it is more important that you understand her distress rather than worry about how much her neighbors really harassed her. When a patient reaches full insight, she may remark that you probably knew all along that her ideas were nonsense. Counter her statement with a question:

"What would you have said if I told you that 6 weeks ago?"

For Richard and Mr. Combs (no insight), the overt goal is to take neuroleptic medication "so that the intruders bother them less." The therapeutic goal is to abolish their delusions.

Restating the overt goal with the patient's growing insight is often a painstakingly slow process. Avoid provocative confrontations and interpretations that may offend them. Give them time to see through their problems and have the overt goal merge with your therapeutic one.

Both overt and therapeutic goals remain elusive if you do not show the patient that you will help him. The more he distorts reality, that is, the more the overt and therapeutic goals differ from each other, the more support he needs. Make him feel that you accept him "unconditionally," as Truax and Mitchell (1971) called it. In their research on the effective therapist—the one who initiates change in his client—they isolated three ingredients: empathy for the patient's suffering, genuineness in the patient-interviewer interaction (see above), and unconditionally positive regard for the patient as a person. These ingredients are not restricted to therapy but also apply to the psychodiagnostic interview, in which an alliance is created to achieve both the immediate interview goal of patient self-disclosure and the more remote goal of patient improvement.

4. SHOW EXPERTISE

Empathy goes a long way, but empathy is not enough. It tells the patient that you care, but it tells nothing about your competence to care. Research has suggested that people rank competence highly in choosing a physician. In the study cited earlier, 205 adults chose "expertise" ("seems knowledgeable in the field, asks me appropriate questions about my problem") as their first and fifth criterion for choosing a physician (Hill 1991).

To establish your expertise, you need to show the patient that you are competent to handle his problems. Use four techniques to convince him that you understand his disorder:

1. Make him aware that he is not alone with his problem; put his illness into social perspective.
2. Communicate to him that you are familiar with his illness—show knowledge.
3. Address his doubt about your professional skills. Your expertise sets you above well-meaning family members or friends and distinguishes you as a professional.
4. Instill hope about his future.

Put the Illness Into Perspective

When the patient describes his problems, you may interject:

"Have you ever known anybody with a problem like yours?"

He may tell you about family members and friends, movies and books concerned with mental illness. Ask him how his own problems fit in. Correct his misconceptions if he has any.

Another patient may claim that he has never heard about a problem like his. Tell him that it is common to hide psychiatric disorders. Ask him what he thinks about his disorder. Discuss with him which features of his illness are common, and which ones are specific to him. Reassure him that many people have similar problems and have gotten well with treatment.

A patient may panic when you mention other patients to him and fear that you will file him away as just another "case." Put his worries at ease and express that his symptoms may be similar to others but his personality to deal with them is unique.

Show Knowledge

Demonstrate expertise to your patient by probing for specific symptoms of his disorder. A patient is sometimes amazed by targeted questions about his condition, wondering: "How did you know that?" Then, he becomes more inclined to trust you and reveal secret concerns such as ruminations, obsessions, or compulsions—since you know anyway.

Another way to establish expertise is to stir up the patient's curiosity about psychology and mental illness that he has read about or seen discussed on television. Discuss famous examples, such as President Lincoln or television personalities for depression (also King Saul if the patient has a religious background). Point out how they relate to him. Use phrases such as:

"You've got a problem about which we have learned quite a bit recently."
"Your problem is common to middle-aged people."
"Recently, we have made some progress in treating a problem such as yours."

Learn from the patient's response what aspect of his problems interests him. Answer his questions in a concise manner; explain heredity, receptor theories, and psychological formulations, or system theory. Your knowledge is reassuring for the intellectual, obsessive, or educated patient who bases his trust in you more on how much you know than how much you care (for him).

What do you do if you do not know the answer to a question? Admit your ignorance freely. Tell him whether the answer is known, but you don't know it, or whether it is not known at all. Admitting to the limits of your knowledge usually increases the patient's confidence in your honesty. Most patients do not expect you to be omnilegent or omniscient, but if one patient does, discuss his false expectations with him.

Deal With Doubt

Whenever you encounter doubt about your expertise, decide how to deal with it (see Chapter 3: Techniques; also compare Othmer and Othmer 2002):

"What caused you to ask this question at this time?"
"Do you have concerns whether I really understand your problems?"

Use openness, counterquestioning, and consider even interpretation when you sense a deeper-seated doubt. If you handle the patient well, he will experience you as an expert. Most patients respect skillful management of their difficulties. We will talk more about this in Chapter 3.

Instill Hope

Often psychiatric patients have suffered from their symptoms, signs, and failures for months or even years before they seek or find effective help. For instance, substance abuse patients may have tried unsuccessfully on their own to cut back on their use or quit the habit altogether. Patients with major depressive disorder have a negative outlook on the future due to the nature of their disorder. Therefore, it is essential to address their view of the future and to instill hope. Tell them what they can expect if they cooperate with your diagnostic assessment and the treatment based on it. Most patients are better off with diagnosis and treatment than without it, a point to be emphasized, without raising unrealistic expectations.

5.   ESTABLISH LEADERSHIP

While empathy grows from your compassion with the patient's suffering, and expertise from your knowledge of his problem, leadership originates from your ability to motivate and guide him. Out of 15 criteria, patients ranked criteria of leadership third and fourth after expertise and empathy (Hill 1991). Establish leadership at the moment you meet your patient by taking control of your interaction with him. Express interest in his welfare. Motivate him to change. The acid test for leadership is his acceptance of your explanations and his willingness to comply with your treatment plan.

Some interviewers overstep their authority. They perceive the patient as a subordinate who should obey. Some patients accept this demanding, or even punitive demeanor, and feel strongly guided rather than imposed on. Obviously, such an interaction fosters dependence. An interviewer who assumes that he knows best, that he does not owe any explanations, and that if the patient does not like it he had better seek help elsewhere jeopardizes genuine rapport. He patronizes rather than guides the patient.

Most authoritarian interviewers are unaware of their lack of empathy or willingness to explain. They are often insecure and hide their self-doubt behind an authority role. If your patient responds to you with resistance or anxious obedience, examine whether you were too threatening or demanding.

Not only may you get hung up on the authoritarian role, but sometimes the patient pushes you there, even against your will. He may put you on a pedestal and then protest against the authority he has endowed you with— or he may be afraid of you, trying to impress or please you in fear of retaliation, or may admire you as a model or idol to identify with. Make the patient aware of his attempts to push you into the authoritarian role and point out to him his unrealistic expectations, thus counteracting false expectations possibly followed later by disappointments.

The grandiose or suspicious patient, or one with antisocial personality disorder, may defy your leadership, try to disarm you, and demonstrate his disrespect. He may grasp the opportunity to launch remarks such as:

"I have to see about this."
"I usually get a second opinion."
"I don't trust doctors. I've fired them before."
"You either deliver, or else."

Confront him with his behavior:

"You seem to have difficulties in accepting some ideas from me."
"Sure, you should get a second opinion . . . but is it really my opinion or my person that gives you problems?"
"When you fire doctors it makes you feel as if you are in control. Don't you wish you could also fire your problems?"
"Do you really distrust my care or your ability to respond?"

Discuss his difficulties in accepting your leadership. For instance, point out the pattern of the difficulties that he has reexperienced with every counselor before and now with you. Tell him you and he have to find out what may cause his uneasiness. Praise him that he was able to show his concerns. Tell him that his openness will help along the exploration of his psychosocial problems.

6. BALANCE THE ROLES

Patients and therapists enter the interview room with a set of expectations, often played out in roles. In some cases, the patient will want you to assume a role, such as the authoritarian, or the empathic listener, or the savior, or the law enforcement officer. If you are aware of the roles that the patient asks of you, you'll be better able to gauge how to respond to his presentation of himself.

The therapist is also playing roles. As you have seen with the different styles of interviewing, the therapist can fall into traps, jeopardize rapport, and sink the interview.

How can you use roles to better interview the patient and establish rapport? How can you catch yourself playing a role with a patient that is detrimental to the therapeutic goals, or to rapport?

THE ROLES OF THE INTERVIEWER

The skillful interviewer balances the roles of empathic listener, expert, and leader throughout the interview. Ideally, he switches these roles according to the patient's needs. However, such flexible interchanges—even though ideal—do not always occur. Many interviewers lock into one stereotype and let that dominate their interviewing style. Therefore, it is necessary to monitor the roles that you and your patient may slide into, adjust to them, or change them if necessary.

The Empathic Listener

The empathic listener puts his patient at ease, is sensitive to his suffering, and expresses his compassion.

Being empathic does not mean being overly lenient, or behaving like a permissive mother with a spoiled child. Interviewers, or therapists, who fail to set professional boundaries may wait for patients when they are late, tolerate forgotten appointments, reduce charges, invite them to dinner, or even get intimately involved. In a desire to comfort patients, interviewers may neglect to set limits when indicated, to hospitalize when necessary, or to recommend more intensive treatment measures such as electroshock treatment when all other treatment has failed. At an extreme, they become compassionate friends or like a family member developing emotional closeness without professional distance. These interviewers fall short as expert and leader.

When you recognize that you overemphasize empathy, start to set limits, assume leadership, and bring your expertise to bear whenever it appears in the best interest of a well-run, economic, yet informative interview.

The Expert

The expert may feel that empathy is a waste of time. What the patient needs is the interviewer's know-how and not compassion. His basic attitude: It is not so important that you want to help—but that you *can*. The expert may ride the high horse of knowledge with an aura of self-proclaimed infallibility. Aloof, he may not care whether the patient follows his recommendations or not, because it is the patient and not him who has to suffer the consequences.

If you are such an "expert," if a warm, friendly tone is missing in your interview, you need to try to become sensitive to the patient's suffering. Review transcripts from your interviews and determine whether you had empathy and communicated it to the patient. Also, see whether you were supportive and provided guidance where appropriate.

The Authority

From the beginning of an interview, the authoritarian interviewer insists on being in command and expects the patient to follow.

>"Compassion?"

she may ask with a thin smile of surgical indifference.

>"What about the patient's respect? Expertise is surely enough—and which patient recognizes it anyway?"

Therefore, she expects a patient to put his trust in her hands without having to waste time answering irritating questions.

Patient and interviewer clash if the interviewer insists on her authority and the patient is unwilling to yield. The following took place between a fourth-year psychiatric resident and a 28-year-old patient in the second session of a diagnostic interview. The resident had asked the supervisor for help with this patient whom she had diagnosed as dependent personality. The resident shook hands with the patient and his wife, and introduced the interviewer:

Novice: This is the clinic director. He will sit in today [she neither explained why, nor asked the patient's permission].

     P: I'm sorry to be late, but we had some car trouble.

Novice:	Well, you know the rules of this clinic and have accepted them. We have to charge you for the time that you were late, because I was here and had the time set aside for you.
P:	I understand. By the way, I also brought my wife because she may be able to explain to you better than me what kind of a dilemma we are in.
Novice:	I thought we had agreed that you should depend more on yourself and not use others to fight your battles.
P:	But I have such a hard time to get through to you. You told me that most of my problems result from our living with my parents—I was out of a job for 6 months and we had no reserves. We can stay in my parents' upstairs apartment by paying only for the utilities and repairs. My wife could tell you that my bad feelings don't have much to do with living with them.
Novice:	I don't see how I can help you if you don't want to do what I told you. You may as well find somebody else.
P:	I guess you are right. I thought I was here to understand myself and my problems better, but I feel bossed around and I don't see how that can help me.

At this point the supervisor stepped in, responded with empathy to the patient's problems, and gave him the opportunity to explain himself.

If you are an authoritarian interviewer you may be unaware of your style and how it may affect your patient. Here are some pointers that may help you become aware of this problem and therefore help you to correct it. The patient opposes you and becomes reluctant, she grins or makes undermining remarks. She contradicts you or becomes very obedient, or becomes uncomfortable and monosyllabic, anxious, or insecure.

If you observe any of these behaviors, examine whether you give the patient enough breathing room, empathy, and support. Obviously, there is more than one reason why the patient may become obedient, or hostile, but all of us interviewers are well advised to analyze how much we contribute to the patient's maladjusted behavior.

THE ROLES OF THE PATIENT

Like interviewers, patients often assume roles. These include: the "carrier of an illness," the "sufferer," and the "VIP."

Carrier of an Illness

As carrier of an illness the patient sees himself only temporarily impaired. He puts distance between himself and his disorder. For instance, he will say it is his sleep not him that is disturbed. He doesn't have a problem, just his marriage. He puts his problem into quarantine so that it cannot infect the rest of him. Other than the pain in his back he tries to live a normal life. He does not demand special privileges, or crave sympathy and pity. All he expects is expert medical management. Rapport with him comes easy.

The Sufferer

Such a patient is the opposite from the carrier of an illness. He is consumed by his pain and anguish. His problems flood him like septicemia. He exaggerates his disability. He craves comfort, sympathy, and understanding rather than expert advice. His demands may often become overwhelming and unbearable. He forces you to set firm limits, yet the expression of your empathy often reestablishes his self-control and containment. Chronic depression and some personality disorders favor the development of this role.

The "VIP"

The "very important patient" sees himself as privileged, entitled to attention at any time of day or night. He expects preferred treatment. He searches for the very best in the field, the star physician or psychologist. Establishing rapport with such a patient may become complex and limit-setting unavoidable. The "VIP" attitude can be adopted by anyone, from the very successful to the least privileged. Often you will be impressed by the modesty of very successful people. In contrast, the true "VIP" will phone you at 3:00 A.M. to tell you he can't sleep.

ROLE INTERACTION

Rapport is achieved when interviewer and patient balance their changing roles and act accordingly.

If you or the patient reject each other's adopted role, conflict arises. Monitor the emerging roles and react accordingly. A few patients may resent your expertise as too "brainy" and may long for guidance and leadership: "You are the doctor, don't explain my problems to me; tell me what to do!" In short, he may search for the authority he can follow, who tells him what to do. Depending on your judgment, you may confront him with that need or you may comply and provide authority.

The following example shows how the interviewer avoided a role conflict when Bernie, a 54-year-old, divorced male, openly rejected both the interviewer's leadership and expertise.

1. I: What can I do for you?
 P: Before I tell you anything, I want you to know that I'm here to get a second opinion. People have told me that you are pretty knowledgeable. But don't expect me to believe what you tell me or do what you advise me.
2. I: If you feel like this, why did you come to see me?
 P: I just want to know what you have to say. If I like it, you are on.
3. I: Okay [silent].
 P: What do you have to say?
4. I: Nothing yet. Except that you don't think much about my ability to help you.
 P: That's right.
5. I: You may be right, but I wonder what makes you think that way.
 P: Nobody else could help me before. I lost my job 7 years ago.
6. I: Because nobody else could help you, you don't have confidence in me either?
 P: Right.
7. I: I can't promise you anything; I may fail also but I will try to help you.
 P: We'll see.

The interviewer does not defend the role the patient assigns to him, nor does he counterattack, but explores the background of the rejection (Q. 2–5). Bernie's response reveals the reason for his hostility (A. 5). When the interviewer admits that his treatment effort may also fail (Q. 7), the intensity of the patient's rejection abates.

If a patient verbally attacks you, the strategy is not to accept the role he has assigned to you—the target for his aggression—but to step aside and to assess the reasons for his aggression. Accept these reasons as the patient's legitimate concerns and communicate this acceptance to him. By not responding to aggression with defense or counterattacks but with analysis of the reason, the patient may start to reflect rather than act out.

Dependence on the Interviewer's Leadership

A patient's dependency needs may be as disturbing to rapport as a rejection of the interviewer. Tom, a 27-year-old student of theology, consulted the interviewer.

I: What kind of problem brought you here?
P: I don't know whether I should push myself or not.
I: Well, you are bringing up an interesting question. Should you push yourself?

P: Yes, what do you think?

I: I would like to understand why you feel I can give you better advice than you can give yourself.

P: Well, I just want to know if I can hurt myself by pushing too hard.

I: Was that why you asked me?

P: Yes. I think so . . . [pause] but you are right. I just can't make up my mind about anything. I always look for somebody to tell me what to do.

I: But do you really do what you are told?

P: I don't know. I have to see whether I agree.

I: That's right, you have to find out for yourself.

The patient attempts to put the interviewer in the role of an advice-giving authority. As in the previous example the interviewer explores Tom's reason. Tom's responses allow the interviewer to direct him to reflection and self-reliance.

Avoid giving advice to the doubting patient who is suffering from depression and instead offer empathic listening. When you listen you allow a patient like Howard to sort out his strengths and weaknesses, and come to a decision himself.

P: I hang around the house. I can't stand it. My family avoids me. Should I go back to work?

I: Can you?

P: I don't know, I would just sit there and stare at the desk.

I: Yes?

P: . . . and I would be so embarrassed if all the people that work for me see me sitting there not doing a thing.

I: I understand how you must feel. I know you want to work and support your family, but if you try, you fear you may fail.

P: Maybe I should have patience until I feel a little better.

I: It seems to me you don't want to take the risk of failing.

In contrast, it is sometimes therapeutic for a patient if you do accept the authority role. For instance, when the patient is pondering a realistic plan but is still filled with self-doubt because of a depression—your support and encouragement for his plans may make the difference.

Marge, a 45-year-old, white woman, had suffered from depression for several months without getting relief in spite of intensive therapy.

P: I realize I'm depressed. I don't want to leave the house. I don't feel like hunting for a job. But staying at home and waiting for the kids to come home from school seems to make me more depressed.

I: Hmm . . . and makes you more aware of it?

P: You seem to understand. I think it would be better for me if I pushed myself and took a job!
I: Well, pushing yourself may neither shorten nor lengthen your depression, but I feel it may help you to tolerate your depression better.
P: That's right.
I: I feel that it is a good sign that you want to push yourself and want to go out.
P: I feel I could try it.
I: We will see how it works.

The interviewer accepts the role of adviser and supports what he feels is appropriate, without violating the patient's ability to make her own decisions. To invite reflection rather than to support reasonable action may have set the patient back.

In short, assume the role of listener when the patient complains, or shows ambivalence and confusion about her goals. Assume the role of expert when she lacks knowledge about her condition and needs information about her disorder. Assume the role of adviser when she has made reasonable decisions, but hesitates to act on them.

The skeptic may argue that the professional interviewer will develop a style and adopt techniques that suit his own personality. Such an argument sounds persuasive but cannot be backed up by facts. Rutter et al. (1981) showed that two experienced interviewers in his clinic could change their style at will. They adopted four different styles, called *the sounding board, active psychotherapy, structured,* and *systematic exploratory.* Among styles, the number of closed-end questions, open-end questions, requests for feelings, interpretations, and expressions of sympathy varied vastly and were statistically significant. Rutter et al.'s (1981) results show that interviewing styles are both teachable and learnable (also Cox et al. 1988).

Why all this fuss about rapport? The 5 minutes you invest at the beginning of the interview to deepen rapport guarantee a high return at the end.

CHECKLIST

Chapter 2: Rapport

The following checklist allows you to rate your skills in establishing and maintaining rapport. It helps you to detect and eliminate weaknesses in interviews that failed in some significant way.

	YES	NO	N/A
1. I put the patient at ease.			
2. I recognized his state of mind.			
3. I addressed his distress.			
4. I helped him to warm up.			
5. I helped him to overcome suspiciousness.			
6. I curbed his intrusiveness.			
7. I stimulated his verbal production.			
8. I curbed his rambling.			
9. I understood his suffering.			
10. I expressed empathy for his suffering.			
11. I tuned in on his affect.			
12. I addressed his affect.			
13. I became aware of his level of insight.			
14. I assumed the patient's view of his disorder.			
15. I had a clear perception of the overt and the therapeutic goals of treatment.			
16. I stated the overt goal of treatment to him.			
17. I communicated to him that I am familiar with his illness.			
18. My questions convinced him that I am familiar with the symptoms of his disorder.			
19. I let him know that he is not alone with his illness.			
20. I expressed my intent to help him.			
21. The patient recognized my expertise.			
22. He respected my authority.			
23. He appeared fully cooperative.			
24. I recognized the patient's attitude toward his illness.			
25. The patient viewed his illness with distance.			

	YES	NO	N/A
26. He presented himself as a sympathy-craving sufferer.	_____	_____	_____
27. He presented himself as a very important patient (VIP).	_____	_____	_____
28. He competed with me for leadership.	_____	_____	_____
29. He was submissive.	_____	_____	_____
30. I adjusted my role to the patient's role.	_____	_____	_____
31. The patient thanked me and made another appointment.	_____	_____	_____

CHAPTER THREE

STRATEGIES TO GET INFORMATION: TECHNIQUES

1. **Complaints**
   Opening Techniques
   Clarification Techniques
   Steering Techniques
2. **Resistance**
   Expressing Acceptance
   Confrontation
   Confrontation With Consequences
   Shifting
   Exaggeration
   Induction to Bragging
3. **Defenses**
   Recognition
   Handling of Defenses

SUMMARY

Chapter 3 describes three sets of techniques to get information from the patient. The first set deals with cooperative patients who openly describe most of their problems. The second set is directed toward those patients who conceal part of their problems from the interviewer. The third set of techniques is geared toward patients who unknowingly distort their perception of themselves and others.

▲ ▲ ▲ ▲ ▲

I listen. Most people don't. Something interesting comes along—and whoosh!—It goes right past them.

—Ted Koppel, *Newsweek,* June 15, 1987

▼ ▼ ▼ ▼ ▼

Examiners for the American Boards of Psychiatry and Neurology rate a candidate's interviewing technique by whether she can open up a topic with a broad, open-ended question, pursue it by becoming more and more focused, and finally close up the topic by detailed and specific questions. This succinctly summarizes the general technical approach to psychodiagnostic interviewing.

How is this done? What are the necessary skills? How do you ask all the right questions? How do you make the patient tell you about his behavior, especially what he sees as his problems (Lovett et al. 1990)?

Patients show varying abilities to cooperate. Some are very compliant and arrive in your office ready to reveal their complaints. Others actively obstruct your efforts to find out their problems; they may feel ashamed, hostile, or scared. Still others unwittingly distort their perceptions and revelations of their problems.

A patient generally communicates his problems in one of three ways: 1) by pouring it all out (complaints); 2) by revealing some problems but concealing the embarrassing items (resistance); or 3) by obfuscating the most embarrassing part to you, and even to himself (defenses). There are strategies to deal with all three situations.

When the patient communicates by *complaining,* the interviewer only has to help the patient talk, describe his problems in detail, and explore all aspects of them. Three sets of approaches accomplish this: opening, clarification, and steering techniques.

Resistance is more difficult to deal with. Acceptance and confrontation are the most useful techniques in getting a patient to overcome resistance. Indicate that you notice and understand his resistance but, at the same time, try to convince him that it is advantageous for him to give it up.

The use of *defenses* by the patient is the most difficult to handle. In many psychodiagnostic interviews, defenses can be ignored if they don't interfere with your need for information. Occasionally, however, you have to confront or interpret the defense mechanisms in order to maintain rapport or to reach a diagnosis.

With each type of patient (and some cooperate at times while not at others), the interviewer needs to adjust strategies to obtain information. The following techniques help to show how to elicit cooperation from patients.

1. COMPLAINTS

The patient who comes voluntarily to a mental health professional harbors a reason for his visit, usually a problem with his functioning, with personal interactions, or with self-conduct and self-satisfaction. When he talks about these problems, the professional listens for the suffering behind the words, and for the patient's complaints (see Chapter 2: Rapport). The patient generally expects empathy for his suffering and expertise to identify the source of his malaise. Technically speaking, he expects a diagnosis and a treatment plan (see Chapter 6: Five Steps to Make a Diagnosis).

Therefore, the professional needs three sets of techniques to accomplish the following goals: 1) elicit all complaints (opening techniques); 2) translate them into symptoms, long-term behavioral traits, or problems of living (clarification techniques); and 3) cover the territory and move from one set of complaints to another (steering techniques). If the interviewer accomplishes these goals, she will arrive at an appropriate diagnosis and be in a position to recommend a treatment plan.

Opening Techniques

While interviewing a psychiatric patient you have to find a balance between letting the patient tell his story in his own words and obtaining information necessary for a diagnosis. If you allow him to tell his story without constraints, he may expound endlessly; if you ask specific questions, your "inquisition" may distort his story. Here are strategies to balance both passive listening and active questioning.

Using a broad, open-ended approach when you begin your dialogue will allow the patient to present his problem in his own words. Useful questions are:

> "How can I help you?"
> "What can I do for you?"
> "What kind of problem brought you here?"
> "Where shall we start?"

Such a "patient-centered" approach invites topic selection by him, gives his view of the problem, and should produce his chief complaint. Broad, open-ended questions are the least suggestive and allow the patient to emphasize and elaborate what he sees as important.

Some interviewers only ask open-ended questions. They rarely follow up on clues or ask for specifics. Such an interviewer may find out, for instance, that the patient was depressed, but will not uncover the length, depth, or symptoms of the depression, unless the patient had volunteered this information. She may also know that the patient had sleep disturbances, but may not have inquired further about the nature of his insomnia. While some advocate this approach, it may prevent obtaining information necessary for diagnosis and timely and efficient assessment.

Occasionally, you encounter the opposite problem. These interviewers unnerve the patient with rapid-fire yes or no questions, getting information but never arriving at the chief complaint. In a mock board interview, one of our candidates had to interview a white, middle-aged male and used the following approach.

C: I'm Dr. A. You agreed to have this interview.
P: Yes.
C: OK. How old are you?
P: 47.
C: Do you have any siblings?
P: What do you mean?
C: Brothers and sisters.
P: Yes.
C: How many?
P: Three.
C: Are you the youngest?
P: No.

For half an hour this candidate bombarded the patient with closed-ended questions, collecting a myriad of small details, which she was not able to assemble to a clinical picture or a diagnostic impression.

These two styles may sound extreme. Yet, the first one is not rare. Milder forms of the second one also occur at the beginning of each student rotation on psychodiagnostic interviewing. There are advantages and disadvantages to both types of questions.

Open-ended questions generate genuine, individualized, spontaneous answers. Most interviewees are motivated to tell you what is bothering them. They want you to help them and thus, with your prodding and direction, will be able to get to their main complaint. Hopkinson et al. (1981)

analyzed naturalistic interviews and found that open-ended questions with few interruptions at follow-up rather than closed-ended questions facilitate emotional expression.

The downside of open-ended questions is that they can elicit answers that are lengthy, unreliable, vague, and incomplete. You may feel inundated with information, yet still lack the details needed for diagnosis.

The advantage of closed-ended questions is the fact that they generate quick, clear, reliable answers about a circumscribed topic. Using a battery of closed-ended but detailed questions can help the interviewer develop a systematic interview that leads to fuller coverage of patients' mental state than a free-style interview. Cox et al. (1981) report that a directive style is more effective in obtaining data about the absence of certain key symptoms. They further found that frequency, severity, context, duration, and qualities of symptoms or problems are better assessed by directive questioning, but did not work better for the assessment of new symptoms or family problems.

Shortcomings of closed-ended questions? Sometimes they may force false-positive answers, and inhibit the patient's freedom to express himself. For overly compliant patients—those who wish to please the interviewer— the closed-ended question may yield little in the way of important information. Finally, the responses can conform to your preconceptions and thus not yield a truthful picture of the patient's perception of reality. Table 3–1 shows the pros and cons of open- versus closed-ended questions.

The best approach is to combine questions along the continuum of broad to sharply focused questions. Introduce a new topic with a broad, open-ended question; follow up with targeted ones; and finish with a series of narrow, sometimes closed-ended questions—the yes/no type. Yes/no questions can be used to verify, specify, or challenge a response. If you want to avoid closed-ended questions altogether, use sharply focused but open-ended questions. Instead of

"Do you have trouble falling asleep?" [expected answer: yes or no],

ask:

"What happens when you try to fall asleep?"

The patient knows that you expect him to talk about sleep onset, but he still has the chance to surprise you with an unexpected answer.

"I have the weirdest experience. I often see monsters. It is as if I start dreaming when I try to fall asleep." [hypnagogic hallucinations—a classic symptom of narcolepsy]

Table 3–1.   Pros and cons of open- and closed-ended questions

Aspect	Broad, open-ended questions	Narrow, closed-ended questions
Genuineness	High They produce spontaneous formulations.	Low They lead the patient.
Reliability	Low They may lead to nonreproducible answers.	High Narrow focus; but they may suggest answers.
Precision	Low Intent of question is vague.	High Intent of question is clear.
Time efficiency	Low Circumstantial elaborations.	High May invite yes/no answers.
Completeness of diagnostic coverage	Low Patient selects the topic.	High Interviewer selects the topic.
Acceptance by patient	Varies Most patients prefer expressing themselves freely; others become guarded and feel insecure.	Varies Some patients enjoy clear-cut checks; others hate to be pressed into a yes/no format.

Thus, the questions change from a predominantly patient-centered to an interviewer-directed format as a topic gets covered. (For more on the different topics of an interview, see Chapters 4, 5, 6, and 7.) Obviously, this progression can be changed and altered to suit your needs.

Depending on a patient's type of disorder or personality, he may favor one or the other type of question. The obsessive patient prefers closed-ended and circumscribed questions, the hysteric personality broad, open-ended ones. Depending on rapport (see Chapter 2) and phase of interview (see Chapters 7 and 8), choose the appropriate type of questions, their combination and sequence.

After a topic has been initially broached, clarify its boundaries, its specific content, and its connections to other topics. Using clarification techniques will help you with this task.

Clarification Techniques

Some patients answer questions clearly; others are narrow, disjointed, vague, or circumstantial in their response. In such situations, the interviewer needs to help the patient to explain himself more clearly. There are various techniques used to encourage the patient's clarity of response. We have termed these: specification, generalization, checking symptoms, leading questions, probing, interrelation, and summarizing.

Specification

The interviewer needs specific, precise, and explicit information, but the patient answers in vague or one-word responses. It is best to switch to a more closed-ended form of questioning as in the following example (Q. 3–6):

1. I: How is your sleep, Mr. Warner?
   P: Lousy.
2. I: What's lousy about it?
   P: Everything.
3. I: Do you have any problems with falling asleep?
   P: Yes.
4. I: How long does it take you to fall asleep lately?
   P: Sometimes an hour, sometimes 3 hours, sometimes I can't sleep all night.
5. I: Are there nights when you fall asleep all right, but you wake up a few times?
   P: No.
6. I: Do you ever wake up early in the morning and then can't go back to sleep?
   P: No.

Questions 3, 5, and 6 are closed-ended but elicit accurate answers. Their validity has to be judged in the context of the total interview. For example, if your patient complains:

"I often feel bad."
"My sleep is lousy."
"I'm not eating as I should."
"My sex life is the pits."

feed the vague words "bad, lousy, not eating as I should, is the pits" back to him (Q. 2, 4 below). If feedback fails, reflect back your understanding of his answer (Q. 5 below). If he responds:

"That's not it!"

let him describe either the most recent or most severe occurrence of the event from beginning to end (Q. 6–8 below).

The following interview shows how this technique was used with Lora Carr, a 43-year-old, white, married female with a diagnosis of fibromyositis, a nonspecific illness characterized by pain, insomnia, tenderness, and stiffness of joints.

1. I: What brought you here, Mrs. Carr?
   P: I feel tired all day.
2. I: Tired?
   P: Because I don't sleep well.
3. I: What's wrong with your sleep?
   P: It's light and restless.
4. I: [interviewer focuses on "restless" first and ignores "tiredness"] Well, in what way is your sleep restless?
   P: I guess, I don't know . . .
5. I: You mean you toss and turn?
   P: No, I don't think so.
6. I: When was the last time that your sleep was restless?
   P: That was last night.
7. I: Why don't you describe your sleep, starting with the time when you went to bed?
   P: I went to bed at 10:30 P.M. and then I was up again a little after midnight.
8. I: Yes?
   P: Then at 1:00 or 1:30 A.M. again. It took me a half hour to get back to bed and then I woke up at 4 A.M. again, and I don't know when I fell asleep. In the morning I had the hardest time getting up.
9. I: So restless sleep for you means waking up a lot during the night.
   P: That's it.
10. I: [now, the interviewer shifts to the second part of the problem, the tiredness] You also said that you feel tired all day.
    P: That's right.
11. I: Does it mostly happen after your restless nights?
    P: No, not necessarily. Some nights I sleep real well and I'm still groggy until 11 o'clock in the morning.
12. I: So then you really seem to have two problems: waking up in the middle of the night and feeling tired during the morning hours.
    P: Yes, that's what's going on.

To this patient, restless sleep means having intermittent insomnia (Q. 9). The interviewer then examines the relationship between intermittent insomnia and daytime tiredness, and learns that they are independent. This kind of questioning also helps the patient feel that she is being heard and understood. If the interviewer were to respond glibly or make presumptions about what the patient was saying, the patient might shut down the communication.

Generalization

Sometimes a patient will offer specific information when the interviewer needs a sense of his overall recurrent pattern of behavior.

Mr. Allen, a 48-year-old, white, married dairy farmer, had his first depressive episode approximately 2 years prior to this visit. He has experienced a relapse and returns to the clinic.

I: Mr. Allen, tell me, what kind of problems have you had lately?
P: Well, I'm having some problems with my sex life.
I: What about it?
P: Last night I had a terrible problem. We flew in from W. to see you. We checked into the hotel, had a nice meal, but later in bed, I just could not get it up.
I: Do you usually have this problem?
P: My wife is very understanding. She's a good lover.
I: So then you really don't have any sex problem?
P: Last night, as I said.
I: What sex problems do you have regularly, if any?
P: I can't come, no matter how hard I try. It tires my wife out and I get frustrated. But that was not my problem yesterday. I could not get it up yesterday.
I: Were you impotent before you felt depressed again?
P: I did not have any problems then.

The patient has a tendency to bring up a recent, single event that is not representative of his usual symptoms. Therefore, the interviewer repeats his question, but emphasizes the longer time perspective, by using terms like "usually," "regularly," "most of the time," or "often." If the patient again refers to specific circumstances or situations you may have to explore each situation to appreciate the overall problem.

Checking Symptoms

When a patient's story is vague, the interviewer can present a list of symptoms to help her detect any psychopathology. Depressed patients, for instance, often lack precision and verbal fluency, which prevent an effective expression of their thoughts and feelings. In that case you may ask for symptoms. If a depressed patient still gives vague answers, you may suggest some symptoms and have him agree or disagree. Cross-check these symptoms to avoid being suggestive. This technique of checking symptoms is used in the following interview.

Joe, a 47-year-old, married manager of a small factory, does not provide diagnostic clues in his first seven answers. The interviewer becomes more directive and translates the patient's vague complaint into symptoms.

1. I: Hi Joe. How have things been going lately?
   P: Well, I don't think my wife is really satisfied with me. She says: "Why can't you be your old self again, the way you were when I first met you and when I married you?"

  2. I: She thinks you have changed?
     P: Well, we are going to meetings of these Amway people. These are just fabu-
         lous people. They try to help you whenever they can. You really have to
         meet them.
  3. I: Your wife thinks you have changed? How does that show in these meetings?
     P: These are fabulous people. They are outgoing and so upbeat. They seem to
         be so optimistic. I met one of them last Monday morning at 8:30 A.M. at the
         post office. It was one of those gloomy mornings. I asked him how he was
         doing. He said, "Super, super." He really seemed to glow. There was only
         one other time that I have seen people act that way. That was in our church.
  4. I: So, in what way are you different? What does your wife have in mind?
     P: Well, I don't really know. She is always understanding, but lately she gets
         impatient with me.
  5. I: You mean you cannot tune in with these people?
     P: Right. They stand up, give a long talk, and tell you how to motivate others.
  6. I: How are you different?
     P: I got up and told them how fabulous they are.
  7. I: What's wrong with that?
     P: I don't know! At work they say: "What's wrong with Joe? He was always in
         a good mood."
  8. I: So your mood has changed?
     P: I believe the people at work made funny remarks about me.
  9. I: What do you think is wrong with you?
     P: At work, they seem to think that I'm different now.
 10. I: It seems that your mood has changed.
     P: Yes, I was always out with the people and joked with everybody and they
         laughed and said: "There's nothing that can get him down."
 11. I: That has changed now?
     P: [starts crying]
 12. I: Are you down in the dumps?
     P: Yeah.
 13. I: And the people at work, you seem to withdraw from them?
     P: Yeah. I want to be left alone.
 14. I: And with the Amway people you just can't get up and give a pep talk?
     P: No, I am just not up to it.
 15. I: Are you unable to find the right words?
     P: That's right. I just want to tell them how understanding they are. But I can't
         even do that. I start crying.

The interviewer first lets the patient tell his story, but the open-ended
approach proves ineffective. He attempts to get the patient to be more specific in Q. 2–6, but still does not get a precise description of the problems.
Finally, the interviewer *checks for symptoms* (Q. 8, 10, 12–15). Even though
checking for symptoms suggests a complaint and supplies words from the
interviewer's rather than the patient's vocabulary, this approach is some-

times the only one that allows you to collect diagnostically useful information within a reasonable time frame.

Leading Questions

Leading questions suggest to the patient a specific answer. For instance,

"Of course, you have never considered suicide, have you?"
"You never heard a voice, did you?"

Such a formulation may lead to denial of symptoms in anxious and dependent patients, even though they did in fact consider suicide or hear voices, but it may provoke a contradiction in oppositional patients who have not considered suicide or heard voices but feel offended by your suggestion or lead. Of course, leading questions can still elicit a valid and truthful answer.

If you intend to obtain reliable and relatively undistorted information, avoid leading questions. However, if you intend to influence the patient in a specific direction, you may select the questions that best suit your purpose. For instance, if you want to express your trust in a patient's cooperation with your treatment plan, you may say:

"You will try to take the medication as prescribed, will you?"
"You will try to go to a crowded mall and see if you still experience panic, will you?"

If you plan to provoke the patient to contradict your assertion, you may formulate a *leading question* accordingly. Thus, most interviewing techniques can be considered neither good nor bad, but rather suitable or unsuitable to accomplish a particular purpose.

Probing

Some patients assign a bewildering significance and meaning to their experiences without explaining why. The interviewer must then try to uncover the reasons for such claims. This is accomplished by a technique we term "probing." Probing is used on many levels—from determining the patient's degree of insight into his delusional state to finding out more about a topic that the patient seems to want to hide.

For the delusional patient, or the one out of touch with reality, probing is an essential tool for helping the patient to tell his story without feeling confronted. There are some easy ways to spot such a patient: he displays abnormal behavior during the interview; he ascribes magical meaning to an event; he says that someone else sent him to see you; he shows superstitious thinking, clairvoyance, or overvalued ideas. Probing helps to detect the underlying logic of his thinking by exposing misinterpretations. Begin probing if you suspect the patient is delusional. Probing helps to identify the patient's level of insight (see Chapters 2 and 4). If the patient says:

"I don't know why I'm here."
"The police brought me."
"My wife made me come."

ask:

"Why do you think they brought you?"

If he denies knowing anything, continue to probe:

"Why did you go along with them?"

Probe with these "why" questions when the patient tells his story in a bewildered and perplexed way. Ask for his interpretation of his experiences:

"Why do you think these things are happening?"
"What do you think it means?"
"Is it possible that what happened shows us that you are ill?"
"Do you think strange things are going on?"
"Are things not what they appear to be?"

The following case shows how probing was used effectively.

Mr. Stone, a 48-year-old, white, divorced man was brought in by the police because he had been speeding and ignoring the police sirens. When arrested after a brawl, he made accusatory statements such as "the police prevent fair elections." This and similar utterances got him to the emergency room of a Veterans Administration hospital. The interviewer first uses continuation (Q. 1–6, see Steering Techniques below) and then probing (Q. 7).

1. I: What brought you to the emergency room, Mr. Stone?
   P: The police.
2. I: How did you get involved with them?
   P: Oh, it's a long story. I live in [small town in Kentucky] and for the last 2 years I was thinking of running for mayor.
3. I: Okay.
   P: During the day I work as an accountant. The only time I have to prepare myself for the mayor's job is at night.

4. I: Yes, go on.
   P: In the evening, all of a sudden, my neighbors began coming over. They started to come over nearly every night. They asked if I had time for a beer. I kind of went along with them.
5. I: What happened then?
   P: Two nights ago I thought, "This time I'll check up on them." Everything was quiet. My next-door neighbor even had his lights off. But I thought, "They can't trick me." I got my gun out and shot in the air. And when my neighbor opened the window, I told him that I knew that he was watching.
6. I: Alright, what happened then?
   P: He said that I was talking nonsense and that he was going to call the police. I said I wouldn't let him do that. So I jumped in my car and drove off. When I got on the highway, I was stopped by a police car. They said they were stopping me for speeding. I told them I knew why they were really stopping me and I started to get away. But they caught up with me. Finally, they brought me here this morning.
7. I: What do you think this means?
   P: Well, can't you see? Can't you see the plan?
8. I: Well, maybe you can help me along, so I can understand better what's going on.
   P: The neighbors came over, I think because they wanted to steal my time so I couldn't prepare myself for the election. I never told them that I planned to run, but they must have known anyway.
9. I: Why is that?
   P: Because I got some hints.
10. I: What kind of hints?
    P: When I came home I looked through the window, before I entered my house, and I saw a shadow.
11. I: What do you think this shadow was?
    P: I think somebody was in the house looking through my things.
12. I: What do you think the police had to do with this?
    P: My goodness, don't you understand? They don't want me to run for mayor. They want me locked up. They figure if I get in, I'll clean out that snake pit and reveal all the corruption that's been going on for much too long.

Probing is useful for scanning the patient's thought content for ideas of reference and delusions (Q. 7–12). The interviewer avoids challenging the patient's interpretations because the patient's way of presenting his experience reveals that he has little insight into his reality distortions.

Probe also when the patient admits to a psychiatric symptom such as a hallucination or delusion. For example, if a patient answers a query about having heard voices or seen visions with "yes," get the precise time, place, and frequency of this occurrence. The patient may give a positive answer about hallucinations, only to elaborate that such experiences occurred while he was asleep or while drifting into or out of a sleeping state.

Probing is not limited to the patient's interpretation of events. It is a handy tool to elicit emotional responses to other life events. In situations where the patient talks about his marriage problem, conflicts at work, or difficulties with his children in a somewhat distant, neutral way, jump out of the groove of collecting further details of the conflict and ask directly for his emotions:

"How did it make you feel when ... happened?"

Hopkinson et al. (1981) report that in 55% of such questions and remarks, the request for feelings is rewarded. These requests should be made in a nonemotional way. Interviewers who remain neutral have a yield of 61% while those who express their own feelings during such a request harvest only 45%. The direct request for feelings yields an unexpected bonus: nearly 18% of these requests also produce spontaneous self-disclosure by the client, which contrasts with 2.5% for all other interventions.

This favorable statistic drives home the point: If you want to know what patients think and feel, ask. Is there any better justification for probing?

Interrelation

Explore illogical connections that your patient offers in a psychodiagnostic interview. As with the technique of probing, the patient may reveal distorted, disordered, and delusional thinking. If your patient relates two seemingly unconnected elements, tell him: "Wait! I don't understand what A has to do with B. Please, help me see the connection between them!"

> Beatrice, a 39-year-old, white, married mother of five children, is suspicious of her colleagues. When asked about experiences at work, she mentions her son's car accident and relates it to the recent change in her work schedule.

1. I: How are things going at work now?
   P: I don't know. The others seem to avoid me.
2. I: Is there a reason?
   P: I don't know. There might be. Last week when they switched me from the morning to the afternoon shift, my son had a car accident.
3. I: What does that have to do with changing your shift?
   P: They planned the accident.
4. I: What does changing your shift have to do with your son's accident?
   P: The accident was late in the afternoon. That was the first day I had to be at work in the afternoon.
5. I: I still don't understand how your working in the afternoon and your son's accident are related.

P: Can't you see? They wanted me to be at work when I got the message about the accident, so they could see my reaction. They probably hoped that I would go to pieces. But I didn't give them that satisfaction. I didn't say a word to anyone when I got the telephone message about the accident.

The elements of Beatrice's story are *interrelated* by her delusional interpretations. The interviewer reveals these delusions by asking the patient how switching her work shift and her son's car accident are interrelated (Q. 3–5).

In the above dialogue, the interviewer asks for logical links but does not discuss the patient's emotions. If he desired a more emotional discharge, he could have continued the interview by saying:

6. I: You must have felt devastated when you realized that all your colleagues were plotting against you.

Such an empathic remark elicits in 80% of the cases a strong emotional expression by the patient (Hopkinson et al. 1981). What is the value of such an emotional discharge? It allows the interviewer to judge whether the patient harbors guilt, feelings of persecution, or hostility. Intellectual interrelating may reveal disordered thinking, emotional interrelating disordered affect.

Summarizing

Summaries are useful for clients whose responses are vague or circumstantial, show loose associations, or flight of ideas, such as patients with bipolar illness or cyclothymia. Summaries focus the patient's attention and reflect back to him what you think he has said. It is helpful to use his vocabulary. Be aware that summaries can lead the patient and you may put words into his mouth.

Ron, a 24-year-old, single, male graduate student first contacted the interviewer by telephone with some mild push of speech (see Glossary: Speech).

1. I: You told me on the phone that you feel terrible. Just tell me a little bit more about these feelings.
   P: Last Sunday is a good example. It started all of a sudden when I talked to Joan on the phone Saturday night. Then I felt just terrible all of a sudden. On Sunday I did not want to get up. Finally I did, and ran my 10 miles. I try to have two 10-mile days and two 15-mile days a week.
2. I: In what way do you feel terrible?
   P: Just worked up and nervous.
3. I: So how did the rest of Sunday go?

     P: I thought the run would clean up my system, which it usually does, but I still felt all tense and panicky. I could not get anything done. This feeling also affects me when I'm with girls.

4. I: You mean that you have difficulties when you date?

     P: Yes, sexually. I can't relax.

5. I: You have trouble getting an erection?

     P: Yes, it tends to be that way.

6. I: Do you have this problem all the time?

     P: No, it's very bad when I feel tense and rotten. It fluctuates.

7. I: So you have frequent, short periods when you feel tense and rotten, cannot relax, and have sexual problems?

     P: That's right. I feel down, can't concentrate on my work, and don't want to do anything.

    In his first answer the patient describes "terrible" feelings of short duration. Since he fails to elaborate (A. 2), he is encouraged to go on and to focus on the new topic: the problems with girls (Q. 4). Notice how the interviewer summarizes the patient's statements (Q. 7) and gets his approval.

8. I: For how long have you had those feelings?

     P: As long as I can think back.

9. I: Does it ever get so bad that you think you would harm yourself?

     P: Usually not. I may think about it. Life is precious, but I can understand the tension that some people may have who just go out and take a gun and start shooting people. I would know how to do away with myself. I'm investing in guns. A .45 would take my whole head off.

10. I: Have the terrible feelings ever been so bad that you seem to hear voices?

     P: [silent, thinks for a while] No, I don't think so.

    The interviewer checks for psychotic symptoms and suicidal ideation. Since hallucinations are absent (A. 10) and suicidal thoughts are presented in a theoretical form and not as a compelling preoccupation (A. 9), the interviewer decides that the patient is presently not psychotically depressed but suffers from moderate depressive mood swings. He therefore explores the presence of normal (Q. 11) and elated mood (Q. 12–16) to check whether the patient is suffering from bipolar disease with rapid mood swings (rapid cycler or cyclothymic disorder), or with long periods of euthymic or normal mood.

11. I: Have you ever felt normal?

     P: Yes, but I really don't know what normal is. I feel very good in between. I can work at a job and go to college, and I'm into investments. I do real well with my money.

12. I: So you have a lot of energy?

P: Yes, I do. But I'm mainly tense and irritable and high-strung. But I can also feel very good about myself.

13. I: How is your sleep during those times?

P: Well, for a few days I'm always up and ready to go.

14. I: You mean you stay up all night?

P: No, I usually sleep 6–8 hours, but I'm wide awake and ready to go in the morning.

15. I: Did you ever do anything foolish during these highs?

P: What do you mean?

16. I: Well, spending a lot of money, getting too involved with girls, or doing things that you really regret later?

P: Well, no, I never do anything that is really crazy.

17. I: So you have short highs that make you tense and irritable, but also make you feel good at other times. But those feelings never interfere with your sleep or make you do irresponsible things.

P: That's it.

The interviewer *summarizes* his impression of hypomania and gets the patient's approval (Q. 17). He then returns to the assessment of normal mood (Q. 18–21).

18. I: I know I asked you before, but are there any normal times when you are neither down or high-strung?

P: You mean, when things just go easy and I don't feel driven or have to kick myself?

19. I: That's right, when things kind of fall in place and seem to run by themselves.

P: Yes, last year, I had a pretty good semester.

20. I: Do you feel good then for several months?

P: Usually not that long. Just a couple of months and I start down again.

21. I: Let me summarize. What you describe to me sounds as if you are on a roller coaster, going up and down. The downs seem to be more troublesome than the ups. But the deep downs rarely last longer than a few days. And there don't seem to be many straight stretches or periods when you feel normal.

P: That's it. That's exactly how I feel.

The interviewer summarizes his diagnostic impression of a mild bipolar disorder or possibly cyclothymia (Q. 21).

Another summarizing method especially good with patients who might be easily intimidated is to enlist their help as follows: "I want to see if I have a good idea of what we have discussed; so I'm going to repeat my understanding of our conversation in my own words and I want you to correct any errors I make."

The seven clarification techniques—specification, generalization, checking symptoms, leading questions, probing, interrelation, and summarizing—carve out the contours of symptoms and assess the interconnections of elements within a topic; they are mostly patient-centered. Steering techniques, which are explained next, help the interviewer to direct the patient's attention from element to element and one topic to another. The interviewer is like the captain of the ship who tells the steersman, the patient, which course to follow. Steering is more interviewer-directed than clarification techniques.

Steering Techniques

A vast territory must be covered in order to make a valid diagnosis. How do you get from one topic to the next—redirecting the patient without suppressing him? Steering techniques offer a way in which to keep the interview on a desired course. The techniques include continuation, echoing, redirecting, and transitions.

Continuation

Continuation is the simplest steering technique. It encourages the patient to go on with his story and indicates the course is right. It tells him that he gives diagnostically useful information. This technique includes gestures, nodding, keeping eye contact, and statements such as:

> "What happened then?"
> "Tell me more."
> "Okay."
> "Anything else?"
> "That's interesting."
> "I want to hear more."
> "I think that's important."
> "Go on."
> "Keep on talking."
> "Hmm."

The advantage of this technique is that you let the patient describe his problems in his own words; no symptoms are suggested.

In the following interview, Gary, a 31-year-old, white, single security guard, talks about recent changes in his feelings, which indicate elated mood such as seen in mania, or amphetamine and cocaine abuse. Since this information is diagnostically useful, the interviewer invites continuation whenever the patient stops talking.

1. I: What kind of problem brought you here?
   P: For the last 10 days I haven't been able to sleep.
2. I: Hmm.
   P: I just can't fall asleep. I may only doze off for 1 to 2 hours toward morning.
3. I: Yes.
   P: And I don't even feel tired during the day at all [raises voice].
4. I: [nods]
   P: Last weekend I was home with my folks. It seemed that they bugged me a lot. We got into several arguments and I started slamming doors again.
5. I: Any other problems?
   P: Well, I called my friends and tried to arrange something for Saturday evening.
6. I: [raises eyebrows]
   P: Both of my friends told me, "You are shouting again on the telephone. Are you getting high?"
7. I: Did anything else happen?
   P: Yes. We went out and I was very attracted to girls. I got so stimulated, I had to go to the bathroom twice to masturbate.
8. I: Hmm.
   P: Well, when I came home I had all these fantasies about having sex from behind and I could do it without having to worry about babies.
9. I: What happened then?
   P: Well, I masturbated throughout the night and had wild fantasies. I felt sky-high, but I only had two or three beers.
10. I: Tell me more.
    P: I'm so restless. I try not to talk so much, but it is hard to do. One of these days I feel medication will help me, or I will help myself. But I'm just not there yet.

Directive interventions are avoided, which allows the patient to talk about himself, choosing his order of importance rather than that of the interviewer.

Echoing

Echoing repeats the part of the patient's answer on which you want him to elaborate. This technique is different from continuation in that you selectively emphasize certain elements of the patient's statements, thus enticing him to follow the highlighted parts rather than any other. This technique can be used when the patient offers several leads but you want him to follow a specific train of thought.

> Bernadette, a 36-year-old, white, married, stay-at-home mother, describes her problems in a circumstantial and flighty way. The interviewer echoes reported problems and chooses to ignore her prepared statement.

1. I: How are things going?
   P: They are not going well at all. In fact, I have made a list with all the prob-
       lems that I have had over the last 2 weeks. I have written them down every
       day. My husband agrees with me and he and I think that I may get sick
       again.
2. I: You may get sick again?
   P: Yes, I think so.
3. I: What makes you think so?
   P: I don't get my housework done and I'm terrible with my husband and the
       children. It must be awful to live with me. But let me read from my notes,
       day by day. Do you want to have them?
4. I: You say you are terrible with your husband.
   P: I'm short and abrupt with him. I have no patience at all. I bite his head off
       when he hasn't done anything. But I have it all written down here.
5. I: So you are pretty short with him?
   P: Yes, and I'm also terrible with the children. I shout for no reason at all and
       I'm so tense and irritable. It says here in my notes that I even spanked my lit-
       tle son when he just asked me the same question twice. It seems to be worse
       when I don't sleep well.
6. I: You can't sleep?
   P: I wake up by 4:30 A.M. I can't sleep but I don't want to get out of bed either.
       I get tense and upset. But I have it written here [points to her diary] much
       more systematically. Don't you want to hear it?
7. I: I want to hear it from you. You can leave me the notes for later.
   P: Okay, it won't be very organized. I have a terrible time getting my thoughts
       together. I can't stay on one topic for any length of time. My husband says
       that if I go on like this I will end up in the hospital again.
8. I: So you are all over the place?
   P: Yes, I am. I start cooking, I start sewing, I call up some people, I start clean-
       ing and I don't seem to finish anything. Nothing gets done.
9. I: So you start many things without finishing them?
   P: Yes. That's typical for my negative highs.

The interviewer selectively *echoes* some of the patient's formulations to
elicit symptoms of her mood disorder: loss of energy, irritability, early morning
awakening, distractibility, increase of activity, and experience of a negative
high. Without checking for symptoms, he obtains a symptom profile typical
for an episode with mixed manic and depressive symptoms as seen in
roughly 30% of bipolar patients. The echoing technique is useful in patients
with distractibility and push of speech.

Redirecting

The redirecting technique tells the patient to stop diverging from the main
course and asks him to return after he has strayed from it. Used when pa-

tients ramble, get lost in irrelevant details, or discuss other people's problems, *redirecting* is indicated in patients with flight of ideas, tangential speech, push of speech, and circumstantiality.

> Stacy, a 25-year-old, white, female graduate student, has a hard time staying on one topic. The interviewer redirects her to make her talk about herself. This creates a conflict between his own and the patient's goals.

1. I: What brought you here?
   P: I think I'm having a crisis. I went to the emergency room last night, and this morning and then this afternoon again. They told me to come back to see you.
2. I: What seems to be the problem?
   P: I'm living with Frank. He told me to throw all my medication away. You know he's a mental patient himself. But anybody has to get sick who plays music all night, smokes pot, and takes drugs.
3. I: [interrupts] Stacy, why don't we stay with your own problems?
   P: Okay. Well, last night I called home. My mother was not there, just my sister. You know she's dating this black guy and . . .
4. I: Let me interrupt you. Let me ask you why you went to the emergency room yesterday.
   P: Okay. After I talked to my sister I got so upset because I think she's ruining her life. My parents don't like what she is doing at all . . .
5. I: [interrupts] So you were upset with her?
   P: Yes, and I started drinking beer, and had pizza. And then I remembered that I should not do these things when I'm on Parnate.
6. I: So you went off your diet?
   P: Yeah, but then I got frightened that my blood pressure might shoot up so I went to the emergency room. My mother will be mad . . .
7. I: Stacy, let's talk about going off your diet. You were upset you said?
   P: Yes, I have not been doing well at all lately. My thoughts seem to race. Last weekend I stayed in bed for 2 days and I've been up since then. I talked to Frank. You know Frank is . . .
8. I: Stacy, let's go back to your own problems.
   P: Well, I wanted to have sex with Frank. He said: "You are getting sick again. I want you to go back to your own apartment." You know he can be a real stinker. Now he's decided to be straight.
9. I: So Frank tried to kick you out?
   P: He's really worried about me and sees to it that I take good care of myself.
10. I: So this time he wanted you out?
    P: That made me so upset. I called home and just my sister was in, which did not help matters. It reminded me of what she's doing to herself.
11. I: So you were upset? Before you got upset, were you already pretty restless?
    P: That's right. I think it's me and it hasn't really anything to do with Frank or my sister. I'm afraid the voices will come back too. Yesterday it seemed that things were starting to have another meaning again.

The interviewer interrupts Stacy continuously to redirect (Q. 3, 4, 5, 7, 8) and focus her on giving a description of her problems and symptoms. In spite of the interviewer's efforts, the yield is small in comparison to the length of the interview, as the above example shows.

Transitions

During an interview, many topics (see Chapters 4–6) have to be covered. You have to entice the patient to change topics. Therefore you need different types of transitions: smooth, accentuated, and abrupt. The choice of transition depends on the patient's mental status. An inattentive patient, for instance, may focus better if a new topic is accentuated, whereas a paranoid patient may become suspicious.

Smooth Transitions

Smooth transitions lead easily from one topic to the next by giving the impression that their connection is self-evident. Here are two types:

Cause-and-effect relationship: You assume that a reported event may affect the patient's functioning. Examples are substance abuse and its effects, life events and their consequences, or a physical ailment and its impact.

> Greg, a 16-year-old, African-American high school student, talks about his problem with glue sniffing.

P: Glue has ruined my life. All I can think about is getting a plastic bag over my head and sniffing some airplane glue.
I: Has this sniffing affected your school work?
P: Yes, it's just terrible. I do not even want to go to school and when I go, I'm in a daze.
I: Has it affected your health?
P: I feel dizzy, my heart beats real fast, and I pass out.
I: Has this sniffing interfered with your sleep?
P: Yes, sometimes I sleep during the day and can't sleep at night.

The interviewer directs the patient from glue sniffing to symptoms of depression and their severity by causally relating them. Such a transition works if the causal relationship is evident to the patient. With a delusional patient suspicious of anything new, smooth transitions work best. Otherwise, the response will be:

"What does that have to do with it?"
"What a stupid question!"
"I am not going to answer that nonsense."
"Why are you asking me that?"

The smooth cause-and-effect transition worked well with a 27-year-old, white, single assembly-line worker with delusional disorder. The interviewer uses the patient's complaint and connects it with questions that assess the premorbid personality.

I: You told me that people at work have plotted against you. You say this has really changed you. Tell me what kind of a person you were before all this plotting started to mess you up.
P: I was somewhat of a loner, but I always had one or two friends. Now I have nobody.

A cause-and-effect transition motivates the patient to answer, since his view of his problems is accepted by the interviewer (whereas his usual experience is that his view is rejected).

Temporal relationship: The transition between symptoms is smoothed by relating symptoms to the same point in time.

I: Kathleen, when you had the panic attacks, did you notice any other changes?
P: Yes, my sleep was real bad. I woke up in the middle of the night and could not get back to sleep.
I: What about your appetite at that time?
P: I forced myself to eat, but I lost several pounds anyway.
I: And how was your social life then?
P: I wanted to hide in the house and not face anybody.

In this example, the smooth transition ties symptoms together that belong to the same syndrome. In other cases you may use time as a reference point to change to an otherwise unrelated topic. For instance, when a patient tells you about his medical problems, but you intend to assess his social history in more detail, you may say: "When you had all those medical problems, how did you get along with your wife and how were things at work at this time?"

Accentuated Transitions

Accentuated transitions emphasize a shift in topic; they set the previous topic apart from the new one, such as:

"Now let's explore . . . " (medical history for example).
"Let's shift to another area."

An accentuated transition may be introduced by summarizing what you have learned before switching to the new topic, such as:

"I now know how glue sniffing has affected your life. Let's talk about something different now. Did you have any disciplinary problems when you were in school?"

You may use an accentuated transition as a partition between the phases—as explained in Chapter 7—of the diagnostic interview and as an introduction to testing mental status functions (see Chapter 5). Here are illustrations of the latter:

"I think we have covered a lot of territory and I feel that I understand most of your problems. Before I give you my recommendations, I would like to cover one more point that does not really seem related to any of your problems. I'd like to get an idea of how well you can respond to some test questions that tell us something about your memory and concentration."

"We have not yet discussed how your memory or thinking may be affected by your problems."
"Would you mind if I asked you a few standardized test questions so I can get a feeling of how well you can concentrate?"

Without explaining such a shift in topic to the patient who, for instance, presents with a marriage problem, he may be surprised if he is subjected to a test of concentration, such as the so-called "serial 7s" backwards (subtracting 7 from 100). However, if you prepare him, he may cooperate.

Accentuated transitions revive the patient's attention and make him aware how many different topics have been covered. Withdrawn depressive patients or schizophrenic patients may liven up. Distractible manic patients refocus their attention. The circumstantial obsessive-compulsive patient may be stimulated by the new topic and cooperate better.

Abrupt Transitions

Abrupt transitions introduce a new topic with little warning. They are often clumsy and awkward and usually ill-advised:

"Now, I am going to examine you."
"Let's see, what's the date today?"
"Now I want to ask you a few questions that you may think are really stupid."

"What I wanted to ask you is this . . . "
"Okay, there is something else . . . "

However, abrupt transitions are useful with patients who lie or simulate symptoms in that they catch them off guard.

> Mr. Martens, a 43-year-old white male, was admitted to a Veterans Administration hospital because he claimed severe memory disturbances due to exposure to Agent Orange during the Vietnam War.

1. I: Hi, Mr. Martens, do you remember me? I talked to you last week.
 P: Yes.
2. I: How was your weekend?
 P: I was out on pass.
3. I: How did it go?
 P: I can't remember . . .
4. I: I want you to remember three things: eyedropper, brown, and justice. Would you repeat them for me?
 P: Yes . . . eyedropper, brown, and justice.
5. I: Did you watch any television during the weekend?
 P: Oh yes, about the Middle East. Some mess they have over there.
6. I: Does that concern you specifically?
 P: Yes, I worry about war, especially in the Middle East.
7. I: Which leaders do you fear?
 P: I don't remember their names.
8. I: How is your wife?
 P: She left when I came home.
9. I: Can you remember the three things?
 P: Brown, and . . . and . . . I don't know. But it may come to me if I wait awhile.
10. I: What is the name of the Iraqi leader?
 P: I don't remember.
11. I: Do you know who Saddam Hussein is?
 P: Isn't he an Iraqi leader?
12. I: I am sorry to hear this about your wife. What did you do after she had left?
 P: I wrote her a letter. I told her that I was very disappointed that she left when I came home and I also told this bitch that if she wanted to desert me she should go right ahead. But then I told her that I still love her and that I would like things to work out between us.
13. I: Do you remember the three things?
 P: No, just brown, as I told you before.
14. I: Last week, Dr. X also asked you to remember three things. Do you recall what they were?
 P: No.
15. I: One of the three things was an animal. Do you remember which one?
 P: No.

16. I: You did not remember then either. What did you tell her?
    P: I told her elephant.
17. I: That's right. But she asked you to remember lion.
    P: Yes, it's coming back to me now.

The interviewer jumps back and forth among three topics: television news (Q. 5, 7, 11), marital problems (Q. 8, 12), and recollection of three items (Q. 4, 9, 13–17). The patient claims he does not remember what happened during the weekend but he recalls the television news. He starts to talk about the Middle Eastern conflict, but then claims forgetfulness (A. 10) when he seems to realize that such a recall involves memory. Mr. Martens also recalls the content of the letter that he wrote to his wife. It appears that he was not aware that his memory was tested, because otherwise he would have realized that this recall contradicts his claimed global amnesia.

Regarding the formal memory testing (recall of three items), he claims to have forgotten the items the examiner gave him, but remembers the faulty answer (elephant) he gave the previous week. This inconsistency is not compatible with severe anterograde memory disturbance.

Abrupt transitions have the effect of a cross-examination (Othmer and Othmer 2002). They prevent the patient from keeping track of what he wants to portray. They reveal inconsistencies. They are the lie detectors of an interview. Mr. Martens is only cooperative on the surface. He does not address his need for compensation or attention that may underlie his simulations. His behavior leads us into the next set of techniques, used for patients with resistance.

2. RESISTANCE

Resistance, in this context, refers to the patient's conscious, voluntary effort to avoid a certain topic. Resistance can surface in several ways. The clearest form is open refusal:

"I prefer not to talk about it right now."
"I don't want to discuss this with you."
"Let's talk about something else."

An indirect form of resistance is the patient's attempt to distract you from pursuing a topic: he may answer your questions only briefly, or not at all, or he starts talking intensely about something else, or he is vague, shows reluctance in his facial expression, or pauses before answering. Finally, he may try to sidetrack you with expressions such as:

"This really doesn't bother me."
"It's not one of my main concerns."
"There are more important things to worry about."

Bear in mind the two common reasons for the patient's resistance: 1) his wish to maintain an image, and/or 2) his uncertainty about the interviewer's response and fear of the interviewer's rejection or ridicule. In the initial interview, most patients try to present themselves in a good light, and do not want to embarrass themselves, or be judged as "crazy." Patients are uncertain how the interviewer may respond to the disclosure of "senseless" obsessions, "silly" fears, or "strange" hallucinations and may initially try to avoid revealing them.

The interviewer has to recognize and deal with the resistance. You have to choose whether you want to tolerate it or persuade the patient to overcome his resistance. If resistance is limited to one particular topic and does not interfere with rapport, you may respect the patient's privacy and move to the next topic. Otherwise, you often have no choice but to address his resistance.

Use one of six strategies: expressing acceptance, confrontation, confrontation with consequences (see below: Handling of Defenses), shifting, exaggeration, and induction to bragging.

Expressing Acceptance

When a patient shows reluctance to talk but not open refusal, it often indicates a concern about ridicule. If the interviewer expresses acceptance of the patient's thoughts and feelings, the patient will feel understood. Free of any moral evaluation, acceptance neither condemns nor praises the patient. To help him to overcome his resistance, encourage him, verbalize what he seems to imply, express that you understand him.

> Sharon, a 25-year-old African-American law student, comes to the outpatient clinic. She has agoraphobia but hesitates to talk about it. The interviewer helps her to overcome her resistance by offering understanding and expressing acceptance.

1. I: What problem brought you here, Sharon?
   P: It's really all so ridiculous that if I tell you, you will just laugh.
2. I: Try me.
   P: I know you will. Why should I try?
3. I: You are afraid I would not understand you and laugh at you?
   P: Yes, that's how I feel.

4. I: It must be a terrible feeling, that you can't talk about what's bothering you. I wish I could help you feel better.

   P: How can you, if it's something so ridiculous?

5. I: It is not ridiculous for you. You are serious, Sharon. And you feel scared.

   P: You really understand?

6. I: Well, you have not told me, but I can feel your fear. It must really torture you.

   P: You are right and it is so ridiculous. Whenever I walk over to the campus all these people stare at me. They sit in front of their houses and they all look at me.

7. I: They look at you? That must make you feel uncomfortable.

   P: I seem to be the only person that walks on the street. All the blacks like to sit in front of their houses in summer. I just feel better when I have reached the campus.

8. I: So you really feel terrible being out there in the street, walking by those houses and having the people stare at you.

   P: Yeah. I hate it. I'm just so scared. I get all these good grades in law school, but I'm so anxious I can't even talk to my relatives when they come over to the house.

9. I: I understand how you feel. It sounds like you are running the gauntlet and I can understand your ordeal. You're doing the right thing by talking to me about it. That's the only way I can understand your feelings and help you.

The phobic patient is often not only fearful about certain objects or situations, but also about the fact that she has to talk about her fear. *Expressing acceptance* helps the patient overcome such fear and can resolve resistance to reveal her fears about her panic and phobia.

Confrontation

Confrontation focuses the patient's attention on the resistance. It heightens his awareness and invites an explanation. Use this technique when you observe either behavioral clues of resistance such as avoidance of eye contact, blushing, repetitive swallowing, overly controlled affect, tension, restlessness, or if the patient uses monosyllabic and censored speech, distraction tactics, or dissimulates, that is, minimizes symptoms, or rambles excessively.

The interviewer confronts Mildred, a 34-year-old, white, single secretary, with a behavioral clue. Mildred talks about social isolation and frustration at work. While talking she stares at the interviewer, becomes restless, pauses repeatedly, then resumes talking.

1. I: Mildred, I have noticed that you often look at me without blinking.

   P: What do you mean? [her posture becomes stiff]

2. I: I mean you look at me for a long time without blinking.

   P: I guess it's just a habit [patient blushes].

3. I: Are you aware of it?
   P: So you noticed [pause]. I was afraid you would. I have had this eye problem since I was 15 years old and had an eye infection [gives a long-winded history of her eye infection].
4. I: So what did this infection do to your eyes?
   P: Since the eye infection I think about blinking when I look at people.
5. I: Can you explain?
   P: I always wonder when it would be natural to blink.
6. I: Hmm.
   P: When I look at somebody I always worry about when to blink. If I look too long and don't blink, people think I am staring at them. But when I make myself blink, I think it's unnatural because I did it voluntarily.
7. I: Why didn't you want to talk about it?
   P: It's so embarrassing, you must think I'm crazy.

When confronted with her staring, Mildred minimizes the significance of her behavior (A. 2). Persistent *confrontation* (Q. 3, 5, 7) yields a full explanation of her signs and symptoms and she gives up her resistance. This confrontation opened up the discussion of her obsessions and compulsions.

> Mr. Nelson, a 57-year-old, white, married lawyer, was confronted with the irrational reason for his resistance.

1. I: What kind of problems would you like to talk about?
   P: I am thinking over and over whether I would be able to go to sleep tonight. Just tell me if it can hurt me if I take 10 mg of Ambien when I can't sleep.
2. I: In what way do you think it will hurt you?
   P: My body may be short of enzymes and the drug could accumulate.
3. I: What do you fear could happen?
   P: My breathing may stop and I may not wake up. Tell me if there is a chance this can happen. I worry about these things. But if I don't take the drug I may not be able to sleep. So I'm really in a bind. Damned if I do and damned if I don't.
4. I: Are these the only thoughts that come to your mind time and again?
   P: Yes, these worries.
5. I: Are there ever any other thoughts? Do you have any other repetitive worries?
   P: Like what?
6. I: Some patients wonder how many tiles are on the floor or how many chairs are in the room and they feel they have to count them. Did you ever have any similar experiences?
   P: I don't want to talk about those now.
7. I: So you can only talk about your worries, but not about the other thoughts?
   P: Right.
8. I: What is so different about these other things?
   P: They are so silly and so embarrassing.

  9. I: So you don't want to embarrass yourself, but it is very important for me to understand your problems fully.

     P: I can't come back to you if I tell you about them. I feel too embarrassed. As a lawyer I should not have these problems.

10. I: So lawyers are immune to certain illnesses?

     P: Okay . . . I think again and again if I have wiped myself. And I always have to turn my back away from people so that they can't smell it. I know it's non-sense. I wash myself, but it tortures me over and over again.

Initially, Mr. Nelson talked about worries over insomnia (Q. 1–4). A worry is similar to an obsession with respect to its intrusive nature and emotional discomfort, but unlike an obsession, it is ego-syntonic, that is, the patient identifies with a worry but not with an obsessive thought. Taking the worries as a clue, the interviewer inquires about obsessions but the patient resists this exploration openly (A. 6–7). Confrontation with the resistance (Q. 8–10) achieved the revelation of his obsession and related compulsion.

Mrs. Finch, a 38-year-old, white female, admitted to being nervous at night but denied any other problems. She was confronted with her dissimulation of symptoms:

  1. I: What has been troubling you, Mrs. Finch?

     P: At night I'm nervous.

  2. I: How do you feel during the day?

     P: I'm just fine, just nervous at night, that's all.

  3. I: Fine?

     P: Yes. Fine [patient looks to the ceiling and appears to listen to something, then looks down].

  4. I: Are you hearing something?

     P: No, they don't bother me anymore.

  5. I: Bother you anymore? What do you mean?

     P: I'm over them now.

  6. I: You mean you don't hear them anymore?

     P: [patient looks up to the outlet of the air conditioner, shakes her head and mumbles]. Shut up. No, no, no.

  7. I: You mean they don't talk to you anymore?

     P: I told you that they don't bother me anymore [angrily looks up to the ceiling].

  8. I: Since we have been talking together I noticed that they must have been talking to you through the air-conditioning unit.

     P: Why do you say that?

  9. I: Well, you just looked up there, made an angry face, and talked back to them.

     P: So you heard them too? My sister always says that I am talking nonsense. But my mother and my sister just won't leave me alone. They sneak up on me and say all those mean and awful things.

10. I: So you hear them through the air-conditioning duct even though they are miles away?
    P: Sure, they're sneaky.
11. I: But, you told me that you are not hearing any voices.
    P: That's right. I'm not imagining anything. You know, if I say I hear voices, you will think I'm crazy and imagining things.

Confrontation with her behavior—listening and talking back to the air-conditioning duct—brought out the patient's hallucinations.

Confrontation With Consequences

To use this technique you have to be aware of the patient's intentions, because this technique relies on gratifying the patient's needs. If the patient is desperate to get some result (leave the hospital, get her child back from foster care, see a lawyer), the prospect of satisfaction may help overcome her resistance. This strategy is useful for patients who stubbornly refuse to interact with you.

> Mrs. McQueen is a 23-year-old, white, married female who was brought to the emergency room by her husband because of repeated wrist cutting. Her husband reported that the patient had been a sloppy housekeeper for most of their marriage and had neglected their two children, spending time with a friend instead of taking care of the family's needs. When he criticized her she threw temper tantrums and recently started to harm herself. Mood, sleep, and appetite were unchanged; according to him she had no hallucinations or delusions. At the emergency room the patient was shouting and had outbursts of anger; she fell into a state of muteness when committed at her husband's request.
>
> The patient is lying on the bed with her head buried in her hands. She refuses to acknowledge the interviewer but glances briefly through her fingers.

1. I: Hi, Mrs. McQueen. I'm Dr. O. I would like to talk to you.
   P: [no response]
2. I: Can you tell me why your husband brought you here?
   P: [no response]
3. I: Do you know that your husband plans to commit you?
   P: [no response]
4. I: Do you think he is right in doing so?
   P: [no response]
5. I: Would you like to get out of here?
   P: [no response]

6. I: I take it that under the circumstances it may be best for you to have some rest. You seem to say: "Leave me alone, until I am ready to talk." Why don't I do that. I'll come back next week and talk to you. Do you want me to let you stay here until next week and then come back?

   P: [shakes her head]

7. I: You mean you don't want to take a week of rest?

   P: [shakes her head]

8. I: Do you want me to stay and talk to you?

   P: [no answer]

9. I: Okay. Maybe I should come back later. Is that alright with you?

   P: [no answer]

10. I: Do you want to stay?

    P: [shakes her head]

11. I: Do you want to get out of here?

    P: [nods]

12. I: Okay, if you want to get out of here, we have to get a few things straight.

    P: [talking through her fingers] You are lying. You won't let me go.

13. I: I have to. I can't hold you if there isn't any reason to hold you. This is not a prison.

    P: [gets up from her bed and starts to walk toward the elevator, which is in the vicinity]

14. I: We can't let you go like this. If you want to go, we have to sit down and find out why your husband really wants you here and why you cut yourself. Why don't I give you time to calm down and come back this evening to talk to you?

    P: I don't want to wait that long. I'll talk now.

Because of the patient's immature, even childlike acting out, a personality disorder seems likely. The interviewer feels that the patient's main urge is to go home. He pretends, however, that she may wish to rest before cooperating and arbitrarily suggests 1 week of rest (Q. 7). He assumes that she is not severely depressed and suicidal, but that the self-mutilating behavior is used as a tactic in her marital quarrels. This assumption cannot, however, be confirmed without the patient's cooperation. Since she refuses to stay (A. 7), the interviewer knows that he has tapped a motive strong enough to use for bargaining. He points out that silence will not speed her release. She realizes the consequences of her behavior and becomes more cooperative.

When you decide to resolve the patient's resistance rather than to tolerate it, show the patient the advantages of giving it up. (For more details about this technique, see Othmer and Othmer 2002, Chapter 12: The Plus-Minus Approach.) Telling her that it is to her advantage may pressure her and increase resistance; breaking down resistance with force is not beneficial for rapport. Therefore, create an atmosphere in which the patient feels supported, can gain insight into her behavior, and experience freedom of choice rather than coercion.

Shifting

Shifting focus means approaching a problem from another direction. It is a technique to get the patient to talk about something he doesn't want to reveal. Instead of forcibly pursuing one line of questioning, let go and get at it from a different angle. It's like coming through the back door. You shift the vantage point.

> Mr. Dan Reuben is a 50-year-old, white, married schoolteacher, father of three children. As an outpatient he is seeking consultation because of his fading energy, inability to sleep, and worries about the cost of college education for his two oldest sons. The interviewer brings up the topic of suicidal thoughts.

1. I: It seems to me that you are carrying quite a burden. Are you able to hold up?
   P: Hmm . . . don't know.
2. I: Have you ever thought of giving in?
   P: How do you mean that?
3. I: I mean has it ever crossed your mind that it is not worth living any more with that much pain?
   P: You mean suicide?
4. I: Yes.
   P: I think that is a terrible sin. It's murder.
5. I: Yes. From a religious point it is . . .
   P: [interrupts] It would be an evil deed.
6. I: Have you thought about it?
   P: One should not even think about it—and I don't want to talk about it.
7. I: You are in enough pain as it is. I don't want to burden you more with talking about those thoughts.
   P: [the patient's eyes fill with tears]
8. I: It seems to me one of your worst worries is your oldest son, whether you can pay those high college costs—and he is such a gifted fellow.
   P: Oh, it's the worst—thinking that I worked all my life so hard as a teacher and can't even give my kid the education he deserves. I feel I let him down . . . and also my other son who is ready to go to college. I let them down, both of them.
9. I: I see. You feel you can't provide what they need.
   P: Right. They would be better off without me. My life insurance would get them through. Isn't it awful?
10. I: That you are worth more to them dead than alive?

P: Yes. I talked to my agent. If something happened to me, even if it is suicide, they would pay. I always thought the worst way to die would be with a rope around your neck [starts crying].

11. I: [nods]

P: Now I feel that's what I deserve. It even feels like peace just hanging there.

Shifting the vantage point often frees the patient and gets him ready to discuss the very topic you were after. In the above example, the thought of committing suicide increases the pathological guilt of the depressed patient to an unbearable degree. Therefore, the thought cannot be pursued. However, the idea of decreasing his guilt through deserved punishment by hanging can be pursued with the patient, and this pursuit reveals the patient's suicidal thoughts. For the logical person, not afflicted by depression, the patient's behavior appears contradictory. However, when you understand delusional guilt, you understand why shifting the focus worked.

Exaggeration

An anxious, obsessive, or very conscientious patient is often reluctant to admit to minor wrongdoings or failures. He fears the interviewer will reject him if he becomes aware of his character flaws. If you sense such reluctance, decrease the patient's concern by putting it into perspective. If a patient, for instance, slapped her child in anger and is concerned that this was child abuse, you can say:

"You did not bruise or suffocate her?"

Or, if a patient is reluctant to elaborate on shoplifting a candy bar when a youngster, you may exaggerate:

"You didn't really rob Fort Knox?"

When his behavior is compared to major harm or crime, the patient usually feels relieved and laughs, and experiences clearly that he has not reached your tolerance level where he has to fear rejection. He feels assured instead and can overcome his reluctance to talk more.

Induction to Bragging

Patients with sociopathic tendencies often like to make a good impression on the interviewer. They fear that their antisocial acts may tarnish their image, and therefore may attempt to censor the description of such acts. While the exaggeration technique (see above) may also work for these patients, a better technique still is to induce them to brag. For instance, when a patient resists talking about his high school troubles, you may challenge him with:

"Were you a good fighter?"

Such a statement often induces him to tell you how he knocked his baseball coach over the head with a bat when he refused to use him in the lineup, or how he tried to beat up another boy in school who seemed to be interested in his girlfriend.

Or when your patient is lying and cheating but tries to conceal these traits from you, you may encourage him by saying:

"You seem to be sly like a fox—you seem to get away with murder."

Such statements telegraph to the patient that the interviewer is willing to accept the patient's foibles. Since the patient with an antisocial personality often believes that he was justified in his actions, he feels that your statements indicate your understanding and acceptance. Your statements tell him that he does not have to fear your criticism and may even gain your praise.

At a later stage you may have to explain to him that accepting his problems neither means that you encourage him to further pursue antisocial acts nor that you condone and like what he has been doing. It just means that you are willing to give him enough space and attention that he can tell his story with the affect typical for this personality disorder—pride in bragging and interest in impressing others with his deeds (compare Chapter 10).

3. DEFENSES

Defenses cannot be fully observed because they postulate specific psychological mechanisms as the underpinnings of observable behavior patterns, signs, and reportable symptoms. Given the concept of disorders as sets of symptoms and signs that satisfy diagnostic criteria, defense mechanisms do not seem to belong in a discussion of diagnosis. Yet being familiar with defense mechanisms helps you understand some of the content and meaning of your patient's psychopathology. In addition, the patient's defenses also may interfere with rapport and history taking.

An in-depth assessment and analysis of defense mechanisms is predominantly used in psychodynamic and psychoanalytic interviewing (Vaillant 1986; McWilliams 1994); this book will give only a brief introduction, and will emphasize the descriptive aspect.

DSM-IV-TR defines 31 defense mechanisms in Appendix B:

- acting out
- affiliation
- altruism
- anticipation
- apathetic withdrawal
- autistic fantasy
- delusional projection
- denial
- devaluation
- displacement
- dissociation
- help-rejecting complaining
- humor
- idealization
- intellectualization
- isolation of affect
- omnipotence
- passive aggression
- projection
- projective identification
- psychotic denial
- psychotic distortion
- rationalization
- reaction formation
- repression
- self-assertion
- self-observation
- splitting of self-image or image of others
- sublimation
- suppression
- undoing

Recognition

Defense mechanisms consist of three components: 1) an observable behavior (often a symptom); 2) an impulse or intent not acceptable to the patient constituting an emotional conflict and stressor; and 3) a process that links the patient's observable behavior (or symptom) to the unacceptable intent. The unacceptable intent and the link to the overt behavior or symptom are accessible only by the therapist's inferential interpretation, which may or may not be corroborated by the patient.

When you try to decipher the underlying defense mechanisms of overt behaviors or symptoms, you sharpen your skill in recognizing and understanding psychopathology. If you can confirm, by the patient's corroboration, the link between apparently symptomatic behavior and an initially unacceptable, embarrassing, aggressive, or libidinous impulse, you have identified the defense mechanism.

You will become sensitive to the presence of defense mechanisms if you look for behaviors that indicate unrealistic and unacceptable goals, extreme in their intensity, self-incriminating, accusatory, or self-serving in their intent.

Table 3–2 summarizes the triple facet of the 31 defense mechanisms listed in DSM-IV-TR. The defense mechanisms are arranged along a continuum. At one end (listed first in the table) are the defenses that reflect the highest adaptive level. At the other end (listed last in the table) are defenses that show the lowest adaptive level, namely defensive dysregulation.

To give examples for each of these 31 defense mechanisms and show how they can interfere with the diagnostic interview would exceed the scope of this text. The following will provide a few examples of how to handle defense mechanisms during a psychodiagnostic interview.

Handling of Defenses

Defense mechanisms distort the patient's perception of himself and his environment. In an insight-oriented therapeutic interview the therapist attempts to make the patient aware of his defenses, their underlying mechanism, and their unconscious origins, with the expectation that the patient will replace his defensive behavior with a more reality-oriented behavior. In a psychodiagnostic interview the interviewer handles defense mechanisms to the extent that they interfere with rapport and history taking.

Handling defenses is different from handling resistance. The patient is usually aware of his resistance and voluntarily conceals information. The patient who uses defense mechanisms is often not aware of them and has

Table 3–2. Defense mechanisms on seven levels (DSM-IV-TR)

Defense mechanism	Observable behavior or symptom	Emotional conflict and stressors	Process
High adaptive level			
Affiliation	Formation of work and trouble-shooting teams; striving for cooperation	Isolation, imperfection, responsibility	Sharing of anxiety and rewards
Altruism	Unconditional offer of help	Defeat in competition	Replacing aggression and competition by support
Anticipation	Predicting probable events and planning countermeasures	Sudden, overwhelming threats	Projecting events and coping strategies
Humor	Highlighting amusing aspects of threat	Failure, loss, or destruction	Converting anxiety of threat to comedy or irony
Self-assertion	Expression of impulses in socially acceptable form	Fear, anxiety, and anger	Transformation of fear, anxiety, and aggression into socially acceptable expressions
Self-observation	Reflection on own feelings, impulses, and thoughts	Fear, anxiety, failures, aggression	Enhancing awareness of feelings, impulses, and thoughts
Sublimation	Socially acceptable behavior	Unacceptable feelings or impulses	Rechanneling of impulses into socially acceptable expressions
Suppression	Avoidance of discussing painful problems, wishes, or feelings	Painful event, sadistic or sexual impulse	Intentional blocking of recall

Mental inhibitions level

Displacement	Phobias	Fear and threat by an object, or love and hate for an object	Transferring a feeling from its actual object to a substitute
Dissociation	Multiple personality, fugue, amnesia	Promiscuous, hostile, or irresponsible behavior, painful events	Temporary alteration of consciousness, memory, perception, and identity
Intellectualization	Abstract thinking, doubting, indecisiveness, generalizations	Disturbing feelings and thoughts	Removal of the emotional and personal components of an event
Isolation of affect	Obsessions, talking about emotional events without feeling	Painful emotions and memories	Separation of content and affect, removal of affect
Reaction formation	Devotion, self-sacrificing behavior, correctness, cleanliness	Feelings of hostility and disinterest	Substitution by wishes or feelings opposite of the true feelings
Repression	Gaps in memory	Threatening memories, feelings, fears, wishes	Banning thoughts and feelings from recall
Undoing	Compulsive behavior	Sadistic wishes, unacceptable impulses	Symbolic negating of an impulse

Minor image-distorting level

Devaluation	Derogative statements about others or self, "sour grapes" about a goal	Positive qualities of others, unattainable goal	Ignoring of positive and exaggeration of negative qualities of self, others, or object
Idealization	Exaggerated praising of self or others	Negative qualities of self or significant others	Ignoring of negative and exaggeration of positive qualities of self or others
Omnipotence	Self-glorification, presumption, entitlement	Inferiority feelings, failure, low self-esteem	Converting inferiority into superiority feelings and actions

(continued)

Table 3–2. Defense mechanisms on seven levels (DSM-IV-TR) (*continued*)

Defense mechanism	Observable behavior or symptom	Emotional conflict and stressors	Process
Disavowal level			
Denial	Stubborn and angry negation of some reality obvious to others	Painful reality	Refusal to acknowledge the awareness of some reality
Projection	Ideas of reference, prejudice, suspiciousness, injustice	Hostility, other unacceptable attitudes, wishes, desires	Attributing one's own feelings to others
Rationalization	Self-serving explanations and justification of behavior	Socially unacceptable impulses, low self-esteem	Giving false, but socially acceptable explanations for behavior
Major image-distorting level			
Autistic fantasy	Daydreaming	Unsatisfied impulses and wishes	Imagined wish fulfillment
Projective identification	Accusing others of causing distress, hostility, and anger	Hate, anger, and hostility	Converting own hostile impulses into justifiable reactions to other persons' aggression
Splitting of self-image or image of others	Idealization alternating with devaluation of self or others	Experience of negative and positive qualities of self or others	Stripping off either all positive or all negative qualities of self or others

Action level			
Acting out	Violent acts, stealing, lying, rape	Sexual and aggressive impulses	Nonreflective, uncontrolled wish fulfillment
Apathetic withdrawal	Decreased emotions, activity, and social interactions	Needs, impulses, wishes	Responding to needs with increasing passivity
Help-rejecting complaining	Depicting oneself with self-pity as unsalvable victim	Hostility and reproach toward others	Converting hostility into victimization
Passive aggression	Procrastination, lack of follow-through	Aggressive, hostile impulses, resentment	Expression through inactivity
Level of defensive dysregulation			
Delusional projection	Persecutory delusions	Overpowering, unacceptable and uncontrollable impulses	Attributing own impulses to others in spite of contradicting reality
Psychotic denial	Negation of obvious reality	Overpowering, painful reality	Profound annulment of obvious reality
Psychotic distortion	Obviously unrealistic statements and claims and irrational actions	Overpowering, unacceptable impulses and reality	Profound misperception and misinterpretation of external reality and feelings

no voluntary control over them. The pathological behavior takes over and interferes with the interview. Handling defenses means neutralizing their impact but not analyzing and interpreting them.

In the following section, we describe a set of five management techniques that will help you to handle defenses: bypassing, reassurance, distraction, confrontation, and interpretation.

Bypassing

Common sense expresses the wisdom of this popular technique in proverbs such as:

> "Let sleeping dogs lie"

and

> "Don't rock the boat."

Every interviewer will meet the patient who clearly shows distorted reality perception. A widow may claim that her husband was the best, one wouldn't find a second like him. The record may show that this idolized man was an alcoholic who physically abused her. For the diagnosis of her depression, it may not be essential to confront her with her denial and idealization, at least not in the first interview. It would be better to bypass or ignore her defenses. Her defense mechanisms may, however, be discussed in the report of her mental status examination.

Reassurance

Reassurance attempts to decrease the patient's anxieties and suspicions and to increase his self-confidence by offering support. Reassurance works by viewing a defense mechanism from the patient's vantage point. This empathic approach will give the patient the feeling of having an ally. It is most effective when the patient appears overwhelmed by his problems.

> During a depressive episode, this 45-year-old, widowed father with bipolar illness is ready to give up job hunting and caring for his two children.

1. I: How can I help you, Russ?
   P: [shakes his head and does not say anything]
2. I: What's on your mind?
   P: I don't even know why I came!

3. I: What is it, Russ?
   P: [no answer]
4. I: You seem to be really down.
   P: [stares at the floor]
5. I: You look depressed . . . and hopeless.
   P: What's the use. Even if I find a job and I get some money saved and get everything straightened out I get high again and blow it all, and nothing is going to stop me. I went through this before, but it was not as bad as it is this time.
6. I: I think you have learned a lot from the past. This may help you with next time! I believe next time you will come for treatment when you get high.
   P: Do you really think so?
7. I: We both have to work at it. I know you can do it. Things will look better again. You will come out of it, we can talk about it and get you through. Let's talk about your depression now.
   P: If you think so.

Notice that the patient's self-punitive behavior is not addressed and interpreted, but is instead counteracted by the interviewer's support. Rather than assessing special problems, the interviewer feeds him supportive and reassuring statements (Q. 5, 6). The patient livens up when he hears that his therapist does not share his hopelessness, but sees a better future for him. Reassurance utilizes the patient's dependency needs. This technique is most effective if the patient perceives you as empathic.

Distraction

This technique works for patients with abnormal mood such as in mania, retarded depression, or intoxication. Such states cannot be changed by addressing underlying defenses. They can be overcome by a stimulus strong enough to get the patient's attention, such as calling his name, shouting, or touching him. The stimulus can be repeated, or combined with other stimuli. Ask short and closed-ended questions. You most likely cannot obtain continuous interaction, but you may get short answers.

> Mr. Wilson is a 57-year-old, white, divorced male with a history of mania. He reports to the emergency room in an excited state and smelling of whiskey. He is upset with a nurse who had asked him to stay in one of the examining rooms until the interviewer arrives. He is screaming tirades of protest. The interviewer stands in the doorway and observes the patient for a while. His presence is ignored.

1. I: Mr. Wilson, can I talk to you? [patient pays no attention and continues to shout in the direction of the nursing station]

P: In this damned place everybody thinks they can push you around. But not me. I'll show this bitch.

2. I: [louder] Mr. Wilson!

P: I've never been treated by anybody like this. And I won't take it from this bitch either!

3. I: [with an intense pressed voice] Hold it!

P: [startled, turns around and looks at him, surprised]

4. I: [looks him in the eye] I want to help you. Will you talk to me?

P: Who are you?

5. I: I'm the doctor on call. My name is Dr. O. I see you have had some problems.

P: This bitch told me not to leave the room. What do you want? Just stay away from me. I know your kind. First thing you do is give me a shot.

6. I: Mr. Wilson, let's sit down. I want to know what's eating you.

P: I don't want to sit down.

7. I: Fine with me.

P: I am just too mad to sit down.

8. I: Can I get you a cup of coffee?

P: No, you stay here [patient gets out his cigarettes].

9. I: Here is an ashtray for you.

P: [lights a cigarette and sits down]

10. I: Mr. Wilson, can I talk to you? Mr. Wilson, I want to help you. Tell me how I can best help you.

P: By leaving me alone!

11. I: Fine, but you were alone. All you did was holler. Is this what you came for?

P: No, I wanted to tell somebody about the problems I'm having in the halfway house.

12. I: Alright, let's sit down, and you tell me about it! [sits down] Okay.

To get attention the interviewer addresses the patient with a short command (Q. 3). In response, the patient directs his hostility toward him (A. 5). When the interviewer asks him whether he came to the emergency room to holler, the patient becomes aware of his self-defeating, acting-out behavior.

Patients who are very excited, who show pronounced push of speech and flight of ideas, or who are intoxicated or delusional may not be distractible. They may need pharmacological intervention before rapport can be established.

Confrontation

Confrontation is used to draw the patient's attention to a particular behavior, with the expectation that he will recognize and correct it during the interview.

Carol is a 38-year-old, white, female outpatient. The interviewer had reviewed with her the circumstances that led to her separation.

1. I: How is your relationship with your husband now?
   P: [looks frightened and hostile] Why do you ask?
2. I: Well, I just want to know if you are still in touch with him.
   P: [more hostile and angry] Of course [the patient gets up and takes her coat].
        I'd better go now!
3. I: Carol, you are getting angry.
   P: Because you know damn well that he is still calling me—goodbye! [walking
        toward the door]
4. I: Carol, you seem to think that I must be in touch with him [superficial inter-
        pretation].
   P: Aren't you?
5. I: You are angry with me and you don't trust me? [confrontation]
   P: Nobody is on my side. Not even you. And you are supposed to be my doc-
        tor.
6. I: So you feel I am against you too? [confrontation]
   P: Aren't you?
7. I: I am on your side, but I notice it is difficult for you to believe me. [support-
        ive statement and confrontation]
   P: [turns around, hangs her coat over her chair] I don't know, I try to trust you.
8. I: What is really bothering you about your husband's telephone calls?
   P: I hear the clicking sound in the system. I know he has his tape recorder on
        and he's recording me again.
9. I: And you think I'm in with him and know about it?
   P: Isn't that why you ask about the calls?
10. I: No, I did not ask you about the calls. I asked you whether you are still in
        touch with him and that made you very upset and suspicious.
    P: It did. I feel everybody is in with him, even my parents who say that they
        hate him. Sometimes I don't trust them either.

Reading the patient's delusional suspicion and confronting her with it prevents breakdown of rapport. The interviewer combines two techniques:
first, he confronts her with her distrust (Q. 3, 5, 6), and second, he shows
her support and empathy (Q. 7) by assuring her that he sides with her,
which makes her reflect upon her suspicion (A. 7). The combined use of
these two techniques works only because the patient has some insight into
her suspiciousness (perhaps she is projecting?). Otherwise, she would have
refused to discuss the topic any further or left the office.

   From a descriptive point of view Carol's beliefs are ideas of reference
that border on persecutory delusions, with the exception that some insight
is preserved. From a dynamic point of view these ideas of reference are
conceived as a result of projection.

   During a diagnostic interview, you have to deal with these reality distortions in order to maintain rapport. You have to decide from case to case
whether it is more appropriate to accept such ideas of reference as the pa-

tient's reality or confront her with them. If she includes you in her delusion, you have to confront the patient with the delusional nature of her thinking. She may not recognize her perception as a reality distortion, but she may be able to continue the dialogue with you and remain connected. However, if the delusion is fully developed, confrontation will fail to make the patient recognize her reality distortion. The interview may break down.

The success of a confrontation is not only dependent on the patient's insight. Choose a vantage point for your confrontation that helps the patient understand his inappropriate behavior and at the same time makes him feel your empathy. More about this aspect in the section below on interpretation.

Interpretation

Interpretation states your understanding of the patient's defensive behavior. You suggest to him the meaning of his thoughts or the intent of his behavior. Usually, interpretation follows confrontation, because you have to make a patient aware of his behavior before he can understand your interpretation. Interpretation conveys to the patient that you try to read his behavior and that you invite him to discuss it with you.

A correct interpretation explains the patient's behavior satisfactorily in the context of all other behaviors. Unfortunately, there is no sure way to be correct. You may feel your interpretation is correct when the patient agrees with it and voluntarily elaborates, when it is in agreement with your clinical experience, or when nothing else in the patient's behavior contradicts it. In each case, you might be right or wrong. You have probably made an effective interpretation if it stimulates emotional dialogue or elicits new information.

You may make a brilliant interpretation, but its usefulness depends on the patient's acceptance. If a patient is unaware of his behavior, an interpretation is usually counterproductive. He will feel criticized and misunderstood, and defend himself against such "accusations," resulting in the deterioration of rapport. In a patient with persecutory delusions, for example, interpretations may lead to a complete breakup of the interview. He may think that you read his mind and control him. Rather than feeling understood, he feels manipulated and walks out. Therefore, it is important to evaluate him for persecutory tendencies before you attempt to use interpretation.

Interpretation is useful with patients who do not initially level with you, or have difficulties expressing their thoughts and feelings. It is used to get the patient more involved and make him realize and understand his attitudes and perceptions, and to encourage his investment in the interview process and his treatment.

Hopkinson et al. (1981) found that interpretations by the interviewer were followed 44% of the time by the patient's emotional expression. If the interviewer precedes his interpretation by his own expression of feelings, his client responds in kind in 75% of his interpretations; if he does not, his yield is only 26%. The interviewer needs to interpret a patient's defense in a clear and empathic manner. He has to ensure that the patient is ready to hear that interpretation and make use of it.

Interpretation will be demonstrated on the defense mechanism of projection. At the same time the three components of a defense mechanism (see above) are illustrated: observable behavior, unconscious impulse or intent, and the patient's behavior that links the two.

> Joan, a 28-year-old African-American law student, enters the interviewer's office and, after some introductory small talk, asks:

P: Why are you looking at me like that? It makes me feel as if I'm naked.
I: What do you mean?
P: The way you look at me . . .

Unaware of having looked at the patient in any particular way, the interviewer suspects that the patient has a perceptive disturbance that could be described as an idea of reference (the first, that is, the observable component of a defense mechanism). He decides to probe for the unconscious intent (the second component of a defense mechanism).

I: Do you feel that other men look at you that way, too?
P: Some do. When I walk home from law school.
I: Anyone in particular?
P: Well, one of my teachers. His name is Raoul and he is from South America. He looked at me like that in class.
I: Did he ever say anything personal to you?
P: I'm kind of embarrassed to talk about it.
I: We may both learn something important about you, if we can understand your embarrassment.
P: Well, I kind of thought he was a good teacher. Once, I stayed after class to show him one of my poems. He seemed to enjoy talking to me about it, and took it home with him.
I. Hmm.
P: I asked him if I could come back after the next class to talk about it some more and he agreed.
I: Well?

P: I went back and he analyzed my poem. I was so pleased that I asked him whether I could meet him. He looked at me and I felt all excited and opened my coat. I was naked underneath. He looked at me with a twinkle in his eye and a smile on his face and said: "Joan, I'm your teacher and I'm also married. Do you understand? I don't want you to feel bad about it. I'm flattered that you feel that way about me."

I: So he understood.

P: I was so embarrassed that I just ran out.

The second component of the defense mechanism, a libidinous intent, emerges. The interviewer infers that the patient may have felt a similar impulse toward him. He attempts to establish the link between the overt behavior and the intent—the third component—namely that the patient projects her intent onto the interviewer, thus sparing her the responsibility for her own erotic wishes.

I: You seem excited when you talk about Raoul.

P: I'm so embarrassed.

I: Do you remember how we got on to this subject?

P: I don't understand your question.

I: Do you remember how we got into the discussion about Raoul?

P: You confuse me. I don't know what you mean.

I: Well, you asked me about the way I look at you.

P: Hmm.

I: And it seemed you felt that I looked at you like Raoul did.

P: Well, that's what I thought.

I: Could it be that you feel toward me as you did toward Raoul?

P: Oh no, that's nonsense. You are jumping to conclusions and that really makes me angry. You are my doctor. I respect you as my doctor. But I don't feel anything else for you. I like you, but not like that.

The patient's resistance to the interpretation is obvious. Without her corroboration, the assumption of projection remains inferential. The interviewer attempts to make the erotic thoughts more acceptable to Joan, thus making her projections less necessary.

I: So you are not really aware of having those thoughts? What would be so bad about them anyway?

P: That you are my doctor. And I also have a boyfriend. He's really something like a fiancé.

I: I don't understand. What do you mean "something like a fiancé"?

P: Well, my mother wants us to stay together.

I: What about you?

P: Well, he's real nice, but he's older and he doesn't have an education and he's awfully jealous.

I: So, if you look at other men, you kind of betray him and also defy your mother's wishes?

P: Now you talk like my psychologist did.

I: Well, I try to understand how you feel and why you were so embarrassed with Raoul. Also why you feel that other men look at you in a certain way.

P: You think it's me?

I: Hmm.

P: You think I'm embarrassed about my wishes?

I: Yes, and that's why you pin them on me.

P: There you go again [laughs]. Maybe, you're right after all. Do you think that's why I have those panic attacks and why I feel uncomfortable when I walk home or when I'm at a restaurant?

I: What do you think? [pause] Patients with panic attacks and agoraphobia sometimes feel that others look at them in a sexual way, and it is often their own sexual feelings that make them think so. But this is just the content of their panicky feelings, not their cause. Even if we talk about these sexual feelings for many hours, and even when you become comfortable with describing these feelings to me, you will still have your panic attacks and still feel anxious in a restaurant. But you may find a different thought content for your panic attacks.

There are four aspects to interpretation: timing, vantage point, scope, and impact on the patient.

Timing: The timeliness of an interpretation is usually easy to judge. When a patient becomes curious about his own behavior, he is ready to explore its meaning.

Bill, a 23-year-old biology student, talks about his relationship with his parents and superiors.

1. I: You are telling me that you still live at home.
   P: Not really. Let's put it this way: I live in the same house as my parents do.
2. I: What does that mean?
   P: It means that I share quarters with them, but I was through with them a long time ago.
3. I: You mean you can't get along with your parents?
   P: They are narrow-minded bourgeois.
4. I: So your social life is not really at home.
   P: Nope.
5. I: How is your life at work?
   P: My supervisor is a real knucklehead. He can't see what isn't in the books—typical product of an American college.
6. I: Did you have better experiences in high school?
   P: I always seem to meet the morons.
7. I: How did you get through college? Did you have a scholarship?

P: I lost my teaching scholarship. John G. told me I'm not doing what I'm sup-
    posed to. The heck with it, it was not worth it anyway. But, so far, I've made
    some money in computer programming.
8. I: So far?
P: I don't know if I still have my job. I did some programming of plays for a
    football coach, but that guy is so authoritarian, he has to have it his way. He
    can't listen to anybody.
9. I: Do you play football yourself?
P: No. I was on the swim team.
10. I: You are not swimming anymore?
P: The coach kicked me off. I was in the locker room when I was supposed to
    be in the pool. Somebody missed $50 after practice. The coach was mad at
    me because I didn't follow the rules.
11. I: [laughs]
P: The rules are really stupid. I just needed to get some medication out of my
    locker and this ass nails me.
12. I: [laughs again]
P: You are laughing. I must come across as a real troublemaker.
13. I: Hmm.
P: Isn't that what you think? You must think this guy can't get along with his
    swim team coach, the football coach, or with his teachers.
14. I: And with his bourgeois parents.
P: I forgot that one. You must think I can't get along with anybody. And that's
    right. I fly off the handle for any old reason. I wonder what ticks me off?
15. I: Authority . . . teachers . . . coaches . . . parents.
P: Hmm, it sure looks that way . . . Hmm.
16. I: Does it feel that way?
P: It feels like I'm always hitting something . . . lashing out.

The interviewer confronts the patient first with the common thread that
runs through different situations (Q. 3, 5, 7, 8, 10). The patient recognizes
the similarities in his problems with others (A. 13). He starts to wonder about
it himself by raising questions about his behavior (Q. 14). This is the time to
attempt an interpretation of the patient's rejection of authority figures (Q. 15).
He can then continue to talk of difficulties in following rules, and of possible feelings of revengefulness and vindictiveness (as seen in patients with
sociopathic tendencies). This example demonstrates the rule of timing. Make
an interpretation when the patient recognizes his behavior as irrational and
starts wondering about its meaning.

Vantage point: The way you deliver an interpretation is important. Interpretations may be made from your own or the patient's vantage point. With
an interpretation from the interviewer's vantage point the patient may feel
criticized, annoyed, angered, and compelled to resist. An interpretation made

from the patient's vantage point is more likely to be accepted—provided it is correct. Here is an example:

> Leslie, a 38-year-old white female, just divorced from a man her age, reported that she has a tendency to date men in their fifties or older.

Interviewer's vantage point:

I: You were acting on sexual impulses originally directed toward your father.
P: [bewildered] I never had sexual feelings for my father, but I do for these men. They turn me on.

Patient's vantage point:

I: There must be something about these older men that comforts you, Leslie.
P: [pause] I feel more wanted. I feel I don't have to compete all the time with other women.
I: You feel accepted and there is no threat to this acceptance.
P: Right, it relaxes me. I can respond without feeling that I'm taken in. I can believe that the man really means it. I feel I can trust him more than a younger man.
I: What about other women?
P: I feel ahead. I feel first in line.
I: Yes, I see. It must feel like being the darling.
P: [surprised] You are right. It just struck me . . . like daddy's darling.
I: Didn't you tell me before that you always had the feeling that your father seemed to like you more than your sisters and brothers?
P: That's right; but I did not mean that that's the reason why I like older men.
I: I know and that is not what I'm really saying. But you felt comfortable with him. You know he meant well. He loved you.
P: He really liked me.
I: And did not just try to have you get into bed with him.
P: That's right.

The patient had wondered about why she focused her attention on older men. She was ready to explore the reason for her feelings, which justified the interpretative approach. The interpretation worked because it focused on the elements in her relationship with her father that were closest to her awareness (daddy's darling). This allowed her to recognize her emotional gain in choosing older men after her painful divorce.

Scope: An interpretation can be made regarding a narrow concern, such as an isolated behavior, or larger issues, such as lifestyle and lifelong patterns. Large-scope interpretations may damage the patient's self-esteem and your rapport with him.

Narrowly defined interpretations are used with Karen, a 42-year-old, depressed, white female who talks about her diet. She denies dysphoria, obsessions, and compulsions.

1. I: How do you feel usually?
   P: I'm doing fine. I feel great and I'm proud to be down to 118 pounds from 142.
2. I: So you are on a diet.
   P: Yes, I am watching my calories very carefully.
3. I: How do you do that?
   P: I have coffee in the morning and then at lunch a rare hamburger without bread, but with lettuce. I have a steak for dinner. Once in awhile I get so hungry that I eat a whole quart of ice cream. Afterwards I feel depressed and guilty about it. I also try to be rigid with my smoking.
4. I: What do you mean?
   P: Before I smoke a cigarette I have to wash my hands.
5. I: Can you tell me why you do that?
   P: It's just a habit. I like to have clean hands when I smoke.
6. I: You mean you are afraid of dirt on your hands?
   P: No, but I make breakfast and lunch for the kids.
7. I: And you think some food is still on your hands?
   P: Yes, they may still be greasy. Fat has many calories.
8. I: But why do you wash your hands before every cigarette?
   P: I can never be sure whether I have really washed them completely the time before.
9. I: So you are thinking of still having calories stick to your hands?
   P: [silent] . . . I may get them in my body accidentally from the cigarettes.
10. I: So these thoughts bother you!
   P: I feel so silly . . .
11. I: It sounds like calories are like bacteria, they can hurt you if they get in your body.
   P: No . . . I guess that's it . . . calories are poison, they make you fat.

In this interview, short interpretations in the form of questions (Q. 6, 7, 9) help reveal obsessive thoughts and compulsions. Confrontation (Q. 10) helps the patient to realize her avoidance of these topics.

Interpretation on a large scope is used to make Janet, a 28-year-old, white, single nurse, aware of how mood swings have affected her choice of partners, and eventually caused the breakup of these relationships. The interviewer points out how she picks fun-loving fellows (often individuals with antisocial personality disorder, alcoholism, or other substance-related problems) during her manic episodes and gets disgusted with their irresponsible behavior during her depressive episodes.

1. I: How are things going now, Janet? Are you still with Bob?
   P: Yes, but things are not going as well. Last summer when I asked Bob to move in with me it was just great. We had so much fun together and I really enjoyed having sex with him. And now I don't know what happened. I resent him.
2. I: What is it that you resent?
   P: He's not working. He doesn't even seem to want a job.
3. I: Hmm.
   P: He starts drinking in the morning and it's my money he's using.
4. I: You really sound resentful and angry.
   P: It makes me feel worn out. I oversleep; I don't get my work done, which is unusual for me.
5. I: I remember when you worked two shifts last summer.
   P: I never ran out of energy. Even on my second shift I was faster than everyone else. It didn't bother me then that Bob was that way. It was all fun, and now it's just a drag. I don't think that anybody should hang around like that, live off a woman, and be too lazy to do anything.
6. I: Well, something has changed in you.
   P: Yes, I am depressed again.
7. I: That's right. Last summer you had your high. You were much more fun oriented. Living out that fun was much more important to you than having a responsible partner.
   P: That's right.
8. I: And you had done the same thing the year before with Frank. You started living with him in August, had a great time, and then got all upset in the spring when he did not want to work, just wanted to party.
   P: Yes, sounds like the same thing.
9. I: When you are high you are like a child, where fun is written in capital letters. And when you are down, you raise your finger like a parent. You see the wrongs in your playmates who still behave like fun-seeking children.
   P: Yes, that's exactly it.

The interviewer first encourages the patient to tell her story and voice her resentment (Q. 1–5). He then starts to interpret her relationship with Bob (Q. 6). Because of her initial positive responses (A. 6, 7) the interviewer continues with his interpretations, which the patient readily accepts.

Impact on the patient: Interpretations have an emotional impact on the patient. She may gain a new awareness of her situation and feel overwhelmed.

Angela is a 46-year-old, white female. She realized that she took verbal and physical abuse from her alcoholic husband because of feelings of guilt and worthlessness while depressed. The patient had just left her husband and started a job. In spite of past abuse, she still feels a strong sexual attraction to him. The interviewer uses echoing, confrontation, and interpretation to clarify her feelings.

1. I: Where do you stand with your husband, Angela?
   P: When Phil is drunk he gets really mean. Last time he grabbed a lamp and hit me over the head. I had a skull fracture.
2. I: So he is really abusive.
   P: At times he can be so gentle.
3. I: Hmm. So he has another side to him.
   P: Usually he is mean. I cannot stand it anymore. I should have left him 2 years ago when he hit me with the lamp.
4. I: Would you say you have wasted your time during the last 2 years?
   P: After a fight he can make up for it—he is really a great lover.
5. I: So physically you are still attracted to him.
   P: Well, that does not make up for the meanness and abuse. If your feelings get hurt it affects everything else.
6. I: Is that why you finally left him, because he is not worth loving anymore?
   P: Yes, but I made a mistake. Before I left him I should have grabbed him and fucked him. Then I should have said: "Now I'm through with you. Now I'll leave you."
7. I: Whenever you tell me something bad about your husband and I agree with you, you turn around and praise him.
   P: [surprised] Do I?
8. I: I think you still love him.
   P: [cries] But it is a self-destructive love and I know deep inside that I did the right thing, but I feel now terribly lonely.

The interpretation (Q. 8) allowed the interviewer to go beyond the patient's ambivalent vacillations, which hindered the assessment of her feelings about leaving her husband. The patient finally claimed she did the right thing, but that she feels lonely.

This interview shows how an interpretation can overwhelm the patient. The responsible interviewer has to answer the question:

"Can the patient digest an interpretation at this time?"

Enlightening the patient, summarizing her behavior for her, and giving her insight and understanding of it is a goal of the psychodiagnostic interview. But you can only burden her with as much as she can carry through an hour—or she may not return.

CHECKLIST

Chapter 3: Techniques

Indicate which interview technique produced which response listed below; enter the appropriate number on the line provided.

Response:

1 = spontaneous talking   5 = silence
2 = rambling   6 = hostility
3 = answering questions adequately   7 = anger
4 = one-word answers

Interview Technique:

Open-ended, patient-centered questions   _____
Open-ended, symptom-centered questions   _____
Closed-ended questions   _____
Leading questions   _____
Requests to be more specific   _____
Requests to generalize   _____
Requests to give reasons for pathology   _____
Probing   _____
Requests to summarize   _____
Interrelating   _____
Statements to go on and continue   _____
Repeating of patient's statements   _____
Attempts to redirect the patient   _____
Questions assessing psychiatric symptoms   _____
Smooth transitions   _____
Accentuated transitions   _____
Abrupt transitions   _____
Confrontations   _____
Expressions of acceptance   _____
Shifting   _____
Induction to bragging   _____
Interpretations   _____
Addressing of defense mechanisms   _____
Bypassing defense mechanisms   _____
Distraction   _____
Reassurance   _____

CHAPTER FOUR

THREE METHODS TO ASSESS MENTAL STATUS

1. **Observation**
   Appearance
   Consciousness
   Psychomotor Behavior
2. **Conversation**
   Attention and Concentration
   Speech and Thinking
   Orientation
   Memory
   Affect
3. **Exploration**
   Mood
   Energy Level
   Perception
   Content of Thinking
   Medically Unexplained Somatic Symptoms
   Conversion
   Dissociation
   Paroxysmal Attacks ("Spells")
   Executive Functioning
   Insight
   Judgment

SUMMARY

Chapter 4 teaches you how to size up the patient's mental status during the interview. Mental status is a profile of at least 20 psychological functions. Assess them through observation, conversation, and exploration. Chapter 4 will tell you what these disturbances mean, not what they are. If you need to know that, consult the Glossary for definitions. Chapter 5 will explore testing, the final step in the mental status examination.

▲ ▲ ▲ ▲ ▲

Hic Rhodos, hic salta!

According to Aesop, in the sixth century B.C. athletes gathered on the island of Rhodes, Greece, for competition. When beaten in the long jump, one athlete boasted: "At home I did much better." The official's response was: "This is Rhodes; you demonstrate your leaping here."

▼ ▼ ▼ ▼ ▼

In the mental status examination it is the here and now that counts.

When you first meet your patient, you immediately start to perceive a number of signals. These get condensed into your first impression. As interviewer, your task is to analyze these signals as expressions of the patient's present functioning—his mental status. It gives you the cross-sectional view of his strengths, weaknesses, and dysfunctions.

A complete picture of the patient's level of functioning in the here and now (and the previous 24 hours) gives you information critical to diagnostic accuracy. In Chapter 6, we will provide the other key ingredient: obtaining the historical development of the patient's dysfunctions. The integration of both provides the basis for your differential diagnosis.

The task in assessing the mental status is to be able to stay alert to the patient's behavior during the interview, as you are working at different levels of communication. Staying vigilant to changes in the patient's behavior throughout the interview can be a challenge. With ease you will soon learn to monitor at least 20 functions: Appearance, level of consciousness, psychomotor behavior, attention, concentration, speech, thinking, orientation, memory, affect, mood, energy, perception, thought content, insight, judgment, social functioning, suggestibility, abstract thinking, and intelligence (Fish 1967; Kaplan and Sadock 1989; Mesulam 1985; Joynt 1992; Strub and Black 1993; Taylor 1993).

TOOLS

In this chapter, we will explore three methods to assess mental status: observation, conversation, and exploration. Testing, which is the last step in assessing mental status, is addressed in Chapter 5.

By observation you register the various behaviors and interpret their meaning. For observation you do not need the patient's cooperation. In contrast, conversation and exploration depend on the patient's full or partial cooperation. Thus you have to establish rapport with the patient so that he will reveal the information you require.

Within each phase of the interview process, you should be monitoring the mental status. In this chapter, we will show you what to look for, what certain signs can indicate, and how to put this information together into a complete mental status evaluation. Let's start with a general description of each method.

Observe all aspects of the patient's behavior and presentation, such as appearance, consciousness, psychomotor activity, and affect, as they unfold in the first minutes of the interview. For those patients who refuse to speak, observation is often your only available assessment method. Any disturbances that you observe are called signs.

Conversation refers to undirected, casual communication with the patient. During conversation, you appraise his condition when he is somewhat off-guard, unaware the psychiatric examination has begun. As you converse, you may assess the patient's orientation; speech; thinking; attention; concentration; comprehension; and remote, recent, and immediate memory. The verbally abusive, hostile, or guarded patient may refuse exploration but not conversation.

Exploration offers a method for tapping into the patient's internal experiences that are not on display, such as mood, motivation, perception, thought content, insight, and judgment. To discern them, the patient must be motivated to talk. If he is willing to talk about his problems, you are assessing symptoms.

Observation, conversation, and exploration take place throughout the interview. With some patients, these three methods might be used seamlessly in sequence, as in the following example:

> This 35-year-old veteran was brought to the emergency room by the police. He looked disheveled, walked unsteadily, and the smell of alcohol lingered about him. His forearm showed a tattoo.

I: Can I take a look at the American Eagle on your arm? [observation]
P: Be my guest. [obviously the patient comprehends what the interviewer is saying and gives a goal-oriented response]
I: Isn't that what the marines had on their berets? [conversation]
P: You don't know what you are talking about.
I: Have you had it for a long time?
P: I don't want to talk about it.

I: You mean you are sick of it? [by trying to guess the patient's underlying feelings, the interviewer invites the patient to talk about himself—attempting to start exploration]

P: The hell—sick of it!? I got it in Nam. We had just survived an ambush and we all got drunk when we did it. Next day I was kicked out. They court-martialed me for stealing and sent me up shitrow.

I: You mean they did you wrong? [exploration with focus on suffering]

P: Everybody did. I just grabbed a few things to make some bread and get some dope. It was hard to keep going without it.

I: So, in Nam you started to take dope. Are you still doing it?

P: No. It's now mainly booze.

I: Does it get you in trouble?

P: I wouldn't be here, would I? Just leave me alone, would you? Before I kick your ass.

I: So Nam really got you into some trouble. Let's see how I can help you out.

P: Yeah, that was quite a war.

Conversing about the observed tattoo, the interviewer learns that the patient is irritable, hostile, and easily provoked by exploration. He has a labile affect, but can comprehend and answer questions. When he feels he becomes the subject of interest in the verbal exchange, he resumes his hostile behavior. As interviewer you have to learn to back off from exploration and return to conversation if the patient becomes hostile.

1. OBSERVATION

Astute observation of a patient can yield many insights about her. This nurse's report shows how much can be learned through observation.

> A 22-year-old, white, married woman had just been admitted to the inpatient service. Rachel M. was lying in bed on her stomach with her face buried in the pillow. She neither answered questions nor responded to any commands. When I mentioned the doctor would arrive shortly, she did not take any notice. After I left, I peeked through the door window. She got up from her bed, went to the adjacent bathroom, and returned with her hair brushed and makeup on her face, only to resume her position on the bed, face down.

Obviously Rachel M. is alert, comprehends, and remembers the nurse's remarks. Her motor movements are grossly intact without posturing or stupor, and she can carry out goal-oriented actions.

As this example shows, observation starts before you talk to your patient. Look at appearance, alertness (level of consciousness), psychomotor behavior, and affect. (To appraise affect, you need—besides facial expression—also the patient's thought content, which we will discuss under 2. Conversation.)

It does not take elaborate techniques to observe and evaluate appearance, hygiene, race, or ethnic background. But the interviewer has to avoid stereotypical evaluations of patients, assuming, for example, that the adolescent with three earrings in one ear exhibits flamboyance when this dress code is endemic among 14-year-olds. Maintain a sense of context about your patient and avoid drawing conclusions until you've carefully considered each aspect of the mental status. You'll then have a more accurate picture of what is, after all, a unique individual sitting across from you.

Appearance

At the moment you meet the patient, you will note, of course, sex, age, race, nutritional status, body type (see Glossary), hygiene, dress, and eye contact. You may observe aspects that are associated with the presence or onset of psychopathology.

Sex and Age

Sex and age are often relevant for the diagnosis, as there are disorders associated more often than not with these factors. For example, in females, anorexia and bulimia nervosa, somatization, and mood disorder are more common; in males, antisocial personality and alcohol abuse are more common.

In young patients, anorexia nervosa, somatization disorder, antisocial personality, and schizophrenia are seen more often; in older patients degenerative dementia. A patient who appears older than his stated age may have a history of substance abuse, cognitive disorders, depression, or physical illness.

Race and Ethnic Background

Race and ethnic background are more than demographic descriptors. They can be one source of stress or of adjustment reactions, and can influence the onset and prevalence of mental disorders. Some cultures ascribe different meanings to behavior; the person with psychotic delusions may be seen as possessed by spirits. For some Asian-American cultures, in which problems are to be dealt with within the family, bringing a problem to a therapist is a deeply shaming experience. Individuals with this cultural background may wait a long period of time before they consult with a mental health professional, and may show greater signs of deterioration in psychological functioning.

Discrepancy between your background and your patient's can influence your interaction. If you differ from the patient in race, culture, or nationality, he may react with caution or distrust. Here is an example.

> After a serious suicide attempt (hanging) while on a hospital ward, an African-American female, lesbian nurse had been resuscitated. Her male resident doctor, an immigrant from Israel, talked with her after the incident and inquired about present suicidal thoughts or plans. The patient denied them emphatically and repeatedly. He believed her. However, the patient admitted to an African-American female staff nurse that next time she would not fail and it would be soon. The distance in race, gender, and nationality produced dramatically discrepant assessments.

What can you do to minimize your stereotypical assumptions about behavior? Gain information about the meanings of behavior in different ethnicities and cultures. Ask your patient to help you understand how his behavior is viewed by his family, or in his country.

Studies have shown that ethnic background is associated with certain psychiatric disorders. For instance, there is more drinking among the Irish, some native-American tribes, the French, and Italians, but low rates of alcoholism among Asian Americans (Goodwin and Guze 1989).

Nutritional Status

Poor nutrition can be the result of a psychiatric or medical illness, for example, anorexia nervosa in young females; anorexia due to alcohol and substance abuse; schizophrenia; depression; or medical illness such as cancer, diabetes, or endocrinopathy.

In contrast, obesity may point to an eating disorder; somatization disorder; a mood disorder with hyperphagia; or use of psychotropic drugs such as mirtazapine (Remeron), lithium, divalproex sodium (Depakote), sedating neuroleptics (thorazine, thioridazine, as well as clozapine; Cohen et al. 1990), and olanzapine (Zyprexa). If there is a question in your mind as to etiology, you may need to directly address the patient's eating habits (section 3: Exploration).

Hygiene and Dress

Self-neglect can indicate the presence of certain psychiatric disorders such as dementia, substance and alcohol abuse, depression, or schizophrenia: a

3-day-old beard, food stains on clothing, soiled shoes, body odor, or dirty fingernails. In contrast, extreme neatness and red hands may disclose excessive hand washing as seen in obsessive-compulsive disorder.

Dress may reveal social and professional status, engagement in leisure or work activity, adjustment to the season, attitude toward society, or an extreme mood state such as mania or depression. Some patients with bipolar disorder advertise their mood state by their appearance:

> When manic, a 65-year-old lady dressed in bright red, wore lots of jewelry, dyed her hair copper, and painted her lips fiery red. When depressed, she let the gray hair grow out, dressed in dark colors, and used no makeup.

In general, a flamboyant outfit, mismatched clothing, and loud makeup can indicate hysteric or manic symptoms, or a cognitive disorder. Highly eccentric, nonconformist, or flagrantly inappropriate attire can be a sign of psychotic behavior. The interviewer must evaluate as to what is inappropriate. The following examples offer some illustrations: the electrician who wears a tuxedo for his appointment; the middle-aged, female lawyer who comes to see you in a bikini top, blue jeans, and barefoot; a patient wearing dark glasses indoors explaining: "I don't want others to see my eyes and read my mind." Such clues should alert but not prejudice you toward a diagnosis.

Eye Contact

Most patients maintain eye contact and track with their eyes the movements and gestures of the interviewer. Aberrant eye movements can be diagnostic: wandering eyes reveal distractibility, visual hallucinations, mania, or cognitive impairment. Avoidance of eye contact may express hostility, shyness, or anxiety. Constant tracking may disclose suspiciousness. If appropriate, question the patient about these clues. His answers may lead you right into his pathology.

Consciousness

Level of consciousness changes by the ingestion of alcohol, drugs, or by some paroxysmal attacks, including fainting, narcoleptic attacks, petit mal, complex partial, grand mal, and pseudoseizures. Rarely are the latter observed during an interview with either in- or outpatients. You have to ask the patient whether or not he has ever experienced these kinds of attacks (see section 3: Exploration).

Lethargy can indicate a mental disorder due to a medical condition or to delirium, dementia, amnestic states, and other cognitive disorders. Don't assume lethargy is the result of depression, alcohol, or drug intoxication. Only exploration and testing will tell you the etiology (see Chapter 5, section 1. Testing, Level of Consciousness).

Psychogenic stupor can complicate panic, somatization, and mood disorders; schizophrenia, catatonic type; and delirium, dementia, amnestic states, and other cognitive disorders.

Psychomotor Behavior

Psychomotor behavior gives diagnostic clues on alertness, affect, energy level, agitation, and movement disturbance in a wide variety of psychiatric and neurological disorders. The interviewer should note the patient's posture and be alert to autonomic responses and to seven types of psychomotor activity: posture, expressive movements, reactive movements, grooming, gestures, symbolic gestures, and goal-directed movements (see also Chapter 5: Testing).

Psychomotor activity is the medium through which nonverbal communication occurs. Therefore it is important that you register the different types of motor activities and learn to interpret them. From a diagnostic point of view, movements can be grouped into four categories:

1. posture
2. psychomotor movements
3. movements that express affect
4. abnormal complex movements

1. Posture

Posture maintains muscle tone of the body. As a diagnostician, you are interested in the strength of this muscle tone and in the change of posture. Muscle tone reflects a person's energy level and tension. Rapid changes in posture as seen in pacing reflect agitation. You see a high muscle tone in a tense and agitated patient, while the calm or sleepy patient shows a low tone.

Erect posture may express an increase in energy level, and stooped posture a decrease. Mannerisms, catalepsy, posturing, and waxy flexibility are all signs of either schizophrenia, catatonic type, mood disorder not otherwise specified, or midbrain lesions.

2. Psychomotor Movements

Psychomotor movements and speech serve as the expression of thoughts and actions. Distinguish between goal-directed movements, expressive and illustrative gestures, and symbolic gestures.

Goal-directed movements: The patient carries out her actions by goal-directed movements. As diagnostician, you judge whether the goal is reached. For instance, the manic patient may initiate movements but never complete the action or reach the goal. Goal-directed movements decrease in depression, parkinsonism, or neuroleptic-induced parkinsonism. In the latter two, all goal-directed movements stiffen.

You can ask the patient to carry out a physical task to allow you to assess the nature of her goal-oriented movements. Notice the latency of initiation, speed, efficiency, ability of completion, and the level and degree of control. Results will indicate areas of concern. Psychosis may disturb the level of control. A patient may feel that his movements are imposed upon him by an outside force.

A patient suffering from attention-deficit/hyperactivity disorder may explore your office by looking around, getting up, and handling objects of interest. Such a patient stays in that explorative mode. He has difficulties engaging himself in one activity, such as focusing on your interview with him.

Expressive and illustrative gestures: Expressive and illustrative gestures accompany speech. They underline what the patient tries to convey verbally. In the most simplistic way, a person may illustrate the height, the width, or the shape of an object. Children and naive adults enrich their stories with these kinds of hand movements. A more sophisticated person uses illustrative gestures less but expresses her attitude and feelings by gestures. For instance, she may make a fist to indicate her resolve to follow a certain course of action. Unlike illustrative movements, expressive movements do not duplicate the verbal message but complement it.

Symbolic gestures: Symbolic gestures are culture-specific. They do not duplicate or complement speech but replace it. The meaning of the "OK" sign, for instance, is clear without any verbalization in the United States.

Even though movements are assessed through observation, they are initiated and become understandable in the context of speech. Speech may occur as a monologue, or may be overheard while directed toward persons other than the interviewer.

3. Movements That Express Affect

These movements are observable. They are elicited mainly during conversation. Therefore they will be discussed under Affect (see below).

4. Abnormal Complex Movements

Abnormal complex movement patterns include stupor (see above), excitement, and impulsive actions (Fish 1967). You see stages of excitement in patients with agitated depression, mania, and schizophrenia of the catatonic and paranoid types. Catatonic excitement may reduce facial expression but exaggerate, stiffen, and stilt other movements. Senseless, violent, and indiscriminate destructiveness characterizes postepileptic confusion and pathological drunkenness. Impulsive actions indicate a deficit of insight and/or judgment.

Movements with a neuropathological basis are tremors, akathisia, tardive dyskinesia, choreatic, athetotic movements, and tics. Suspect a tremor to be hysterical if it is limited to one limb, irregular, and variable over time. Fear and intention increase the tremor, distraction decreases it. Besides parkinsonian tremor, akathisia and tardive dyskinesia are induced by neuroleptics.

Athetotic movements and choreatic movements indicate neurological disease and are differentiated from catatonia. Both interfere with voluntary actions but disappear during sleep.

Here is an example of a tic:

> A 19-year-old, white male enters the office accompanied by his mother. While she introduces her son, he throws his head three times to the left side and shouts: "Shit, shit, shit."

This movement is a motor tic and it is associated with a vocal tic, the shouting of profanities; these are the essential features of Gilles de la Tourette's syndrome. Children with tics or Tourette's syndrome usually do not experience clinically significant distress or impairment. Tics can be motor or vocal independent of each other and may occur chronically for more than 1 year or transiently for less than 1 year. Distinguish these tics from stereotypic movement disorders that are also repetitive and nonfunctional. Examples are hand shaking, waving, body rocking, head banging, mouthing of objects, self-biting, picking at skin or body orifices, hitting own body—all of which may be associated with self-injurious behavior. These movement disorders start like tics and Tourette's in childhood and often peak in adolescence. Associated with stereotypic movement disorders are often mental retardation, blindness, deafness, and institutional environments. (For abnormal induced movements, see Chapter 5, section 8. Pathological Reflexes and Movements.)

Observation may thus yield a great deal about the patient's current mental status and lead you to hypotheses about dysfunctions that can be further elaborated during conversation and exploration.

5. Movement Disturbances in Some Psychiatric Disorders

Adult patients with attention-deficit/hyperactivity disorder may give you clues if you observe their motor activity. They fidget and squirm in their seat and may get up and look at your certificates on the wall. They may complain that they can't sit still, ask to go to the bathroom, ask for a cigarette break, or ask for a drink of water. They may appear restless.

Agitated depression augments pacing nearly uncontrollably, but impoverishes all other movements. Similar to thought blocking, a catatonic patient shows a blocking of all psychomotor movements. Such a stupor may be time-limited and without general slowing once the block is overcome. A catatonic patient may refuse to answer but respond hastily after you have turned your back to leave the room. This has been called "reaction at the last moment."

2. CONVERSATION

In casual conversation, the patient tends to be less guarded. You have not yet hit his "hot spots," and you can more readily and surreptitiously evaluate a range of items including: attention and concentration, speech and thinking, and affect. Disturbances or weaknesses in any of these areas can point toward particular dysfunctions. Some areas, like affect, are evaluated in regard to speech patterns as well as facial expressions or body movements. Others, like attention and concentration, can be established in the first few moments of your conversation. Whatever you uncover about the patient may point the way toward problems requiring further evaluation.

While observing your patient, you may begin the verbal part of the psychodiagnostic interview with conversation or "small talk" about any topic other than the patient's problems. What can you look for?

Attention and Concentration

When you meet a new patient, ask him about where he has parked or when his appointment was set. This will allow you to determine his level of attention, concentration, orientation, and memory. If his answers are brief, try to follow up and get details. Monitor whether he stays with your questions or drifts off. Is his concentration limited to interesting subjects? Can he concentrate only when he talks, or also when he listens?

Psychiatric disturbances can be revealed during this initial conversation. Patients who may meet criteria for one of the four subtypes of attention-deficit/hyperactivity disorder (American Psychiatric Association 2000, pp. 85–93) may give you clues about their attention deficit, such as failing to describe details, stay on topic, listen to your questions, or organize their psychiatric or medical history when asked broadbased, open-ended questions. They may express dislike when you test their attention (see Chapter 5: Testing). They may tell you they are often forgetful and demonstrate this symptom by not having with them all their medications for you to review or their checkbook to make their copayment. They also may be distracted by noises in the hallway, the phone ringing, or people walking by your window. Also, substance intoxication causes the patient to appear drowsy and inattentive, and depression decreases interest and concentration. Patients with a frontal lobe lesion may be initially alert and attentive but soon lose focus.

Speech and Thinking

Speech is encoded thought; to decode it is to comprehend what the patient is thinking. Speech and thinking must be separated to effectively assess the patient. Speech is executed by the speech centers in the dominant cortical hemisphere. Disturbances in speech may indicate disturbances in thinking but not always. In this section, we will show you what you can find out about the patient through attention to his speech.

Speech

The patient's speech provides a window into his thinking, a feel for the range of affect, and a recognition of disturbances in articulation. To fathom these areas, invite your patient to talk about emotional topics. In responding to emotionally charged subjects, the patient will reveal the range of his affect. What should you specifically listen for? For speech disturbances, listen to articulation, rhythm, and flow; for thinking, monitor word usage, grammar, and sentence structure; for affect, notice latency of response, speed, tone, amount, loudness, and inflection.

In interviews with children and adolescents, check the DSM-IV-TR criteria for phonological disorder and stuttering (American Psychiatric Association, pp. 65–69). Also, impulsivity, as in attention-deficit/hyperactivity disorder, may be displayed even by adult patients, who may cut you off, impatiently jump to new topics, or interrupt if you answer a phone call, seek some information in a book, or make a note in the chart.

Formal aspects of speech: Disturbed articulation (dysarthria or slurring of speech) often indicates a neurological disorder, or intoxication, especially with sedatives, hypnotics, and alcohol.

Disturbed rhythm of speech is called *dysprosody*. For example, scanning speech (that is, pronunciation of words with pauses between the syllables) occurs in multiple sclerosis, staccato speech in psychomotor epilepsy, and mumbling in Huntington's chorea.

Distinguish between speed and flow. When flow is disturbed, patients talk either in fragments or merge their words. If the patient is difficult to interrupt, it may indicate a lack of inhibitory control. Continuous flow of speech, or pressure, is often associated with such push of speech, that is, speech that is difficult to interrupt. Patients with mania or intoxication from alcohol or stimulant drugs may show both disturbances; patients with anxiety, persecutory delusions, or obsessive-compulsive thinking may show pressure only.

Damage to the speech centers of the brain interferes with the ability to speak and causes different forms of aphasia. Speed and flow of speech are affected in these aphasias. Nonfluent speech—with many pauses and without prepositions, conjunctions, and pronouns between the nouns and verbs—is called *telegram style*. The patient struggles to find appropriate words and circumscribes those words he cannot remember. In these cases, the patient has expressive (motor) aphasia, a damage to Broca's area in the frontal dominant hemisphere. It may develop suddenly after a head trauma or a stroke, or slowly with brain tumors and beginning senility (Alzheimer's disease). The circumscriptions help to distinguish between depression and incipient senile dementia. (Older patients frequently forget names. This is senescent forgetfulness, a benign aphasia unrelated to dementia.)

Continuous, senseless word fluency is called *word salad*. Pauses are missing; nouns are substituted with incorrect ones (paraphasia). Unable to comprehend what you tell him, this patient has receptive sensory aphasia. Wernicke's area in the temporal lobe of the dominant hemisphere—responsible for decoding speech—is afflicted.

In paraphasic speech, the patient uses the wrong word, invents new words, or distorts the phonetic structure of words. Neurologists recognize different forms of paraphasia: semantic, literal, approximative, and neologistic.

In semantic paraphasia, the correct word is substituted by another semantically correct but inappropriate word:

"I wrote the letter with my grass."
"I like to drive around in my tent."

In literal or phonemic paraphasia, only one syllable or letter is substituted:

"I wrote the letter with my len."

In word approximation, the correct word is substituted by an incorrect
word, which has some relationship with the correct word:

"I wrote the letter with my writing toy."

And, finally, neologisms are newly created words:

"I wrote the letter with my zemps. On Sundays I like to watch my flom."

Paraphasia occurs also in some schizophrenic patients or in some patients with other functional psychosis without known organic disturbance.
    Here are some pointers for the differential diagnosis of receptive apha-
sia and paraphasic speech indicating disorganized thinking in patients with
schizophrenia, schizophreniform disorder, schizoaffective disorder, or brief
psychotic disorder. Receptive aphasias show:

• poverty of verbs and nouns
• abundance of conjunctions, prepositions, and interjections
• random, nonrepetitive neologisms without fixed meaning
• isolated sentences, unintelligible in their grammatical structure (see
  Chapter 5: Testing).

For interviews with children or adolescents, you will find additional features in the DSM-IV-TR section "Communication Disorders" (American Psychiatric Association 2000, p. 58).
    In contrast, a schizophrenic patient uses the same neologisms over
and over again and attaches a private meaning to them. The grammatical
structure of sentences may remain intact. Besides the use of neologisms,
patients with schizophrenia show other forms of disorganization, such as
derailment, loose associations, and tangentiality. It is rare that the disorganized speech of schizophrenic patients is so extreme that it resembles

receptive aphasia with linguistic disorganization, such as incoherence or word salad.

Incorrect grammar is used by mentally retarded patients, by some patients with schizophrenia, by patients with damage to the speech areas, and, of course, by some non-native speakers of English. Details of agrammatical sentence construction in speech and writing will be given in *Thinking* below and in Chapter 5: Testing.

Speech and affect: Affect is reflected in the patient's autonomic responses; reactive, facial, and grooming movements; and in his speech. Affect is disturbed in various psychiatric disorders. Prolonged latency of response to your questions, for example, may indicate depressed affect. Mania shortens response time. Schizophrenia varies it. Be alert to the differences between depressed affect and low intelligence. The patient with mental retardation or dementia answers quickly to concrete, short, and simple questions but hesitates in his response to more complex questions.

The tone of voice is also an indicator for psychiatric disorders: the manic patient may be hoarse from talking too much; the alcoholic patient may be hoarse from cigarette smoking and throat irritation by alcohol. If not due to a hearing problem, shouting indicates lack of inhibition, and could be caused by intoxication or mania. A soft, hesitant, subdued voice may point to depression and anxiety.

Inflection of speech reflects affect. The depressed and schizophrenic patient may speak in a monotonous voice, while patients with mania or somatization disorder modulate excessively. The anxious and excited patient often talks at a rising pitch that drops with sadness.

Thinking

Thinking is transmitted by speech. You have to separate a speech disturbance from a disturbance in thinking. You also need to exclude a disturbance of comprehension before you diagnose a thought disorder. Three criteria help you to judge thinking: concepts of words, tightness of association, and goal directedness.

Concept of words: Patients with disturbed word concept use words in a concrete and overinclusive manner. You notice such formal thought disorder often during initial conversation, as the following examples show.

1. Concreteness of thinking:

I: What brought you here?
P: A car. I came in a car.
I: I mean what kind of problem did you have?
P: We did not have any. The car was running smoothly. My brother was driving it.

Notice that the patient cannot grasp the question's abstract meaning about his health but interprets it verbatim. Both the mentally retarded and the schizophrenic patient (Goldstein 1964) miss the symbolic meaning of words and limit them to a specific situation. Concrete thinking is therefore not specific for schizophrenia (Payne and Hewlett 1960). Concrete thinking can be tested by asking the patient to interpret a proverb he is familiar with. (See Chapter 5: Testing.)

2. Overinclusiveness: The opposite of concrete thinking, overinclusiveness expands the concept of a word (Cameron 1964):

I: What problem brought you here?
P: The west. Everything that comes from the warm to the cold, from the west, drifted in. I live west from here coming with the wind which blows from the west. All problems are more in the east. My problems bring me from the west to the east.

In this case, overinclusiveness of the concept "problem" leads the patient to elaborate on his belief that there is more trouble in world politics in the East than in the West, and then fits himself into this schema. Since he has problems himself he should go to the East. In addition, this patient shows concreteness of thinking by referring to the wind blowing from warm to cold as an analogy to his own problems. Payne and Hewlett (1960) reported that a battery of tests separated schizophrenic patients from depressed and neurotic patients on a factor called *overinclusion*, but not on factors called *retardation* and *concreteness*.

Tightness of association and goal-directedness: How tightly does your patient connect words and sentences? Different forms are: perseveration, verbigeration or palilalia, clang association, blocking and derailment, flight of ideas, non sequitur, fragmentation, rambling, driveling, and word salad. Logical gaps among sentences are called loosening of association. Tight connections lead to inclusions of very minute details that result in circumstantial speech. Disturbed association frequently leads to a loss of goal-directedness.

In the following examples, two types of disturbed association are described where the goal is totally or partially preserved: circumstantiality and tangentiality.

Circumstantiality. Circumstantial speech has tightly linked associations that in the end reach their goal, but the thinking is sidetracked over a long circuitous route lined with irrelevant details, as in the following interview with Dorothy.

I: What brought you here?
P: I have this feeling. Let me explain this. I remember when I was 8 years old I had a dirty spot in my pants. I may not have wiped myself properly. I always had the feeling that I'm contaminating myself. Wherever I put my stuff it becomes contaminated. I have to avoid it. It does not have to be actual dirt, just the thought that the dirt is there. I would contaminate my clothes. The contaminated clothes can contaminate me. So when I look behind me I want to see if I am clean or if I have contaminated the chair. That is why I look behind me to see if there are any signs of contamination. I know it's silly. Even when I'm not completely clean it will get through my clothes. I have the feeling that I have to look behind me all the time. This is what brought me here.

Dorothy shows perseveration in theme and circumstantiality that is typical for obsessive-compulsive and cognitive disorders. Circumstantiality is also seen in mania where it presents as enrichment with many irrelevant free associations, only loosely connected to the goal of the thought. Therefore, the minute details of the previous example do not fit manic circumstantiality.

Tangentiality. Tangential thinking may show tight or loose associations. The patient's answers miss the goal, but land in close proximity.

I: What brought you here?
P: I have this feeling. I have it all the time. It's all the talk that's around me. Can you imagine how it feels when it spreads? It was first at my job. Then in my neighborhood. It seems it's now everywhere.
I: Does this talk bother you?
P: It has to do with what others think. It shows what they think. It is like loud thinking. You hear it everywhere and you know they think again because they talk.

Goal-directedness and sentence association. The patient who thinks in a goal-oriented manner can give you a coherent history and answers questions to the point. In severe thought disorder the goal is lost and the associations are disturbed. Here are 10 different types of disturbances.

1. Perseveration: The patient repeats the same phrases and words, even if the subject is changed, or he sticks with the same theme:

I: What brought you here?
P: I came for my manic problem. You know, it has to do with my situation. At home, my things disappear. That is the situation, you know. I believe my son-in-law has to do with it. In my situation I don't know what to do. That is the situation.

The patient repeats the term "situation" several times. The repeated word is called a *stock phrase*. In another example of perseveration, the patient is unable to shift from one topic to another.

I: What did you have for breakfast?
P: Cereals.
I: What did you have for lunch?
P: Cereals.
I: For dinner?
P: Cereals.

Perseveration is seen in major depressive disorder, frontal lobe damage, and schizophrenia, catatonic type.

2. Verbigeration or palilalia: Catatonic and sometimes manic patients repeat words or phrases automatically, especially at the end of a sentence.

I: What problems brought you here?
P: My problems brought me here, problems brought me here, me here.

3. Clang association: Clang association is dictated neither by logic nor by meaning, but by similarity of sounds.

I: What brought you here?
P: All the things said the sphinx. Whatever brings and rings and clings.

Some clang associations sound like rhyming, others appear forced as if the patient succumbs to or is obsessed by the need to associate words by clang. It is seen in patients with dementia, with phonemic paraphasia, schizophrenia, and in some manic episodes.

4. Blocking and derailment: In blocking, the stream of thought is suddenly interrupted; after a pause the patient may start with an entirely new thought, called derailment.

I: What brought you here?
P: I had this argument with my neighbors and they started to . . . [pause] Nobody
    should support the mayor.

The patient did not complete his first thought, but stopped midstream. In
simple blocking, he may continue the original thought after a pause. If you
ask what happened when the patient blocked, he will tell you that he suddenly lost his train of thought. This experience has been called thought
omission. Blocking resembles petit mal seizures in children; however, neither the electroencephalographic abnormality nor the blank stare typical for
petit mal have been demonstrated in blocking.

5. *Flight of ideas:* Flight of ideas is non-goal-directed speech due to distractibility. While the patient answers one question, he switches to a new
train of thought, often triggered by a word in the previous sentence.

I: What brought you here?
P: I got here by getting on my feet. But I have hurt my feet while jogging. Do you
    think jogging is good for me? It may not help against heart infarct, aspirin may
    be better. But I don't like to take drugs. Drugs and crime go together.

The patient initially gives a concrete answer. Subsequently he never reaches
his goal of explaining why he came, because he associates freely to important words in the preceding sentence. Here is another example:

I: What brought you here?
P: I was not brought here, but I walked, not with a car. I like new cars, especially
    foreign ones. Do you like the Mercedes? It is the best, but the gas consumption
    is high. You would have difficulties in Russia. There are not many gas stations
    over there. But it would help the economy. I knew it all along that the Russians
    put the cyanide in the Tylenol capsules.

   In flight of ideas—typical in manic patients—you can identify the words
that trigger the connections between subsequent sentences, but they don't
arrive at a goal. Flight of ideas is usually associated with accelerated speech.
You can follow the succession of ideas, which is in contrast to speech of
schizophrenic patients where the content is cryptic.
   We captured flight of ideas visually. A 19-year-old female college student
was asked to draw a watch. In rapid strokes she sketched Figure 4–1 in four
stages.

6. *Non sequitur:* A non sequitur is a totally unrelated response to a question, on a concrete or abstract level:

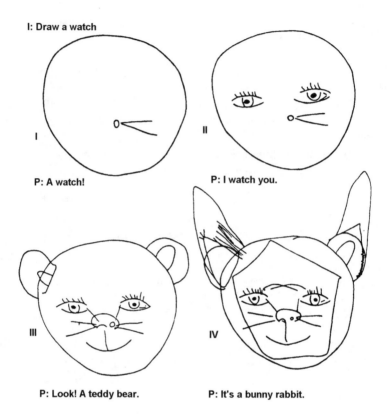

Figure 4–1. Draw a watch.

I: What problem brought you here?
P: There is some evidence but it is not appropriate for my age.

You find this type of thought disorder in dementia and schizophrenia.

7. *Fragmentation:* Patients with fragmented speech talk in phrases unrelated to each other. They show continuous non sequiturs in subsequent
phrases.

I: What brought you here?
P: I have been over . . . There is the street light . . . Can I go . . . No one will
    be . . . Let them all fly . . . Bye and hi.

Fragmentation is not specific for any psychiatric disorder. You may hear it from patients with bipolar disorder, manic episode; schizophrenia, disorganized and catatonic types; or dementia.

8. Rambling: Patients who ramble use groups of sentences that are closely connected but followed by other groups without connection or goal.

I: What brought you here?
P: What a stupid question. Can't you see? But you look cute. Aren't you cute? Okay? Let me tell you, I don't want to repeat it, but I tell you here and now these damned bastards, why can't they leave me alone. I have not done anything. There is the cook. Comes and cooks again. Go away. Just leave me alone.

This type of speech is often seen in patients with delirium and substance intoxication. Watch for other signs of intoxication such as slurred speech, gait ataxia, and nystagmus.

9. Driveling: Patients who drivel speak with preserved syntax and subsequent sentences appear linked, yet the speech cannot be understood.

I: What brought you here?
P: Okay. There was all of the others rounded by the broom, but nevertheless gathering the lomb. So what is the downward onvent creatability? If nothing on those things never recreate a ribboned layer of all times.

In driveling you find no verbigeration and perseveration, but some neologisms. Neurologists have termed this type of speech *jargon agrammatism*. It can be observed in Wernicke's aphasia, but also in chronic schizophrenia.

10. Word salad: In some hospitalized chronic schizophrenic patients the meaningful connection between words is altogether disrupted. Whereas in fragmentation the loosening occurs between phrases and sentences, in word salad consecutive words are not linked by meaning; speech is incomprehensible.

I: What brought you here?
P: The, my, not, rode, for, new, cold, it, what, may, so.

Bleuler called this phenomenon *schizophasia*. It resembles global aphasia (see Chapter 5: Testing).

   A formal thought disorder (disorganized thinking) is not pathognomonic for schizophrenia. Not all schizophrenic patients exhibit thought disorder.

On the other hand, patients with a mood disorder may also display thought disorder. Like most other symptoms and signs, evaluate formal thought disorder in the context of all other psychopathology, psychosocial functioning, and family history.

After completing your evaluation of the patient's speech and thinking, you need to establish his orientation to time and place.

Orientation

To check orientation to place, ask the new patient how he found your office. Severely disoriented outpatients are usually brought in by a family member or friend.

Time is a sensitive indicator of orientation. To check orientation to time, ask when the appointment was made. Ask inpatients when they were admitted and how long they have been in the hospital. In a Board Examination ask when the patient was informed about this examination, and by whom.

The demented patient may attempt to minimize deficiencies and claim:

"For my daily living I don't need to know the date. What a silly question—I don't need to answer that."

Be persistent to learn whether the patient is unable to perform or oppositional.

Patients with mental retardation may also be disoriented to time but without using excuses or denial. Withdrawn or distractible patients may appear disoriented, but will answer correctly if you insist.

If the patient is disoriented, focus on the mental status examination rather than asking him for his recent history; it will be unreliable. If you evaluate orientation initially, you avoid the awkward question at the end of the interview:

"Now before we close, do you know what date it is?"

Memory

During the initial conversation you can check your patient's memory in an informal manner. (A formal quantitative approach is described in Chapter 5: Testing.) For instance, spell your name when you introduce yourself. When he can repeat your name, his immediate recall is probably intact; if he addresses you later by name, his recent memory appears to be working. The same is true if he can describe how he got to the clinic and where he parked. Discussion of past events will reveal possible disturbances of memory.

Patients with memory disturbances focus on events that they can readily recall. Therefore, introduce topics of your choice such as movies, sports events, television series, or political events that you can verify. Without a vested interest in the subject matter, the patient will be less likely to remember the event.

Conversation may, of course, be used at any time during the interview. When you suspect simulation or dissimulation of amnesia, or dissociative amnesia, small talk helps you to detect contradictions between facts and intent. Elisa's case demonstrates how conversation can aid in the diagnostic assessment.

> This 27-year-old, white woman was brought to the hospital emergency room by the highway patrol with the complaint of total memory loss. She had been found wandering the highway, unable to remember her last name or address. She claimed she did not know anything about her past. She denied drinking or head injury and she had no signs of trauma. However she was not sure about substance abuse because she just could not remember. During the interview, she was guarded and mentioned repetitively that she did not remember. When hypnosis was suggested to recover her memory, she declined.
>
> At the end of the interview the examiner accompanied her from the emergency room to the floor and, while walking with her, mentioned that hypnosis is frightening for many people and that he could understand that she might be scared of it. She replied: "That's right. My father once took me to the carnival in Columbus, Ohio, close to the place where we lived. And they had a show there, and some people from the audience were invited to be hypnotized. I can still see how these volunteers were talking and crying like babies." This statement made while off-guard contradicted the massive memory disturbance claimed during the "official" interview.

Distortion of Memory

Psychiatric disorders can distort memory. The depressed patient may claim he has been depressed since childhood, or is a born loser, sinner, or criminal. The manic patient may exaggerate his achievements, or distort past experiences, recalling previous hospitalizations, for example, as an ordeal of restrictive tortures without recalling his aggressive behavior that necessitated physical constraints. The schizophrenic patient may report injustice and persecutions that never happened. The patient with antisocial personality disorder may invent a life history.

False Memory

Déjà vu and déjà vécu occur predominantly in patients with temporal lobe lesions, but also in people without neurological findings (Sno and Linszen 1990). False memory has also been suggested in dissociative disorders in which instances of sexual abuse have been claimed but not verified.

Affect

Affect is the visible and audible manifestation of the patient's emotional response to external and internal events, that is, thoughts, ideas, evoked memories, and reflections. It is expressed in autonomic response, posture, facial and reactive movements, grooming, and in tone of voice, vocalizations, and word selection.

Autonomic responses are mediated by the sympathetic and parasympathetic system. They become visible in turning pale as an anger response, in blushing, sweating, and trembling.

Posture has been described above.

Facial movements involve the muscles around the mouth, nose, and eyes. All nine basic transcultural affects (see below) are reflected in the movement in these muscle groups.

Reactive movements involve the face and the entire body. They are made in response to a novel stimulus. A person looks up when you enter the room, looks over in response to a noise. Thus reactive movements reflect alertness, surprise, and interest.

Grooming movements manipulate the outer appearance. The person may preen his hair, massage his hands and chest, scratch his neck, or poke his teeth or nose. A person carries out grooming movements to maintain or regain composure and a feeling of well-being. For instance, if a patient feels uncomfortable in an interview, he may start to scratch his leg or rub his forehead.

Affect needs to be distinguished from mood. You can do so by considering four features:

● Affect is momentary, lasting as little as 1–2 seconds; mood lasts longer.
● Affect is attached to outside or internal stimuli and changes with them; mood can change spontaneously.
● Affect is the foreground; mood is the emotional background.
● Affect is observed by you (sign); mood is reported by your patient (symptom).

(As mood needs to be described by the patient, it will be discussed in section 3: Exploration.)

Affect has three functions: 1) self-perception, 2) communication, and 3) motivation. In the case of *self-perception*, affect provides us with an emotional value judgment. It tells us whether we like what we experience or hate it. For instance, if you learn unexpectedly that you have been promoted, your heart and breathing rate may increase, you have a warm feeling in your chest, your trunk muscles may firm up, you get a happy expression on your face. This represents your affective response.

Affect expresses our feelings and makes them known to others. It thus *communicates* our emotional response to events, to interpersonal interactions, to behavior, and to situations.

In respect to *motivation,* feelings of anger and rage, for instance, may initiate aggression and destructive behavior; alertness and interest stimulate exploration; fear predisposes to escape. Affect is a precursor to action.

When we show affect we initiate a goal-directed action in a rudimentary and incomplete form. For instance, in disgust we curl back our lips so as not to touch any spoiled food with them; we turn up our nose and exhale heavily so as not to smell the stench. In a boring lecture we whip our legs as if ready to escape. Even to an abstract thought, we respond with our affect as if it were concrete.

What Is the Origin of Affect?

Research has supported Charles Darwin's theory on the innateness and universality of emotional expression, that is, *affect* (Izard 1977, 1979). Izard et al. (1983) found nine basic expressive movements to be innate: disgust, surprise, joy, anger, fear, sadness, interest, shame, and content. Their basic expression develops in the first 18 months of life in a predictable sequence. Thus affect is an inborn means of interpersonal communication that can be disturbed in psychiatric disorders. The recognition of this disturbance provides diagnostic clues.

All nine affects are disturbed in psychiatric disorders: disgust, perplexity (surprise), elation (joy), anger, anxiety (fear), sadness, interest, shame (guilt), and suspicion (content). In a specific psychiatric disorder, one or two of the basic affects may dominate at the expense of some others such as anxiety (anxiety disorders), sadness, disgust and guilt (depression), elation and interest (mania), suspicion (paranoia), and perplexity (cognitive disorders).

How Do You Evaluate Affect?

Watch the flow of gestures and facial expressions. These nonverbal clues emerge before verbal communications and will persist no matter what the content of the words. The patient expresses his feelings in tone of voice, pitch, modulation, and selection of vocabulary. When you can sense how the patient feels, you have learned to read affect.

The innateness of the basic affects does not preclude their manipulation. We do learn to suppress, exaggerate, distort, pretend, and falsify the expression of our emotions, thus using affect for a purpose. We develop our personal style of display, and can do it on demand.

> When Mr. Smith, a successful CPA, became depressed, he still smiled and sought eye contact while talking, but he dropped his smile between sentences or when he felt unobserved. His feet were tapping throughout the interview as if to flee from the situation and his morbid, suicidal thoughts.

Thus affect can contain a double message. Spontaneous affect uses the limbic and extrapyramidal system and precedes the deliberately displayed affect, which may contradict the spontaneous one. You encounter this double message in patients who plan to deceive you by concealing, falsifying, malingering, and fabricating. A thorough study of such double messages is presented in *The Clinical Interview Using DSM-IV-TR, Volume 2: The Difficult Patient* (Othmer and Othmer 2002).

Affect is not only exhibited through facial expression. As Morris (1987) points out, most adults have learned to control their facial expressions but not their legs and feet to convey a desired affect. When interviewing patients who suppress affect, you may evoke it. To do so, ask the patient to talk about sensitive subjects (family situations, personal losses, success or failure at work, frustrations and disappointments, or hobbies).

Primary dimensions of affect are quality, intensity, duration, and appropriateness to stimuli; secondary dimensions are range and control. The expression of specific *qualities* of affect are, for instance, wide-open eyes and a frowning forehead, which will alert you to anxiety, or a restless and apprehensive look, which will alert you to perplexity. Clenched teeth and fists and stiff facial muscles portray anger. A head turned sideways and a patient observing you out of the corner of his narrowed eyes demonstrate suspicion. Smiles, rapid changes in expressions, euphoric glimmer in the eyes interrupted by outbursts of anger give away manic excitement. A stiff facial expression with lively moving eyes, as if looking through a mask, and sparse gestures with the mouth in so-called snout spasm indicate catatonia.

The omega sign on the forehead, corners of the mouth drawn downward, tearful eyes, and drooping shoulders point toward depression (Darwin 1965; Greden et al. 1985). Some depressed patients smile with their lips, but have "dead eyes." A patient with agitated depression sits in her chair wringing her hands, rocking back and forth, repeating the same phrase:

"Please help me, please help me!"

Intensity shows the patient's involvement in a topic. Schizophrenic patients are often unable to feel involved. Interviewing them is like talking to a computer. Nothing appears to touch them; their affect is flat or shallow. The person with schizophrenia, paranoid type, however, may come alive if you challenge his overvalued ideas or delusions (Leonhard 1979 calls this affect *laden paraphrenia*).

Duration: An affective response may perk up for a split second or freeze, it may rise and mellow slowly, or be switched on and off. The affect's relationship to thought content determines its appropriateness. Affect may be inappropriate, for example, the schizophrenic patient who giggles about the death of his mother. Another abnormality in the relationship between thought content and affect is the lack of concern that a patient with conversion reactions may show. Such a patient may claim he is blind, paralyzed, or has no sensations in his body, yet he shows no concern for his future fate, or for the impact of the symptoms on his life. The French psychiatrist Janet has used the term *la belle indifférence* for this sign (Campbell 1981).

The *range* of affect and its different qualities varies from narrow (as in the withdrawn schizophrenic patient, the retarded depressive patient, or the obsessive-compulsive patient) to wide (as in the intoxicated or brain-damaged patient). Some types of affect may dominate over others, such as suspicion in delusional disorder, hopelessness and guilt in major depressive disorder, or irritability and joy in a manic episode.

Judge whether the patient has *control* over her affect. Are her emotions stable and only slightly modulated by the topic of the conversation? Or is her affect rapidly changing in response to the topic (labile affect)? Such changes occur in the intoxicated or manic patient.

The limbic system of the brain colors speech and actions emotionally (Isaacson 1982; Joynt 1992); the right (nondominant) parietal lobe recognizes these emotions and the right frontal lobe expresses them (Ross 1982). By evaluation of affect, the interviewer makes a statement about functioning of the patient's subcortical and cortical brain structures.

3. EXPLORATION

An interviewer can observe and converse with the patient without her consent. But with exploration, the interviewer needs the patient to cooperate and to talk about herself. Exploration requires you to probe more deeply into the meaning behind the patient's words, behaviors, and presentation of facts. You start to explore when you ask:

"What brought you here?"

When she describes her symptoms you zero in; when you observe signs of disturbed behavior you may confront her and explore their meaning.

When do you question her about symptoms and signs? Immediately, if they disrupt rapport or might be forgotten later, or when they lead into the center of psychopathology. The following vignette offers an example of how exploration can reveal pathology. John keeps staring at the nameplate on your desk, seems distracted, and pays little attention to your questions. Ask him why.

P: I try to figure out how many different words I can make with the letters in your name.
I: Do you often play with letters or words in this way?
P: All the time. I blow 3 or 4 hours a day by doing that and other things.

It is best to delay exploration of a sign or symptom if it seems of minor importance, sidetracks you, or is part of a complex psychopathology such as a delusional system.

What kinds of items in the mental status do you need to look for during exploration? Novices and experienced clinicians alike run the risk of being overwhelmed by the wealth of clinical details and therefore may neglect to explore four key symptoms and signs that threaten rapid decline. They are:

1. Suicidal and homicidal tendencies expressing immediate danger (see below: Content of Thinking)
2. Organic conditions, now called general medical conditions that contribute to the development of cognitive disorders (see Chapter 5: Testing)
3. Alcohol and other substance use that leads to intoxication, withdrawal, and long-term toxic effects on the brain and other body systems (see Psychiatric History in Chapter 6: Diagnosis)
4. Psychosis, that is, hallucinations and delusions that interrupt the patient's relationship to reality and render him a victim of irrational thinking and unrealistic perception (see below: Content of Thinking)

These symptoms and signs can be summarized in the mnemonic **SOAP**. In each patient, these four symptoms and signs have to be assessed to make a diagnosis and to initiate a treatment plan.

In general, in exploration you need to focus on discerning mood, quality of mood, stability of mood, reactivity, intensity of mood, and duration; energy level; perception; insight, especially in regard to delusions and hallucinations; and content of thinking—delusions, phobias, compulsions, narcoleptic attacks, grand mal seizures, panic attacks, and so forth. We will cover all of these aspects of the mental status examination in this section.

Mood

An understanding of the patient's mood is critical in that it is the long-term feeling state through which all experiences are filtered. Mood is not necessarily discernible; it will be revealed if the patient is asked directly about it. Sometimes you find an apparent discrepancy between affect and mood; the patient controls his affect by wearing a social mask, but describes depressed mood.

Mr. Brink, a real estate developer in his sixties, slender, tall, wearing coat and tie, entered my office smiling and seemingly in good spirits. He was accompanied by his wife, dressed in designer clothes.

I: Why did you come to see me?
Wife: I heard a friend of mine talk about you and my ears perked up, because I thought about my husband's problems. He was most active until about 14 years ago, when he had a bout with depression. He was treated by a local psychiatrist with several antidepressants, but never responded. He finally got better without medication.
I: How do you feel now? [I asked Mr. Brink]
P: [he smiled and looked at his wife; I continued to look at him] Well . . . I don't know . . . Bad, I feel bad. I put everything off, don't want to do anything. See . . . I can't even speak up. She does all the talking.
Wife: And it was just the opposite before he got sick. It was me who always was nervous.
I: What do you feel when you feel bad?
P: I worry. I worried about coming here. I worried all evening and night.
I: You worried in the evening. Is that different from the morning?
P: In the morning I'm numb. I don't want to get up. I don't want to do anything. I don't want to talk.
I: What feels worse, the morning or evening?
P: I'd have to say the morning . . . like now.
I: Is there anything that will make you feel better for a while?

P: No, nothing, nothing at all.

Wife: Yesterday he was feeling good. His son was over and took him out. And he always enjoys that a lot.

I: Having your son over makes you feel better? [Mr. Brink's face seemed to drop; the lines in his face deepened; he looked ashen.]

P: Maybe for a while [with a doubting, weak voice].

I: Talking about your son cheers you up?

P: Not really. Nothing makes a real difference. Talking usually makes me feel worse.

I: [while I spoke with him, he smiled with thin lips, only to look much older again when the interviewer turned toward his wife] When I talk to you, you don't seem that depressed [I addressed him again].

P: For a short while I can put up a front, but I feel worse behind it.

Wife: He has to do that in his business.

P: I can't accomplish anything. I can't do my work. I just sit there. I don't know what to do first.

I: How does the future look to you?

P: I will never get better. I wish I wasn't around anymore.

Mood has five dimensions: quality, stability, reactivity, intensity, and duration. These can be explored as they emerge in the interview.

Quality

Mood seeks and finds a fitting content, for instance, a depressed mood finds themes of guilt and failure. The quality of mood cannot be determined from observed affect—you have to ask. Good questions to uncover mood are:

"How do you feel most of the day?"
"How do you feel now?"

These questions may yield clear answers:

"good"
"energetic"
"high"
"depressed"
"tired"

or ambiguous ones:

"I feel rough."
"I've been sitting on the swing a lot."
"I've been lying around the house lately."
"Okay, I guess."

To explore ambiguous answers, you can offer the patient a range of responses:

> "Are you more blue, sad, down in the dumps, low spirited or high, up, on top of the world?"

If a patient cannot describe his mood in his own words, you can ask questions about his everyday activities or vegetative functions:

> "Do you enjoy talking to me?"
> "Do you get fun out of your favorite activities?"
> "What are your plans for the future?"
> "Do you get satisfaction from your work and the things you do every day?"
> "How is your sleep . . . appetite . . . sex drive . . . energy?"

Once you find descriptors of his mood, use them as anchors. Reflecting back his expressions of feeling states puts the patient in touch with his inner sense of experience and can help him assess his own mood.

Stability

A patient with stable mood reports he remains tranquil no matter what adversities he encounters:

> "I feel like the rock of Gibraltar, nothing seems to shake me. That's a real new feeling for me."

Unstable mood changes spontaneously or reactively. Spontaneous mood changes can occur during a single day.

> "I feel rotten when I wake up at 4 A.M., unable to fall asleep again. I feel depressed most of the morning hours, but I feel better after lunch, and evenings are the best for me."

This so-called *diurnal variation* is often associated with a mood disorder. These questions may help you:

> "Compare your mood in the morning with your mood in the evening. Are there any differences?"
> "When do you feel better—at breakfast or at supper?"
> "Do you feel better now or later?"

Reactivity

Lack of reactivity is typical for a major depressive episode with melancholic features, moderate to severe (American Psychiatric Association 2000, p. 420). For example, nothing could cheer up Mr. Brink, not even his son's visit. In contrast, some dysphoric patients with substance-related disorders, somatization disorder, or some personality disorders feel better if their social situation improves. Also, patients with major depression with atypical features may show brightening in mood in response to positive events.

Intensity

The experience of mood varies between intense and shallow. Patients experience panic, mania, and substance-induced excitement as intense. In contrast, schizophrenic patients have a flat and shallow mood. A depressed mood can be intense despite a flat affect.

Duration

Duration gives mood its diagnostic value. Dysphoria lasting hours or days is seen in personality disorders, especially antisocial personality disorder and substance abuse, while a depressed episode of a mood disorder lasts 2 weeks or longer. The same is true for elated mood. DSM-IV-TR proposes, for instance, an arbitrary cutoff of 1 week to diagnose a manic episode.

Energy Level

Energy level can be determined in a number of different ways. Monitor how often a patient brings up a new topic, and how well he elaborates on it. Ask him about how easily he can initiate and carry out actions. Ask him whether he has to push himself and drags through the day. Ask him about his last 24 hours. Was it easy to go through daily routines? What about new tasks? Ask whether he plans his day or not.

The depressed patient complains that he cannot plan, decide, initiate, and carry through actions. The obsessive patient worries about her indecision and repeated checking. The manic patient initiates lots of things, but finishes few. The phobic patient is restricted by numerous avoidances. The patient with antisocial personality may appear active, but he pursues pleasure rather than productive work. The schizophrenic patient may watch television all day long.

Perception

Normal perception originates from stimulation of specific sensory receptors. It is disturbed in psychotic patients. Patients with hallucinatory perceptions have images and auditory and olfactory impressions in the absence of verifiable stimulation. Psychotic patients hear voices without people around, sometimes over enormous distances; these voices come and go capriciously, follow the patient, making him feel trapped. Most hallucinating patients realize the "hallucinatory character" of their perceptions without being able to explain it, but they insist that these perceptions are real and not imagined. You can safely ask:

"Do you hear any voices, even when nobody is present?"

Or more empathically:

"Are you bothered or harassed by voices?"

Some patients with schizophrenia are ambivalent whether they should tell you or not. Such patients may deny voices unless you assume that they hear them and ask a leading question:

"What did the voices tell you today?"

If the patient still denies hearing voices, ask him whether the voices forbid him to talk about them.

Insight Into Hallucinations

When you are trying to determine whether a patient has hallucinations, assume that the patient has no insight into their morbid nature. Therefore, ask factual questions:

"Do you hear voices?"

rather than questions that imply morbidity:

"Have you ever been so sick that you heard voices?"

Even though most hallucinating patients realize that others consider their perceptions as "crazy," they themselves do not share that view.
There are five stages of insight:

Stage I: Previously reported hallucinations have now stopped. The patient has full insight into their morbid nature.

"In the past I believed that I heard my mother's and sister's voices calling me names. I must have really been sick. I know they will not do such a thing. And even if they could, they would not do it."

Stage II: Hallucinations were experienced in the past, but are not present now; the patient believes that they were real.

"Some months ago my mother's and sister's voices harassed me. They have stopped now."

Stage III: Hallucinations have been experienced recently but the patient refuses to talk about them. He seems to realize the contradiction between the psychotic perceptions and reality.

"I don't want to talk about my mother's and sister's voices anymore. I just don't care for that nonsense. They don't bother me anymore."

Stage IV: The patient talks about his hallucinations, but does not act upon them.

"I hear my mother's and sister's voices. They are calling me names. I hear them all the time."

Stage V: The patient acts upon his hallucinations. He obeys or responds to the voices.

"My mother and sister scolded me again. I heard their voices, they called me a monkey. I called them up and told them to stop. But they are vicious and lied to me, they denied that they are doing it."

One patient, a recent immigrant, harassed by voices, had murdered his mother and sister because they denied hearing the same voices he heard and refused to stop them. Obviously, this patient did not comprehend that his hallucinations were unique and limited to him. Usually you can convince a patient that no one else is experiencing his hallucinations. This however does not convince him that they are unreal. With treatment patients become more receptive to this argument. If they insist on the reality of their hallucinations, take it as an expression of the severity of their symptoms. Find out whether your patient is aware that the hallucinations are exclusive to him by asking:

"Can other people hear the voices too? Do you think I can hear them?"

Hallucinations usually appear and disappear by passing through these five stages. These stages are clinically important for two reasons: First, to consider discharge, the patient should be at stage I. Clinicians who are unaware of these stages often consider patients at stage III as symptom-free and discharge them prematurely. Schizophrenic patients at this stage are usually not compliant; they often stop their medication and relapse. Second, since nonacute hallucinations reappear in the same order as they disappear, use these stages to titrate medication on an outpatient basis. Clinicians who pay no attention to these stages often miss more vigorous treatment for stages II and III.

Patients talk about their hallucinations in different ways. They may deny them or present them with insight. Here are some techniques to handle this.

1. During stage III: If you suspect that your patient has hallucinations but denies them, ask flatly:

"What did the voices tell you this morning?"

The patient may then describe his hallucinations.

    I: Did you hear voices recently?
    P: No.
    I: When was the last time you heard them?
    P: About 2 or 3 months ago when I was in the hospital.
    I: You have not heard them since?
    P: [hesitates] No, I don't think so.
    I: Tell me, what did these voices tell you this morning?
    P: They told me everything I should do and they told me not to talk about it.

2. During stages IV and V: If a patient calls his hallucinations "crazy," be reluctant to accept this as an indication of insight. Instead, expect it to be lip service and challenge his statement. He may not have true insight in his hallucinations but has learned that others consider them as "crazy." Pursue the topic by asking what he thinks about the nature of his hallucinations. His comments may be quite delusional.

    P: I think I'm getting crazy again.
    I: Why?
    P: I believe some people use waves to transmit their voices into my ears.
    I: Is it crazy for you to hear these voices?
    P: Not for me, only for others.

A patient may ask you whether you believe that he is crazy. Tell him that you believe that he has these experiences, that they are real for him, and that you want an accurate description from him to understand them better.

3. If a patient resorts to delusional explanations, such as:

"My ears seem to be extremely sensitive."
"A radio station is sending these voices."
"The heating duct works as a loudspeaker."

accept his delusional explanations as real and empathize with his experience of harassment. Offer him treatment for his suffering. Don't tell him that the medication will give him insight into the morbid character of the voices or make them disappear, because for him they are real.

4. Patients who emphasize the reality of their hallucinations and belittle others who lack the talent to perceive them should not be challenged, but be allowed to describe in detail their experiences as if they were reports from another planet.

5. Patients who accuse you of maliciously lying when you deny hearing the voices usually suffer from persecutory delusions and may become dangerous. Let the patient voice his accusations and let him explain why he thinks you are withholding the hallucinatory experience and not leveling with him. Thus, focus on the assessment of the delusion rather than a confrontation with reality.

Content of Thinking

Many psychiatric disorders are characterized by a pathological content of thinking. In this section, we will go through the various disorders in thinking and offer some suggestions about how to get patients to reveal their innermost thoughts.

Suicidal and Homicidal Tendencies

Patients are often reluctant to reveal their aggressive impulses. Thoughts about suicide can be graded from 1 to 5:

1. I just want to stop the way I feel, but I have no plan or intent or morbid thoughts to do anything to myself.

2. I often wish I did not wake up in the morning or that a truck would run me over, but I would not do anything to myself.
3. I thought about suicide, but I have no plan or intent to do it. I know I would not do anything like that.
4. I have thought about overdosing or cutting my wrist just to stop my pain. I don't really want to die, but these are my thoughts.
5. I thought about suicide, like starting my car in the garage and sitting in it until it's all over, or doing something more violent like having a single-car accident, hanging myself, or shooting myself.

    a. I know these are just fantasies, and I know I wouldn't do anything like that.
    b. I don't know whether I would ever do that.
    c. It looks tempting to me.

Most patients know that you will have to hospitalize them if they reveal a suicide plan or intent. Therefore, they may refuse to answer your questions, or they may hide their true level of suicidality.

We know some risk factors, such as being male, being over 40 years of age, experiencing social isolation, having previous serious attempts, writing a suicide note, or distributing property. We know that there is an increased suicide risk for various disorders (see courses of disorders in DSM-IV-TR). We also know that we cannot prevent suicide. Patients have committed suicide in psychiatric hospitals, on passes while hospitalized, as outpatients, and as nonpatients.

We use a positive and a negative approach in assessing suicidality. If you use the positive approach, assess the risk factors by starting from a vantage point other than the suicidal impulse, by exploring the value the patient places on his or her own life and the satisfaction he or she gets from living. Such an opening easily leads to discussions of reduced worth and possible plans to end it all. If you use the negative approach, start more directly by asking the patient about suicidal ideas, plans, and intent. Direct, fast-working, and irreversible methods—shooting, hanging, jumping from a high place, and carbon monoxide poisoning—show a patient at the highest risk. Other methods—such as wrist cutting or aspirin overdose—identify someone who is more focused on the attempt than the completion of suicide. (For details on suicide and suicide in alcoholic patients, see Murphy 1992.) The lethal risk of overdosing depends on the substance used.

Homicidal tendencies can often be identified by offering the patient a release of his anger:

"Is there any person in your life who holds you back, who suppresses you, or treats you unfairly? In other words, do you have a foe or an enemy?"
"Is there anybody who let you down or has ruined your life?"

From here you can assess the fantasies and plans a patient may entertain to take care of his or her opponent. Patients may disclose to you whether they go armed to work ready to pull the trigger. Along with patients with antisocial personality disorder, patients with a diagnosis of paranoid personality disorder, delusional disorder, or schizophrenia, paranoid type, may pose an increased risk for homicide.

A patient may ask you whether you have to report him to the police or warn the intended victim if he tells you about the homicidal plans. Your answer depends on the patient's mental status. If the patient is delusional and psychotic, you may say:

"I will help you to solve the problem without your having to commit a crime. I protect you in the hospital. I may also discuss with your (foe) what he has done to you. To do this, I need the name and phone number."

If the patient is not delusional or psychotic, you may persuade him to identify the victim. If the patient, psychotic or not, refuses to identify the victim, you may tell him that you have the duty to warn in order to prevent him from committing a criminal act. The duty to warn may include informing the patient's family members, employer, or the police.

Here are three case vignettes that, to different degrees, may present a duty to warn intended victims (Case 1); to warn officials about a potentially dangerous situation and its prevention (Case 2); and to warn the patient himself about self-incrimination (Case 3). The legal opinion that follows each case vignette is given from a Missouri perspective, because that is the state of the authors' practice. Therapists living in any other state should refer to their respective legislation.

Case 1

Mr. Jesse M., a middle-aged, married, Caucasian male referred to the psychiatrist by another patient, stated: "I'm harrassed at work, and they want to fire me. This is the fourth time in my life that I've risen in my position just to be demoted and fired, or forced to resign. I can't endure this one more time." The therapist obtained written consent from the patient to contact his boss to find out what was going on. The supervisor indeed confirmed Mr. M.'s demotion and transfer to a small office without salary cut. Later, the patient showed the therapist in writing the supervisor's expectations for completing a job and explained to the therapist why this job could not be completed within the alloted time: "They're creating a paper trail to fire me. I can't bear that. I will kill some people on the job if they fire me. I may kill myself afterward if people find out." The patient gave the therapist the names of his enemies. The therapist told the patient that he will get him out of that job situation through immediate short-term medical disability and asked him whether that would help him to solve his crisis for now. The patient agreed and withdrew his threats under these circumstances.

Mr. M. gave the therapist written permission to talk to the plant physician, who agreed to immediate sick leave. Subsequently, the therapist obtained the patient's written permission to talk to the patient's wife. In the patient's presence, the therapist discussed with her the necessity to reveal the homicidal threats to the plant physician, because the granting of permanent disability would hinge on the patient's homicidal tendencies and his psychiatric problems. The documentation of his homicidal plans would expose him as a serious risk at work. The therapist asked the wife whether she was in agreement with his assessment of her husband's dangerousness and if she wanted to consult a lawyer before he used the patient's homicidal, revenge-based tendencies to obtain permanent disability. The wife felt the therapist should go ahead without her consulting an attorney.

The therapist discussed the situation with the plant physician, who agreed with the therapist's assessment and disclosed that Mr. M.'s work group was dysfunctional and that Mr. M. had also talked to him about homicidal ideas. With the plant physician's help, Mr. M. received permanent disability.

Homicidal tendencies had been managed by removing the patient from the work situation and by warning wife and plant physician about the patient's dangerousness. The patient dropped his threats when he realized there was a more satisfactory way out of his situation than homicide. The retraction of the threat made the direct warning of the targets unneccessary. Subsequent psychotherapy revealed the patient's undermining job strategies, underlying personality disorders, and brief delusional disorder. The therapist used this insight to help the patient to resolve social conflicts that the patient had after he was removed from the pressure at the plant.

Legal opinion. The law is clear about health care professionals' duty to warn potential victims of homicidal threats, and/or the persons who can remove the motive for a violent act. The seminal case that recognized a duty to warn on behalf of mental health professionals is *Tarasoff v. Regents of University of California* (551 P2d 334 [1976]). In this case, a family sued a psychotherapist after the murder of their daughter by a psychiatric patient who had disclosed to the therapist his intent to kill the young woman. The California court ruled that when a psychotherapist determines that his patient presents a serious danger of violence to another, he has an obligation to use reasonable care to protect the intended or "foreseeable" victim against such danger (551 P2d 344–345 [1976]). In finding a duty owed to a third party, the court placed emphasis on the "special relationship" between the patient and the therapist, noting that this special relationship may legally create affirmative duties owed to third parties (551 P2d 344–345 [1976]). By entering into a doctor-patient relationship, the therapist assumes some responsibility for the safety of the patient and any third parties whom the therapist knows to be threatened by the patient (551 P2d 344–345 [1976]). Although the therapist in *Tarasoff* had no direct relationship with the victim, the special relationship between the patient/defendant and the therapist was sufficient to create certain affirmative duties for the benefit of third persons.

Case 2

> From his military days, Mr. Kelvin D., a patient with major depression, severe with psychotic features (persecutory delusions), in remission, has approximately 83 pounds of C4, a plastic explosive, safely stored in a steel box in his basement. He had planned to use it to clear out some trees in his remote lake property but had second thoughts about that. The therapist suggested he should get rid of the explosives without legal problems. Only fire or direct ignition, but not physical impact, can cause the material to explode. Although there is no intended victim, an accident could kill many people. After consultation with colleagues, the psychiatrist proposed that the patient contact his lawyer or the county sheriff for a safe transfer of the explosives to a military site.

In this case, it is not clear to what degree the patient's confidentiality is protected and whether a more direct warning by the therapist to the county, the FBI, or other authorities has to be implemented.

Legal opinion.   After the *Tarasoff* opinion, some courts have clarified that a duty to warn exists only to "identifiable" third parties, as opposed to the general public. In *Thompson v. County of Alameda* (614 P2d 728 [1980]), the court held that the duty to warn does not extend to the general public, but only arises when the intended victim is "foreseeable" and "readily identifiable." According to the *Thompson* opinion, no affirmative duty to warn exists when a patient has made "nonspecific threats of harm directed at nonspecific victims" (614 P2d 735 [1980]).

Some states have rejected the *Thompson* holding and extended the *Tarasoff* duty to warn any foreseeable victim, even if there has been no specific threat to a particular victim (see, e.g., Hamma v. County of Maricopa, 161 Ariz 58, 775 P2d 1122, 1128 [1989] [Arizona]; Schuster v. Altenberg, 144

Wis2d 223, 424 NW2d 159 [1988] [Wisconsin]). Other states have enacted a statutory duty to warn similar to the duty recognized in *Tarasoff*. For example, the Nebraska statute is limited to a patient or client's threatened behavior where the threat involves a "reasonably identifiable" victim(s) (NEB REV STAT, para 71-1, 206.30 [1994]). Care should be taken to become fully advised of the "duty to warn" cases and laws in each state where the mental health professional practices.

The law is unclear about past crimes. For a health professional, is there a duty to report past crimes? Is there a duty to warn a patient about self-incrimination and lack of confidentiality of the medical chart?

Case 3

Mr. Karl D., a patient in his fifties, is disabled because of several medical disorders. He also suffers from major depression, severe with paranoid features. He reports that he has had a bad temper all his life, which has come out, for example, in incidents of road rage, in which, armed with a gun, he followed to their homes drivers who annoyed him. He reveals: "I have done bad things in my life that I have not told anybody. I have a good and a bad side in me." When asked about the "bad things," he mentions killing people and having been involved with organized crime. He would like to get all this off his chest, but he wonders whether the therapist would have to report him to the authorities.

The therapist tells him that she has to warn possible victims if he plans to kill somebody now, but that, to the best of her knowledge, a patient's past criminal acts are protected by doctor-patient confidentiality:

I would have to chart what you tell me, and also my therapeutic interventions to deal with your problems like your remorse and guilt. Therapists' records are not well protected. Insurance companies have clauses where the patient's benefits hinge on chart review by the insurance company. Charts can be subpoenaed.

The therapist applies the Miranda rule that warns the patient that what he says can be used against him and that he does not have to incriminate himself if he does not desire to do so. He could also get legal advice.

Legal opinion. The law is not clear regarding a duty to report past criminal acts. In Missouri, there are no reported cases that clearly answer this question. There are, however, some Missouri statutes that create reporting requirements for certain, narrow categories of information, such as child abuse. These statutes do not provide a clear answer for prior criminal acts that do not fall within a mandatory reporting category. Since the courts have not squarely addressed this issue, it would seem reasonable to assume that there is no specific duty of the health care professional to disclose prior criminal acts committed by a patient. If this issue arises, however, the best course for the health care professional would be to seek the advice of health care and/or criminal counsel. The legal advice not only will provide a course of conduct to follow in these types of situations, but also may provide the health care professional with a potential advice-of-counsel defense should the issue be litigated in the future.

With respect to warning a patient about self-incrimination, there is also not a clear answer found under Missouri law. Certainly, the best practice would be for the patient to be fully informed of the ramifications of advising the mental health care professional about past criminal acts or conduct.

As with any issues, the health care professional must exercise extreme caution before divulging patient information or confidences. Most states have statutes and/or regulations that protect the physician-patient privilege and/or the disclosure of confidential information learned from a patient. In such instances where a duty to warn may arise, mental health care professionals must become thoroughly knowledgeable of the laws and regulations of the state in which they practice.

Delusions

Delusions are fixed false beliefs, often about some action that has taken place, such as the neighbors spying and plotting against the patient.

Here are four questions that assess a delusion.

1. What is going on? This assesses content. Asking a direct question such as

   "Do you have strange or crazy ideas?"

   does not work when the patient lacks insight. It is much better to ask:

   "Do other people think that you have crazy ideas?"

   This approach works because most patients talk about their delusional ideas to family members and friends and get rebuffed by remarks like "That's crazy!" Also, tap key areas known as breeding grounds for delusions such as: persecution, injustice, discrimination, guilt, grandiosity, love, power, knowledge, jealousy, illness, passivity, nihilism, poverty, extrasensory perception, supernatural abilities, or victimization by cosmic waves and X rays.

2. Why is it going on? This gives the patient an opportunity to offer his explanation. He may respond by indicating they punish, harm, control, or honor him.

3. Where will it lead? This generates the patient's expectations about the delusion. Common responses are they will attack or they want to drive him crazy.
4. What is he going to do about it? This will give the patient's reaction. For instance, he will defend himself or surrender.

Bleuler (1972) and Schneider (1959) attempted to correlate the content of a delusion with specific psychiatric disorders, especially schizophrenia. Schneider described 11 so-called first-rank symptoms—7 delusions, 1 delusion combined with a kinesthetic hallucination, and 3 auditory hallucinations—that he believed to be pathognomonic for schizophrenia. However, recent research has shown that these symptoms are neither sensitive nor specific for schizophrenia. According to Mellor (1970), only 80% of schizophrenic patients show first-rank symptoms.

Especially chronic schizophrenics with negative symptoms and some acute schizophrenics are free of first-rank symptoms. In contrast, approximately 11.5% of patients with an affective disorder studied by Taylor and Abrams (1973) had Schneiderian first-rank symptoms.

Delusions are not disorder specific. Evaluate them in the context of other psychopathology such as type and age of onset, course, social deterioration, premorbid personality, and association with other mood or cognitive symptoms.

Delusions with depressive themes (Table 4–1) are seen when a depressed patient suffering from delusions is burdened by guilt feelings. Claiming he has always been wicked but that he has only recently been found out, he expects only one possible outcome: harsh and merciless punishment. He says he will plead for mercy and forgiveness or request to be punished as the only way to rid himself of guilt.

Grandiose delusions (Table 4–2) surface without much probing. Ask the patient what the immediate future holds for him and he will present thoughts flavored with messianic glow, coming wealth, power, and indestructible health.

More difficult to explore are delusions of passivity formerly thought to occur in schizophrenia (Table 4–3). Such a patient often wants to hide them from you. Table 4–3 lists Kurt Schneider's eight delusions, which have the following in common:

1. The patient feels under the influence of a strong force such as X rays, electronic surveillance, magnetic fields, or telepathy.
2. This force is overpowering; it makes him think, feel, want, and act com-

pletely out of his own control (feelings of passivity). He experiences other people's feelings and thinks other people's thoughts rather than his own.

3. The reaction to his delusion is submission; he cannot resist; he is the victim.

To induce a patient to describe some of these delusions, start with an open-ended question such as "How do you control your mind, your thoughts, your feelings, and your actions?" If the answer is evasive, become more specific and ask if anybody ever tried to tamper with his thoughts or his feelings, or control or force him to do things against his will. For instance, when you check for thought insertion:

"Is it really somebody else's thought?"

ensure that the patient is delusional and not just describing anxious feelings of derealization, where "things appear as if they are not real." The patient with a delusion of alienation does not have the "as if" experience, but is convinced of living in an unreal world without being frightened by it.

Manic patients may report that other people can read their minds, a claim also voiced by patients with schizophrenia. To make a distinction you can ask for the total delusional profile.

Table 4–1.   Delusions with depressive themes

Content	Patient's explanation	Patient's expectation	Patient's reaction
Guilt	Wickedness of own character; sinful, evil conduct	Harsh punishment	Plea for mercy, self-accusation, surrender
Poverty	Unproductivity, worthlessness, moral weakness	Stripping of all goods and rights, ridicule, expulsion from society	Submission, self-destruction, suicide
Nihilism and death	Result of deprivation and punishment	Helpless and powerless victim	Self-mutilation
Illness	Weakness and worthlessness of mind and body	Permanent disability, death	Seek help, surrender to the inevitable

Table 4–2.   Grandiose delusions

Content	Patient's explanation	Patient's expectation	Patient's reaction
Messianic abilities	Chosen, reborn, special reward for accomplishments	Future admiration, acknowledgment as leader of mankind	Preaching, helping, healing
Wealth	Deserved reward	Public praise and acknowledgment	Use wealth to abolish poverty on earth
Power and giftedness	Deserved reward	Respect	Help and lead mankind, great inventions
Indestructible health, eternal life	Special endowment and gift, chosen	Admiration	Investment in many activities

I: Danielle, what kind of thoughts did you have when you were hospitalized last?

P: I thought other people can read my mind.

I: What was the reason for that ability?

P: My thoughts were so fast, so intense, and so loud that I believed other people must hear them. I wasn't aware of the difference between saying something or just thinking it.

I: So what did you do when you had this experience?

P: I got so frustrated about other people because they did not respond to my thoughts, so I started to throw things at them.

I: How did you get back in control?

P: When I calmed down, I noticed that I had to talk in order to get a response. My thoughts became slower, I could sort them out and put them into words.

Danielle was not a passive victim of outside forces like a patient with schizophrenia would describe herself, but experienced the fast and intense thoughts typical for mania. Throwing objects was not due to hostility, as a patient with schizophrenia would report, but due to her frustration, sensing that her physical limitations constrained her self-expression.

Persecutory and grandiose delusions (Table 4–4) are seen in mood disorders, delusional disorders, schizophrenia, cognitive disorders, and substance-related disorders. Assess the complete profile of these delusions.

Besides persecution and grandiosity, another delusional theme deserves attention: jealousy. Premorbidly, such a patient may have been suspicious and preoccupied with marital infidelity. As the delusion begins to emerge,

Table 4–3. Delusions of passivity

Content	Patient's explanation	Example	Patient's reaction
Insertion of sensations (somatic passivity)	Experience of feeling a controlling force	"My boss gives me evil looks that run down my body and give me tingling sensations in my genitals."	Passive submission
Thought broadcasting	Radio waves, magnetic waves, telepathy	"My head is a radio; it transmits all my thoughts so everybody can hear them."	Lack of control; no action taken
Thought withdrawal	Magnets, a black hole, vacuum suction or evil people steal thoughts	"In the evening they turn on the big wind pump and suck all my thoughts out of my head."	Complaints and submission
Thought insertion	Outside thoughts being forced into mind by micro or radio waves	"Mr. X on TV uses my head to think with."	Passive compliance
Insertion of feelings ("made" feelings)	Outside agent projects feelings onto patient	"My dead sister transmits her anger into me. She shouts and cries, and uses my body to do that."	Patient displays feelings he is forced to feel
Insertion of impulses ("made" impulses)	Impulse manufactured by outside agent and imposed on patient	"The devil turns my head and makes me look at all men's crotches."	Submission to imposed impulse
Insertion of an outside will	Outside force pulls the strings and controls patient's actions	"The university computer sends impulses to all my muscles, makes them move, and controls my actions."	Compliance like a marionette
Delusional perception	Patient gives a delusional explanation to a real perception	"The doctor crossed his legs. Then I knew he wanted me to go home and masturbate."	Compliance with message

Table 4–4. Persecutory and grandiose delusions and their diagnostic correlates

Content	Patient's explanation	Patient's expectation	Patient's reaction	Probable diagnostic correlation
Persecution	Jealousy of persecutors	Battle and friction, but final victory	Careful guardedness, outbreak of verbal or physical attacks	Schizophrenia, delusional disorder
Persecution	Moral failure, sin	Punishment	Self-accusation, surrender to punishing authorities, plea for mercy	Major depressive disorder
Persecution	Misunderstanding of good intentions by persecutors	Acknowledgment of good intentions	Demonstration of good deeds	Mania
Persecution	Bewilderment, inability to figure out the reason for persecution	Hope for cessation of persecution	Fearful or hostile self-protection, complaints, accusations	Cognitive disorders
Grandiosity (delusion of entitlement)	Superiority, elevation above others	Spectacular victory and annihilation of opponents	Hostile and arrogant depreciation of others	Schizophrenia, irritable mania
Grandiosity	Enlightenment, self-improvement, giftedness	Effective as healer and helper	Messianic-like and forceful preaching	Mania
Grandiosity (martyrdom)	Chosen to suffer for the evil of all mankind	Punishment as a symbolic victim	Self-sacrifice	Bipolar disorder, major depressive disorder
Grandiosity (per se)	Past accomplishments, evidence, no need for explanation	Acceptance by everybody without questions	Grandiose mannerisms and claims	Cognitive disorders, general paresis

he may start to interrogate his spouse for hours, during most of the night, claiming that her vagina is moister than usual and that she looks exhausted with bags under her eyes. In the case of a female delusional patient, she may be inspecting her husband's underwear for stains of semen. This delusion is disorder-nonspecific; it may lead to both homicide and suicide (Manschreck 1989).

The bizarreness of the delusional content may have some value in the differential diagnosis of psychotic disorders. For instance, in delusional disorder, the nonbizarre delusions involving situations that could occur in real life, such as being followed, poisoned, or infected, constitute the lead symptom for this disorder. The nonbizarre delusion has to occur in the absence of any of the other psychotic symptoms listed for schizophrenia. The exception is a tactile or olfactory hallucination that may fit the nonbizarre delusional theme, such as smelling the gas that the patient believes she is being poisoned with.

Overvalued Ideas

Similar to delusions, overvalued ideas cannot be corrected by logical arguments, and sometimes they are not obviously false. They can be persistent; their importance is exaggerated. The patient realizes the emotional engagement but justifies it.

Similar to delusions, overvalued ideas center around injustice, discrimination, disappointment, betrayal, jealousy, or grandiose plans, but they are less intense. The following types of questions may elicit them:

"Is there anything going on that concerns you a great deal?"
"Have you been a victim of injustice, discrimination, or unfair treatment?"
"Do you have any important plans or goals?"
"Are you working on an invention?"
"Will you become famous one day?"

Occurring in patients with schizophrenia, mood disorders, cognitive disorders, phobias, obsessions, and personality disorders, overvalued ideas have no specific diagnostic value, but can be harbingers of a delusion.

Phobias

Phobias consist of a specific stimulus, an unreasonable and unexplained anxiety of being exposed to it, and subsequent avoidance behavior or tolerance with severe dread. In the interview it is best to focus on one aspect at a time. Specific phobic objects or situations can be assessed by questions such as:

"Is there anything you dread like: animals, sharp objects, or heights?" (to assess specific phobias)
"Do you feel comfortable talking to a crowd? Does it bother you to be watched by a group of people?" (to assess social phobias)
"Does it bother you to eat in a crowded restaurant, visit a movie theater on Friday night when it is filled to the brim? Does it bother you to wait in line with a huge crowd of people?" (to assess agoraphobia)

Exploration requires you to probe into the meaning behind the patient's words, behaviors, and presentation of facts. Since specific phobias are classified by the type of the dreaded and avoided object or situation, be specific about this aspect. Ask for excessive or unreasonable fears:

"Do you experience any excessive or unreasonable fears?"
"Do you have any anxiety that is ridiculous?"

Finally, ask for avoidance behavior:

"Is there anything you have to avoid under all circumstances?"

Explore whether panic attacks preceded the development of a phobia, which often occurs in agoraphobia. Choose the order that fits best in the flow of the interview. Find out what impact the phobias have on the patient's life. Do they choke his social activities, prevent his advancement, or take an unusual toll on his time? If DSM-IV-TR criteria for a specific phobia are met, specify the subtypes: animal, natural environment, blood-injection-injury, situational, or other (American Psychiatric Association 2000, p. 445). In patients younger than age 18, specific phobias should have persisted for at least 6 months. Besides determining the subtypes of specific phobias, the interview should assess the patient for agoraphobia, with or without panic attacks, and for social phobia.

Obsessions

Obsessions should be differentiated from repetitive, enjoyable thoughts such as sexual fantasies; from overvalued ideas and delusions that beset the patient's mind but are acceptable to him (ego-syntonic); and from depressive worries that are unwanted, but not resisted, because the patient identifies with them.

To explore obsessions is difficult because the patient feels embarrassed. Ask whether he attempts to resist, ignore, or suppress any embarrassing, silly, or time-consuming thoughts. Focus on the common content of obsessions:

"Do you have unwanted pornographic images in your mind?"
"Do you have thoughts of hurting somebody?"
"Do you have dirty thoughts or thoughts of getting contaminated or doubts about having forgotten something?"
"Do you have to have things in a particular order, like symmetrical?"

If he concurs, go on to confirm that the thoughts are intrusive, inappropriate, and resisted by the patient. Do they cause anxiety or distress?

I: Mr. N., do you often have embarrassing thoughts that pop into your mind against your will—again and again?
P: [hesitating] No, not really.
I: Or thoughts that torture you, that you can't resist—that you spend a lot of time on?
P: How do you know?
I: I'm asking you because some of my patients are bothered by intrusive thoughts.
P: Well, I'm embarrassed to tell you, even though the thoughts are not embarrassing; just that I have them, they drive me crazy.
I: Tell me about them.
P: Well, I had to quit my job last month, because I was so slow. Whenever I picked up a tool, a thought came up: Does God want me to pick up the tool? Does he want me to pick it up now? Do I do the right thing? Should I do something else instead? I know it's silly, but I have no control over these thoughts.

Compulsions

Compulsions are meaningless, repetitive acts that the patient feels compelled to perform according to self-imposed rules or obsessions. The patient uses some of the behaviors or mental acts to symbolically prevent a dreaded, distressing event. The most common compulsions are checking, cleaning, counting, demanding reassurance repeatedly, and putting things into order. Since most adult patients have insight, you can ask directly:

"Do you have to perform some acts against your will?"

If he is reluctant, embarrassed, and afraid that you will consider him "crazy," express empathy, as the interviewer did with Mr. S.

I: Have you ever felt compelled to carry out an activity, even though you knew it was nonsense?
P: [hesitates] What do you mean?
I: Some patients have the feeling they have to do things, like counting, unnecessary cleaning, or checking . . .
P: Yes, I do that sort of thing. I have to light my cigarette over and over again.
I: Can you tell me why?
P: There is no real reason. Just a nonsense, stupid thought.

I: Tell me about it.
P: It's really stupid. You must think I'm crazy.
I: Well, I understand your embarrassment. What is that stupid thought about?
P: I think about my father's death. I am afraid he is going to die. If I light the cigarette I think it brings his life back. And then I think it's nonsense. I shouldn't do it and I put the cigarette out; and then the thought comes back and I have to light the cigarette again.
I: You know it is nonsense?
P: Absolutely, there is no connection. It is ludicrous.
I: Why do you do it?
P: I couldn't live should anything happen to him and I didn't try anything to help him. It's not a big deal to light a cigarette. So I just do it.

Usually, children have no insight into their obsessions and/or compulsions. Occasionally, in adults, obsessions and compulsions take on a delusional quality, when patients start to defend their obsessive thoughts as meaningful.

Mr. Benjamin R., a 32-year-old freelance artist, at first was obsessively concerned that his heart would stop beating when he fell asleep. He considered this repetitive thought as nonsense but felt compelled to call the therapist for reassurance. Two years later he made it a habit to call his sister, a nurse, for reassurance every night. At this stage he identified fully with his concern and defended his calling as necessary and therapeutic. The thought could not be considered ego-dystonic any longer—it approached a delusion.

Medically Unexplained Somatic Symptoms

Multiple, medically unexplained somatic symptoms typify somatization disorder. Results of laboratory tests ordered to support the subjective complaints are negative. The following standardized symptom list (Othmer and Desouza 1985) helps to screen such symptoms efficiently. Ask patients for particular symptoms: shortness of breath, dysmenorrhea, burning sensation in sex organs, lump in throat, amnesia, vomiting, and paralysis. Patients with two or more of these symptoms are suspected to have somatization disorder if the symptoms have interfered with their life, are medically unexplained, and occurred prior to age 30. Somatization disorder is defined in DSM-IV-TR by pain symptoms (4), gastrointestinal symptoms (2), sexual symptoms (1), and pseudoneurological symptoms (1) (American Psychiatric Association 2000). Since patients with somatization disorder are colorful in describing their symptoms but contradictory and vague about factual information, you may have to focus on previous medical treatment and hospitalizations to support your diagnosis.

Conversion

Conversion symptoms are medically unexplained neurological symptoms such as paralysis, blindness, or deafness. Spot conversion symptoms by open-ended questions such as:

"Did you ever experience any nerve problems, for instance, with your vision—such as being blind—or with walking—such as being paralyzed?"

Go through a list (DSM-IV-TR) of common conversion symptoms. They occur under stress alone or together with multiple somatic symptoms and often result in "secondary gain," that is, external incentives (DSM-IV-TR). They can be seen in any psychiatric disorder (Othmer and Othmer 2002).

Dissociation

Dissociation "is a disruption in the usually integrated functions of consciousness, memory, identity, or perception" (American Psychiatric Association 2000, p. 519). Five dissociative disorders have to be interviewed for: dissociative amnesia, dissociative fugue, dissociative identity disorder, depersonalization disorder, and dissociative disorder not otherwise specified.

Dissociative identity disorder is relatively easy to assess, if the presenting personality is aware of other personalities (Kluft and Fine 1993). In this case, direct questions yield the answer:

"Do you switch into any other personality?"

If the presenting personality is not aware of alternating personalities, she will negate the question. In that case, you may look for evidence of lost time or memory disturbance:

"Do you have periods of memory loss?"

In addition, family or friends have often witnessed such a blackout and told the patient that she had assumed a different name, dressed differently, spoke with a different voice, and claimed to be unaware of her identity. You may approach the patient from this point of view and ask whether friends have ever told her that she sometimes presents as a different personality. By hypnosis you can often restore lost memory or induce personality switching in such a patient.

The assessment of dissociative identity disorder becomes difficult if the patient presents with hostility and symptoms that resemble psychotic experiences (Kluft 1987). If hostility is directed toward the interviewer, she should attempt to sedate the patient with a neuroleptic rather than attempt to establish rapport, and continue to interview to uncover the dissociative nature of the behavior. Switching the patient to a friendlier personality can be utilized here, provided the interviewer recognizes the dissociation. This switching technique is best used by more experienced interviewers (Othmer and Othmer 2002).

Up to 97% of patients with dissociative identity disorder have a history of child abuse, 83% a history of sexual abuse, 75% a history of physical abuse, and 68% a history of sexual and physical abuse (Putnam et al. 1986; Wilbur 1984). If the patient has talked about experiences of abuse, consider the assessment of dissociative identity disorder. The patient may acknowledge sexual abuse while hiding her dissociative tendency. Kluft reports that of 33 patients, only 5% came in self-diagnosed, 15% openly dissociated during the interview or after months or years of therapy, 40% were highly disguised, and 40% showed subtle forms of classic signs (Kluft 1984, 1985). You may recognize subtle signs of dissociation during your interview, such as fluctuations in rapport, affect, developmental level, attitudes, viewpoints, memory, and behaviors, suggesting the presence of different alternate personalities (Franklin 1990). These observations may open yet another avenue to the detection of dissociative identity disorder, which is now recognized in a variety of cultures around the world.

Paroxysmal Attacks ("Spells")

Frequently overlooked are paroxysmal phenomena. Patients do not consider them as psychiatric but as neurological, or medical symptoms. Assess paroxysmal phenomena directly:

> "Do you have any kind of spells, such as losing consciousness, falling asleep during the day, feeling weak, or dizzy, feeling your heart pound real hard, or feeling as if you were having a heart attack, a seizure, or a memory blackout?"

If the answer is yes, let the patient describe the spells, their symptom profile, duration, when and how often they occur, what triggers them, and their different types. Here is an account of the most common attacks.

Fainting (syncope): "Things start to turn and I feel dizzy and black out when I get up, or have to stand for a long time, or when I get very hot. I may have to lie down. The attack lasts from a few seconds to minutes and subsides as soon as I am in a horizontal position with legs and arms up and head down."

Narcoleptic attacks: These are sudden, irresistible sleep attacks. Patients sleep enough during the night but have several sleep attacks during the daytime. The naps last 10 to 20 minutes but can last up to 1 hour if the individual is uninterrupted. At all times, the patient can be awakened. The attacks are often spaced 90 minutes or multiples of 90 minutes apart. They may be associated with three auxiliary symptoms: 1) Cataplectic attacks: patients report sudden muscle weakness of the whole or of parts of the body such as in arm and jaw. Emotional excitement, anger, or jokes can trigger the attacks. 2) Sleep paralysis: patients wake up during the night and are paralyzed for a few minutes but are able to breathe. 3) Hypnagogic and hypnopompic hallucinations: patients report mostly visual but also auditory and kinetic hallucinations while falling asleep at night (hypnagogic hallucinations) and/or when waking up in the middle of the night or in the morning (hypnopompic hallucinations). These hallucinations incorporate elements of the actual environment. They are reported by 20%–40% of individuals with narcolepsy.

Grand mal seizures: The patient passes out and wakes up confused, weak, with headaches and often generalized muscle aches; sometimes he has injured himself, bitten his tongue, or become incontinent. Others have told him that his arms and legs contracted and relaxed rhythmically when he was passed out.

Pseudoseizures: Patients may report epileptic "seizures," but they admit that they can still hear and see what is going on around them, that they cannot talk, that their body is shaking, and their arms and legs are contracting. They rarely injure themselves, bite their tongue, become incontinent, or confused afterward. Most of these patients are suggestible—they can be induced to have pseudoseizures under hypnosis or in a clinical environment that impresses them, such as an electroencephalographic laboratory.

Complex partial or temporal lobe seizures: The patient reports that he has amnestic attacks during which he carries out certain automatic stereotyped activities such as unintelligible, inappropriate, or irrelevant verbalizations, lip smacking, chewing, swallowing, patting, rubbing a part of the body, or fumbling with parts of his clothing. At the end the patient feels confused, has partial amnesia, and is fatigued. Recovery may last up to 20 minutes before the patient can resume his usual activities.

Panic attacks: The patient reports that he often has attacks that feel like a heart attack. Reported symptoms include: palpitations, pounding heart, or accelerated heart rate; sweating; trembling or shaking; sensations of shortness of breath or smothering; feeling of choking; chest pain or discomfort; nausea or abdominal distress; feeling dizzy, unsteady, lightheaded, or faint; derealization or depersonalization; fear of losing control or going crazy; fear of dying; paresthesias; or chills or hot flushes (see DSM-IV-TR, panic attack). The attacks often start in young adulthood. Individual attacks start suddenly and are most intense within 10 minutes or less. Sometimes physical exertion may bring them on. They can occur unexpectedly without known trigger, or in conjunction with an external trigger such as being stuck in an elevator or an internal trigger such as when a patient experiences palpitations. The situationally predisposed panic attack is similar to the situationally bound panic attack (American Psychiatric Association 2000, p. 431). The diagnosis of panic disorder requires unexpected attacks.

Amnestic attacks (alcoholic blackout):   See Chapter 5, section 3.

Dissociative amnesia: See section 2. Conversation: Memory, and Chapter 5, section 3.

Depersonalization: The patient reports that after experiencing severe stress she often feels not herself, as if she were in a movie or out of her body. She has, however, full insight.

Derealization: The patient reports that the world around her appears unreal and strange. Objects appear larger (macropsia) or smaller (micropsia), and people appear unfamiliar or mechanical. The patient has full insight.

Dissociative fugue: The patient travels unexpectedly away from home or work, assumes a new identity, or is confused about his personal identity. Perplexity and disorientation may occur even though usually there is no evidence of substance use, a cognitive disorder, or a general medical condition. After recovery the patient does not remember what took place during the fugue.

Dissociative switching: The patient suddenly changes tone of voice, facial expression, and psychomotor behavior. Such a switch can occur apparently spontaneously in a patient with dissociative identity disorder; however, the switch may be due to a trigger that escapes the interviewer. A dissociative switch can be induced by the interviewer after having become familiar with some of the patient's identities.

Hypoglycemic attack: A patient reports that he often feels sweaty, tremulous, and hungry 1 to 2 hours after a meal.

Transient global amnesia: The patient reports that he lost memory for nearly an entire day. He had no preceding conflicts; hypnotic sessions cannot recover the lost memory. These attacks occur sporadically in patients over the age of 60 and may be due to circulatory insufficiency of brain structures involved in memory recall, such as the hippocampus.

Transient ischemic attacks (TIAs):   The patient reports a focal neurological deficit which lasts less than 15 minutes such as blindness in one eye, paresis in one arm or leg. These attacks occur in patients with cerebral vascular disease.

If a patient describes one type of "spell," ask her immediately whether this is the only type of spell she has, or if she has several different ones. For instance, a patient suffering from true grand mal seizures may use her attacks as external incentives, and also fake them. A mental health professional who witnesses such malingering may come to the conclusion that the patient does not have true grand mal seizures and may discontinue the seizure medication. Patients suffering from panic attacks are often able to distinguish between attacks that surprise them and those that are anticipated. Therefore it is necessary to invite patients to describe their different spells.

Executive Functioning

Beginning dementia may first affect the highest, most complex and integrated cognitive functions. The authors of DSM-IV-TR have summarized these functions under the term *executive functioning*. They include planning, organizing, sequencing, and abstracting. You can assess executive functioning following either an inductive or a deductive approach.

The inductive approach focuses on basic cognitive functions on which effective executive functioning is based. These basic functions include attention, concentration, shifting sets, and memory. On a more complex level, they comprise abstracting, problem solving, and dimensions of intelligence.

This inductive approach will be demonstrated in Chapter 5: Testing.

The deductive approach targets the most complex functions directly as they become evident in the patient's daily life. Search for evidence of a decline of the patient's intellectual effectiveness by asking specific questions about his daily life rather than utilizing quantifying tests. You may assess planning by asking whether the patient can make and keep a schedule, make and keep a budget, and whether he uses his time wisely. Assess sequencing by asking him to prioritize his daily tasks at work or at home. You may get an impression about his ability to abstract by discussing with him the principles on which he bases his priorities.

A practical way to discuss these functions, especially organizing, is to ask the patient to describe his activities during the last day, week, month and year. Such a task requires intact recent memory. Then discuss with him alternative ways to accomplish the goals that he had pursued during these time periods. Such reflection requires abstracting, reasoning, and decision making. Thus you can spot deficits in executive functioning with this screening method. The analysis of these deficits will direct you toward testing of the underlying basic cognitive functions that may have declined (Royall et al. 1992). Use the Executive Interview (EXIT) and the Qualitative Evaluation of Dementia (QED) for testing (see Chapter 5: Testing and Appendix).

Insight

Get a feeling for your patient's insight into his symptoms right from the outset of the interview (see Chapter 2). Monitor insight whenever new symptoms or problems surface by probing:

> "What do you think about . . . ?"
> "Do you consider this normal for you?"
> "Do you need help for it?"

If he responds with:

> "That's what I'm here for!"

he demonstrates at least some insight. Then counterprobe:

> "What are your strengths?"

This double-barreled approach helps the patient to recognize the border between intact and disordered functions. If he defends his symptoms as reality-based, he has limited insight. As we have mentioned before, patients rarely have insight into persistent, current, non-substance-induced hallucinations and delusions. The reason is simple: insight is based on a cognitive awareness of consensual reality, and this process is disturbed in the delusional hallucinatory state. If a patient hallucinates or displays delusional thinking, the pathological process affects the very function necessary to recognize disordered perception and thinking as disturbed. This lack of insight is called *anosognosia.*

Patients can identify disordered emotions more easily than disturbed cognition. This is true for depressed and schizophrenic patients. The manic patient is more capable of recognizing his behaviors—such as spending sprees, overtalkativeness, or indiscriminate sexual affairs—as disturbed than his persistent feelings of euphoria or irritability. He experiences anxious and depressive moods earlier as disordered rather than elated moods.

Obsessions, compulsions, phobic avoidances, and substance abuse rarely occur without the patient's insight into their pathological nature. With the exception of some of the substance abusers, such a patient has little problem in identifying them as disturbances. He has, however, a problem in controlling or changing them.

Judgment

Judgment is the ability to choose appropriate goals, and to select socially acceptable and appropriate means to reach them. It reflects reality testing, intelligence, and experience. Since judgment requires an integration of outside reality, internal needs, and living skills, it is a sensitive indicator of disturbed mental functions.

Interviewers often evaluate judgment by exploring general knowledge and problem-solving abilities. Clinicians ask, for instance:

"Why do rivers flow into the oceans?"
"Why do the stars come out at night?"
"Why does the government collect taxes?"

The answers demonstrate some aspects of social intelligence but fail to address the gist of judgment.

Questions that require the patient to verbalize his view of his own potential and limits in a social context help to elicit his judgment. You might ask about his future plans:

"How does the future look to you?"
"What are your chances of making a new start in life?"
"Do you think you can create a major invention?"
"Is there any chance that you may become famous?"
"What is the likelihood that you will become a leader of some kind?"

These questions invite the patient to make connections between his present state and his future. They explore the self-perception of his own abilities and assess his estimate of the risks involved in certain actions and how much risk he is willing to take. Here are typical answers from various types of patients to these questions:

A patient with a cognitive disorder describes highly unrealistic plans for his future, selects inappropriate and illogical means to achieve them, and shows disregard for his lack of ability, experience, or track record to reach them.

A patient with schizophrenia often answers a judgment question completely inappropriately, displaying a bizarre delusion. He may say:

"I will stop the battles of stars."
"I will insulate my bedroom so that the X rays from the big machine can't penetrate my body."

A patient with a mood disorder gives divergent answers depending on whether he is depressed or manic. When depressed, he underestimates his abilities, is pessimistic about the outcome of his actions, overestimates risks, and abhors taking them. His future looks bleak, with no possibility of growth or success. When manic, no goal is too high to achieve; he perceives his abilities as unlimited, risks are negligible, and his willingness to take them is high. His future glows in bright colors. Mishaps are quickly forgotten, and even without completion of the tasks, happiness is assured.

An anxious patient recognizes his abilities but overestimates the risks and shies away from taking them. He views his future with guardedness; he expects obstacles and controversies everywhere and does not expect satisfaction.

You can gauge your patient's judgment by comparing it to his past accomplishments. If his goals are in line with his track record, lie within his capabilities and control, the better his judgment; the greater the discrepancy, the poorer the judgment.

Since symptoms of most psychiatric disorders affect judgment, it is best to systematically and intensively assess your patient's judgment in each case. It will improve your psychodiagnostic evaluation. Even mild symptoms can have a profound impact on judgment. When a patient changes his job, location, spouse, career goals, business partners, or investment strategies, evaluate whether such a change reflects an impairment in judgment triggered by a mood, anxiety, or substance-related disorder.

CHECKLIST

Chapter 4: Mental Status Examination

This checklist is designed to give even the perfectionist interviewer guilt feelings about the completeness of his mental status examination. What have you forgotten? To receive the full benefit of the guilt trip, answer each question for those patients that you interviewed without being able to make a diagnosis. Mark the nonassessed items in red. Look up in the glossary any unfamiliar terms.

Fill in the appropriate numbers.

1. The patient's willingness to cooperate allowed me to use the
    following assessment methods (list up to four; also compare
    Chapter 5: Testing):
    1 = observation
    2 = conversation
    3 = exploration
    4 = testing   ____ ____ ____ ____

OBSERVATION

Appearance
2. The following characteristics of the patient's appearance were of
    diagnostic interest (list up to three):
    1 = none
    2 = race
    3 = difference in appearance of age vs. stated age
    4 = nutrition
    5 = body type
    6 = hygiene
    7 = dress
    8 = eye contact   ____ ____ ____

Consciousness
3. The patient's level of consciousness indicated:
    1 = alertness
    2 = lethargy
    3 = sleepiness
    4 = stupor
    5 = coma   _____

Psychomotor behavior
4. The following functions were of diagnostic importance
    (list up to three):
    1 = none
    2 = posture
    3 = expressive movements
    4 = reactive movements
    5 = grooming
    6 = symbolic gestures
    7 = goal-directed movements   _____ _____ _____

5. The following abnormal movements were observable:
    1 = none
    2 = tremors
    3 = athetotic movements
    4 = choreatic movements
    5 = catatonic stupor
    6 = tics   _____ _____ _____

CONVERSATION

Attention and concentration
6. During the interview the patient appeared:
    1 = attentive
    2 = distractible
    3 = apathic   _____

Speech

7. The patient had the following problems with speech
    (list up to three):
    1 = none
    2 = disturbed articulation
    3 = dysprosody
    4 = nonfluency
    5 = pressure of speech
    6 = circumscriptions
    7 = paraphasic language
    8 = neologistic language
    9 = faulty grammar   ____   ____   ____

Thinking

8. The patient had the following thought disturbances
    (list up to three):
    1 = none
    2 = concrete word use
    3 = overinclusive word use
    4 = circumstantiality
    5 = tangentiality
    6 = perseveration
    7 = palilalia
    8 = clang association
    9 = blocking and derailment
    10 = flight of ideas
    11 = non sequitur
    12 = fragmentation
    13 = rambling
    14 = driveling
    15 = word salad   ____   ____   ____

Orientation

9. The patient showed the following types of disorientation
    (list all if present):
    1 = none
    2 = to person
    3 = to day of the week
    4 = to day of the month
    5 = to time of the day

6 = to month
7 = to year
· 8 = to season
9 = to place   ____ ____ ____

Memory during conversation (also compare Chapter 5: Testing)
10. The patient gave the following evidence of immediate recall,
    short-term, long-term, and remote memory:
    1 = repeat your name (or gray, watch, daisy, justice)
    2 = immediately recall the spelling of your name (or four words)
    3 = recall your name (or four words) during the course of
        the interview
    4 = recall events of last 24 hours
    5 = discuss verifiable remote events   ____ ____ ____

Affect
11. Which of the following affects predominated in your patient
    during the interview?
    1 = sadness
    2 = elation
    3 = disgust
    4 = anxiety
    5 = anger
    6 = perplexity
    7 = guilt
    8 = suspicion
    9 = content   ____

12. Which of the nine affects were missing? Use the key
    from question 11.   ____ ____ ____ ____ ____

13. The patient's affect was mostly expressed in:
    1 = gestures
    2 = facial expressions
    3 = posture
    4 = grooming
    5 = reactive movements
    6 = goal-directed movements
    7 = tone of voice
    8 = pitch of voice
    9 = selection of vocabulary
    (Limit of three ranked by importance)   ____ ____ ____

14. The patient regulated his affect predominantly by:
    1 = suppression
    2 = appropriate control
    3 = acting out
    4 = faking
    5 = none of the above   _____

15. How did you judge the intensity of your patient's affect?:
    1 = high
    2 = medium
    3 = low   _____

16. The range of the patient's affective display was:
    1 = narrow
    2 = medium
    3 = wide   _____

EXPLORATION

Mood
17. Name the terms that the patient used to describe the quality of his mood.

    _____

18. How stable was the patient's mood over the past 24 hours? If there were changes in mood, list the type and how they occurred.

    _____

19. How reactive is your patient to good news? Describe at least one good event and the patient's reaction to it.

    _____

20. Give examples that demonstrate the intensity of the patient's mood.

    _____

21. Describe if the patient's predominant mood changed in the past 4 weeks and how long it lasted.

    _____

Energy
22. Describe how energetic your patient is.

    _____

23. Is he organized in his planning?   YES   NO

24. Is it easy for him to get started?   YES   NO

25. Does he procrastinate?   YES   NO

26. Is he persistent in pursuing his goals?   YES   NO

27. Does he complete the tasks?   YES   NO

Perception
28. In case the patient ever had hallucinations, describe their content.

_____

29. Determine the patient's stage of insight (I–V) into the hallucination.

Content of thinking
30. In case the patient ever had delusions, describe their content.

_____

31. Determine the patient's stage of insight (I–V) for the delusion.

32. Classify the patient's delusion according to its content
    as predominantly:
    1 = manic
    2 = depressive
    3 = schizophrenic
    4 = nonspecific   _____

33. Describe the patient's overvalued ideas, if any.

_____

34. Describe the content of the patient's phobias.

_____

35. List the patient's obsessive ideas, if any.

_____

36. List his compulsions, if any.

_____

Medically unexplained somatic symptoms

37. Indicate which of the seven symptoms of the rapid screening test for somatization disorder are present:

    1 = shortness of breath
    2 = dysmenorrhea
    3 = burning sensation in sex organs
    4 = lump in throat
    5 = amnesia
    6 = vomiting
    7 = pain in extremities   ____   ____   ____   ____   ____

38. In the answer to question 37, circle those symptoms that fulfill both onset before age 30 and lack of medical explanation.

Conversion symptoms

39. List them, if any.

_____

Dissociative identity

40. Describe whether your patient ever had amnestic periods in which he assumed another identity.

_____

Paroxysmal attacks

41. List your patient's paroxysmal attacks, if any:

    1 = fainting
    2 = narcoleptic attacks
    3 = grand mal seizures
    4 = pseudoseizures
    5 = complex partial seizures
    6 = panic attacks
    7 = alcoholic blackouts
    8 = psychogenic amnesia
    9 = fugue state
    10 = hypoglycemic attacks
    11 = transient global amnesia
    12 = transient ischemic attacks
    13 = Tourette's tics   ____   ____   ____   ____   ____

Insight

42. Classify the patient's insight into his disorder:

    1 = he recognizes symptoms as part of a disorder
    2 = he recognizes symptoms but provides a rational explanation
    3 = he denies that his symptoms are expressions of a disorder   ____

Judgment

43. Describe your patient's future plans. Are they realistic?

_____

CHAPTER FIVE

TESTING

1. Level of Consciousness: Lethargy, Stupor, and Coma
2. Attention and Vigilance: Distractibility and Perseveration
3. Memory: Amnesia and Inability to Learn
4. Orientation: Confusion
5. Language: Aphasia
6. Knowing: Agnosia
7. Performing: Apraxia
8. Pathological Reflexes and Movements
9. Range of Affect
10. Suggestibility: Dissociation
11. Abstract Thinking: Concreteness
12. Intelligence: Dementia, Mental Retardation
13. Serial Testing of Selected Psychological States

SUMMARY

Chapter 5 describes mental functions and psychological states altered in some Axis I psychiatric disorders. It localizes these mental functions in the brain and proposes brief, bedside mental function tests and common scales for the serial measurement of psychological states.

▲ ▲ ▲ ▲ ▲

Few things are impossible to diligence and skill.

—Samuel Johnson (1709–1784), *Rasselas,*
Chap. XII (1759)

▼ ▼ ▼ ▼ ▼

In each mental status examination you perform, you pay homage to the history of three disciplines: psychiatry, psychology, and neurology. The founding fathers of psychiatry were neurologists who diagnosed and treated both neurological and psychiatric disorders. They introduced the mental status examination. Since then the schism between psychiatry and neurology has widened, and this is reflected in today's mental status examination. The mental status examination conducted by neurologists differs from the mental status examination conducted by psychiatrists, psychologists, and social workers, and the difference reflects the different patient populations with which these groups work.

Neurologists mostly deal with patients who suffer from gross structural, predominantly focal lesions to the brain such as cerebral vascular accidents (strokes), tumors, and injuries. Thus the neurological mental status examination focuses on anatomical areas such as the lobes (frontal, parietal, occipital), right versus left hemisphere, and the cerebellum. In their mental status examination, neurologists therefore concentrate on particular areas, namely shifting sets, apraxia typical for disturbances in the frontal lobe, aphasias and agnosias, and constructional deficits typical for disturbances in the parietal, occipital, and temporal lobes.

Psychologists and psychiatrists deal predominantly with patients who suffer from nonstructural impairment of brain functions such as in mood, anxiety, dissociative, and personality disorders, to name just a few. Standardized evaluation of affective response, obsessiveness, hypnotizability, defense mechanisms, and transference patterns seen during the interview may be included in the customary mental status examination if indicated. In addition, the neuropsychological mental status examination includes several standardized office tests that can be used to systematically evaluate patients for the subtle onset of cognitive disorders. Patients who suffer from three known general conditions are usually tested with respect to neuropsychological functioning:

1. slowly developing dementias due to Alzheimer's disease and vascular dementias;
2. substance-related disorders such as intoxication, withdrawal, deliria, and persisting damage that may be responsible for amnestic states and persisting substance-induced dementia;
3. general medical conditions that lead to an acute disturbance causing a delirium or general medical conditions that lead to a chronic disturbance causing a dementia, such as HIV disease, head trauma, Parkinson's disease, Huntington's disease, Pick's disease, Creutzfeldt-Jakob disease, and others (e.g., Lewy body disease and frontotemporal dementia).

Psychologists have been heavily influenced by neurophysiology with its emphasis on the measurement of psychological and cognitive functions. They prefer standardized, reliable, and valid quantitative measurements of a client's current level of functioning over the qualitative mental status exam of psychiatrists. By virtue of their training, psychologists have developed a high degree of sensitivity to the selection of appropriate tests to quantify their clients' strengths and weaknesses. In contrast, clinical psychiatrists use a categorical approach in their diagnosis that includes relatively brief assessments of concentration, memory, orientation, and other cognitive functions.

This chapter describes tests from all three disciplines. It includes the contributions from the neurological mental status examination, including how to evaluate lobe functions—especially agnosia, apraxia, and aphasia. It includes quantitative assessments for the expression of affect and hypnotizability. Furthermore, it addresses a growing number of standardized, reliable, and valid rating scales to measure depression, mania, panic, anxiety, psychosis, intelligence, and cognitive functions, among others (van Riezen and Segal 1988).

Standardized rating scales are routinely demanded by the Food and Drug Administration (FDA) to document the comparative efficacy of old and new psychotropic drugs. They are the standard for documenting the clinical change in psychiatric disorders.

What Do Tests Do?

A test in the mental health field measures mental functions. Most readers are aware of available tests and how to use them. Testing helps to establish and confirm psychiatric diagnoses. Testing requires the patient's cooperation. Hostile or paranoid patients may refuse. Such a refusal is as diagnostic as a test score.

Any testing has two characteristics: First, it allows you to examine a suspected impairment in a standardized way. Second, it provides you with quantified information about the impairment at a certain point in the patient's history, and can therefore serve as a baseline and measurement of change. It allows you to document improvement, maintenance of status quo, or deterioration.

As we have mentioned, tests differ in their purpose. Neurological testing identifies deficits of higher functions due to brain lesions by showing failure in a circumscribed task. Psychiatric and psychological testing often measures functional disturbances quantitatively by comparing test scores with age-adjusted standards, for example the Wechsler Adult Intelligence Scale (WAIS; Wechsler 1981).

Whom Do You Test?

Tests are used selectively; not every patient gets tested for everything. If a patient functions socially and professionally, presents a reliable history, answers questions in a detailed manner, and behaves appropriately in the interview situation, we assume that attention, comprehension and expression of language, psychomotor behavior, orientation, memory and intelligence, and abstraction are grossly intact. Often in this situation, a psychiatrist will forgo any mental status testing.

Testing is usually done when exploration either fails to establish the patient's level of functioning or reveals impairment. If outside confirmation supports the patient's ability to exercise his executive functions—planning, organizing, sequencing, and abstracting—in a goal-directed and efficient manner, testing may be shortened. However, in most cases a patient consults you for some behavioral problems that affect his social and executive functions, even if he is not suffering from beginning dementia. Therefore, the formal testing of three cognitive functions—orientation, memory, and intelligence—is a core assessment. The assessment of these three core functions is also demanded by third-party payors, such as Medicare (HCFA 1989).

The reason why these tests are often omitted in highly functioning psychiatric patients is twofold:

1. the professional is embarrassed to ask for orientation and memory;
2. she is unfamiliar with a quick, quantitative assessment of intelligence.

This chapter will help to overcome these obstacles to testing.

When Do You Test?

There are two basic times when testing can be done:

1. When a dysfunction first emerges in the interview, as the following example illustrates:

   "You are telling me that you have difficulties with your memory. I would like to examine that problem further. Would you mind if we conduct a short test, so I can get a better feeling for your problems?"

2. At the end of the interview, when it does not interrupt the flow of interviewing. At this point, you may say:

"You have given me an idea about your problems. I wonder whether your problems have ever affected your ability to keep track of time, or whether they interfered with your memory or your ability to solve everyday problems."

Even if the patient says,

"I don't think so,"

you may then say:

"Would you mind if I asked you a few standard questions to document your level of functioning?"

In most cases, the patient will agree. If the patient showed or complained about some difficulties during the interview but you had decided not to test this problem at that time, you may say, for instance:

"You told me you have problems with attention. Would you mind if we test this briefly now?"

How Do You Test?

Before you start, explain to your patient what you test for and why testing is important. Test higher functions—for economical reasons—in a reversed hierarchy from complex to simple (Ludwig 1985; Strub and Black 1993). Complex functions are impaired first; disturbance of lower functions indicates increasing severity. For example, you first examine problem solving and abstraction, and if you detect gross difficulties, you test for memory and orientation. If you find difficulties there, you may want to check attention, vigilance, concentration, and shifting of sets.

In the following layout, we will start with the more basic mental functions first and progress to the complex ones. This approach is usually followed by other authors (Strub and Black 1993; Taylor 1993; Weintraub and Mesulam 1985).

Here is the hierarchy from simple to complex:

1. Level of consciousness: lethargy, stupor, and coma
2. Attention and vigilance: distractibility and perseveration
3. Memory: amnesia and inability to learn
4. Orientation: confusion

5. Language: aphasia
6. Knowing: agnosia
7. Performing: apraxia
8. Pathological reflexes and movements
9. Range of affect
10. Suggestibility: dissociation
11. Abstract thinking: concreteness
12. Intelligence: dementia, mental retardation
13. Serial testing of selected psychological states

1. LEVEL OF CONSCIOUSNESS: LETHARGY, STUPOR, AND COMA

Consciousness refers to the ability to recognize and respond to stimuli. The ascending activating system of the reticular formation of the brain stem and its diffuse projection to the thalamus and the cortex propel the stimuli. The firing rate of the system determines the level of arousal, scored as alert, lethargic, obtundated, stuporous, or comatose. Testing of consciousness is simple (see Chapter 4, section 1: Observation). When you address the lethargic patient with a loud voice, she responds. Her thinking is diffuse and not goal-directed, her movements are decreased, and her awareness limited. Lethargy may occur in deliria due to substance intoxication, medical (metabolic) disturbances, multiple etiology, or NOS disorders.

Stuporous patients barely respond even to persistent and vigorous stimulation, perhaps only by groaning or showing restlessness. Special forms are akinetic mutism and Gjessing's periodic catatonia (see Glossary). The obtundated patient ranks between lethargy and stupor. The comatose patient is unresponsive even if you pinch her. If consciousness is impaired, as in the intoxicated, sedated, or sleep-deprived person, all other higher functions will be affected proportionately.

Psychogenic stupor is the combination of two symptoms of catatonia: motoric immobility and mutism (American Psychiatric Association 2000, p. 316). It is a state of nonresponsiveness in which the patient is alert and can remember what happened during this state. The patient may resist eye opening. Eye closing will not be slow and sluggish as seen in a true comatose state. Cold water applied to the ear channel (caloric test) produces—unlike in true coma—nystagmus. Furthermore, the electroencephalogram (EEG) is normal (Edward and Simon 1992). Psychogenic stupor in a panic state may paralyze the patient with fear. Psychogenic stupor in somatization disorder without incontinence of urine may indicate an avoidance of an un-pleasant situation.

Psychogenic stupor may characterize special forms of bipolar disorder called confusional and motility psychoses (Leonhard 1979). Such stupor affects mainly the reactive and expressive movements and to a lesser extent the goal-directed ones. Incontinence is rare. Pathologically induced movements are absent. A similar stupor can be seen with extreme psychomotor retardation in depression. Some psychogenic stupor is associated with an increase in muscle tone, catalepsy, stereotypies, "deadpan" facial expression, and incontinence of urine.

The increase in muscle tone can lead to an odd facial expression, the so-called *Schnauzkrampf,* where the mouth is protruded due to the increased tension of the oral muscles. When these patients lie down, their head is raised an inch above the pillow because their sternomastoid muscles contract. This has been termed the "psychological pillow." Patients interviewed after such a so-called catatonic stupor may describe the ordeal as a bad dream and report hallucinations and delusions. They usually admit that they could hear the ward personnel or visiting family members talking, and they remember how they were treated. One patient was asked why he did not answer any questions while motionless. He replied,

"because I was in a different dimension."

2. ATTENTION AND VIGILANCE: DISTRACTIBILITY AND PERSEVERATION

Attention is the ability of an alert patient to focus on an outside stimulus. The reticular ascending activating system together with frontal lobe functions are responsible for this ability. Test attention by having the patient repeat up to seven digits, forward and backward, presented to him at one-second intervals (Digit Span Test; Weintraub and Mesulam 1985). The lower level of normal performance is five digits forward and four backward. Failure to meet this standard is called inattention or distractibility. Patients with amnestic disorder perform within normal range.

Vigilance (concentration) refers to sustained attention to stream of stimuli. To test vigilance use the Continuance Performance Test (Rosvold et al. 1956). Ask the patient to tap on the table whenever he hears an A among a series of spoken random letters such as K, D, A, M, T, X, T, A, F, O, K, L, E, N, A, X, D. The number of errors (omission and commission) shows his ability to sustain attention. If he taps after each letter he shows perseveration. The norm equals 90% correct responses during a 10-minute exposure; 80% if complex response is required, that is, tap on A only if A is followed by X.

Low scores on these tests may give you evidence of attention deficit as seen in several psychiatric disorders, such as attention-deficit/hyperactivity disorder, predominantly inattentive type, which often persists into adulthood, even if partial remission of other preexisting symptoms of hyperactivity has occurred (American Psychiatric Association 2000, p. 90).

Perseverance and Impersistence

Perseverance is the ability to sustain a behavior over a long period of time; this is another measure of concentration. Generating lists of three words that start with the letters F, A, and S, respectively, over a 60-second interval has been standardized (Spreen and Benton 1969). Normal high school graduates respond with an average of 36 words over 3 minutes, that is, with 12 words per list. Serial-7 or serial-3 backwards test perseverance and mathematical abilities as well as other functions (Smith 1967, 1975).

Ask the patient to subtract 7 from 100 and repeat the subtraction from each remainder ($100 - 7 = 93 - 7 = 86 - 7 = 79$, etc.). Have patients with an IQ below 80 subtract 3 serially from 30. Record time and number of errors; standards are not available, however, to our knowledge. Attention and vigilance can be assessed in combination by asking the patient to name all the months in reverse order, or to spell words backwards. The inability to do so shows inattention or impersistence.

Motor perseverance can be tested by asking the patient, for instance, to keep his eyes closed, to keep his tongue protruded, or to maintain a lateral gaze. The inability to persevere is called motor impersistence. Patients with frontal lobe damage show such impersistence (Ben-Yishay et al. 1968).

The ability to switch from one behavior to another, called *set shifting*, is measured by visual, auditory, and tactile stimuli. Failure to shift is called perseveration. Examples follow.

Visual: The patient is asked to copy a given pattern, as shown in Figure 5–1.

The patient with visual perseveration cannot continuously shift back and forth between a rounded and a pointed design. He starts the perseveration on the rounded design (upper portion of figure). The same patient is also unable to juxtapose loops; he breaks off the pattern after two loops.

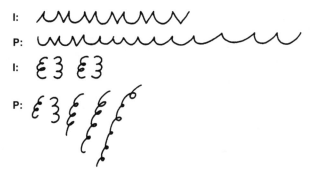

Figure 5–1. Perseveration.

Instead, after his first acceptable try he continues the loops in one direction only and also increases the number of loops.

> *Auditory:* The patient is asked to count the letters of the alphabet A1, B2, and so on. Educated and intelligent patients are asked to count by 3: A3, B6, C9, and so forth. The patient with auditory perseveration may manage initially to pair consecutive letters of the alphabet with consecutive numbers but after D4, for instance, he perseverates on 4.

I: A1 B2 C3 D4 . . .
P: A1 B2 C3 D4 E4 F4 G4

Patients with impairment in the reticular activating system, the limbic, or frontal lobe, fail tests of attention and vigilance, as in delirium, attention-deficit/hyperactivity disorder, severe mania, depression, and intoxication with sedatives. Patients with frontal lobe damage may especially fail tests for set shifting. For more extensive testing use the Halstead-Reitan Battery (Reitan and Wolfson 1985) or Luria's Neuropsychological Investigation (Luria 1966; Golden et al. 1991).

3. MEMORY: AMNESIA AND INABILITY TO LEARN

Differentiate immediate, short-term, long-term, recent, and remote memory.

Test *immediate* memory (recall after 5–10 seconds) by repetition of letters, numbers (see section 2: Attention above), or four unrelated words (brown, honesty, tulip, and eyedropper) (Strub and Black 1993). Immediate

memory requires receiving, registration, acquisition, and reproduction involving the reticular activating system, frontal lobe, limbic system, and central speech area (see Chapter 4, section 2: Conversation, Speech).

You can test visual immediate memory, which is regulated mostly by
the nondominant temporal lobe, by having the patient copy abstract
drawings (Fig. 5–2). The following instructions (Strub and Black 1993)
are useful:

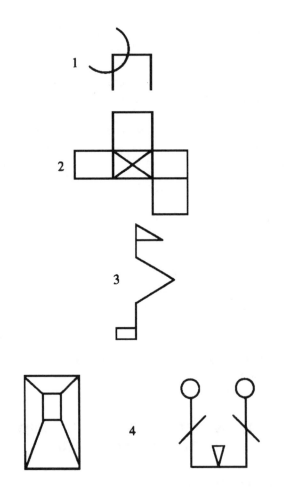

Figure 5–2.   Test items for visual design reproduction test. Reprinted from Strub
RL and Black FW: *The Mental Status Examination in Neurology*, 3rd Edition.
Philadelphia, F.A. Davis, 1993. Reprinted with permission.

"I am now going to show you some simple drawings. I want you to look at each drawing as I show it to you. Be sure to look at it carefully so that you can draw what you have seen from memory. Do not draw the design until I have told you to begin."

After you have said this, hold the first design for 5 seconds in front of the patient. After withdrawing the design wait 5 seconds, then tell him to draw the picture.

Scoring: Score each design on a four-point scale with values from 0 to 3:

0 = Poor: Given for a failure to recall and reproduce the design.
1 = Fair: Recognizable, but distorted, rotated, partially omitted, or confabulated designs.
2 = Good: Easily recognizable with minor errors of integration, omission, or addition.
3 = Excellent: Perfect (or near perfect) reproductions.

The average patient reproduces all designs with a score of 2 or 3. Low scores indicate a deficit in immediate visual memory (Strub and Black 1993).

Short-term memory is the ability to recall information after 5–10 minutes, usually tested after distraction between presentation and recall. Test visual short-term memory by having the patient repeat the figure drawings (Fig. 5–2) 5 to 10 minutes after exposure. Test short-term auditory memory by asking the patient to repeat four words—**brown, honesty, tulip, eyedropper**—and recall them after 10 minutes. Norm equals 3–4 words for normal adults before age 60 (Strub and Black 1993). Patients with stage I dementia of the Alzheimer type remember on average 1.9 words.

You can test complex auditory memory by testing the recall of a story. There are many such stories; we like the butcher story (source unknown). Instruct the patient to pay attention to the following short story, because he will have to repeat it in detail and discuss it. Then slowly read the following:

    1   2   3
On December 18/ 1 week/ before Christmas/
    4   5   6
Giovanni Scapini/ a 51-year-old/ married/
    7   8   9
butcher/ of Italian descent/ from Columbia/
    10   11   12   13
Missouri/ was cutting meat/ in back/ of his/

14   15   16
shop. While working he/ accidentally/
     17   18   19   20
cut off his/ left/ hand./ He got so mad/
     21   22   23
that he picked up/ the cleaver/ and cut off/
     24
his right hand too./

By clinical judgment, the patient should recall at least 12 of the 24 elements and grasp the story's illogical nature; compare the vacation story by Strub and Black (1993, p. 82), which contains 26 elements. In their experience, adults below age 70 can recall 10 elements; age 71–80, 8.2 elements; and age 81–90, 7.6 elements.

To test *long-term* memory (recall after 30 minutes to days) have the patient reconstruct the interview with him, or have him recall the four words, or the butcher story, after 30 minutes. Patients who fail on short-term memory tests usually fail the same test again when asked at a later interval, as shown for patients with alcoholic blackout (Goodwin et al. 1970).

Clinicians often combine short-term and long-term memory as recent memory and distinguish it from remote memory. Recent memory assures everyday functioning and learning. Test it, for instance, by having an inpatient describe his last breakfast, lunch, and dinner and verify it with the staff. Table 5–1 summarizes the memory tests that have been described.

Recent memory depends on registration (cortex), consolidation (hippocampus), storage (convexity of cortical temporal lobe), and retrieval (hippocampus, and both dorsal medial nuclei and pulvinar of the thalamus). Involvement of other structures in memory functions is discussed in the literature, such as the fornix, amygdala, and mammillary bodies, but a generally accepted model of memory has not yet been constructed (Young and McGlone 1992). The dominant temporal lobe regulates verbal learning, the nondominant temporal lobe visual learning.

The symptoms of recent memory disturbance are anterograde amnesia (inability to learn new material) and confabulation (willingness to fill gaps with made-up stories).

The following disorders interfere with recent memory:

1. Alcohol-induced persisting amnestic disorder (Korsakoff syndrome); alcohol depletes vitamin B_1 (thiamine), which damages the mammillary bodies and the dorsal medial nuclei of the thalamus.

2. Head injury with concussion temporarily interrupts hippocampal functions. The anterograde amnestic (disturbed storage) period persists, but the associated retrograde amnesia (disturbed retrieval) shrinks with recovery.
3. Transient global amnesia occurs when the posterior cerebral arteries obstruct the supply to the memory center of the medial temporal lobes.

Isolated disturbances occur in which memory retrieval, but not storage, is affected. Impairment of retrieval can be tested by examining recognition. If a patient cannot recall any of the four words after 10 minutes, give him a multiple choice that includes one of the words in question. For instance, if he misses **tulip, eyedropper,** and **honesty** and remembers only **brown,** ask him:

"Was one of the words watch, stone, **tulip,** or pencil?"

Table 5–1. Dimensions of memory

Time span	Immediate (seconds)	Recent (minutes–months)	Remote (years)
Memory process	Registration	Consolidation	Storage
Localization	Central cortical language center	Hippocampus Pulvinar Medial dorsal nuclei of thalamus	Association cortex
Tests	Repeat: 4–7 numbers forward 4 backward 4 objects Abstract pictures Story	Immediate memory tests Repeat after 10 min Describe last meals	Facts about verifiable past
Types of amnesia	Inattention Central aphasias	Anterograde: Impaired new learning	Retrograde
Disorders			
Fugue	Intact	Intact/Impaired*	Intact/Impaired*
Amnestic	Intact	Impaired	Intact
Early Alzheimer	Impaired	Impaired	Intact
Late Alzheimer	Impaired	Impaired	Impaired

*Depends on how long the fugue lasted and when the patient with the fugue was interviewed.

If he can identify **tulip** he can store but not retrieve. Retrieval is impaired in normal forgetfulness, and in retrograde amnesia.

Test *remote* memory (recall after months or years) by having the patient talk about historical events, such as World War II, the Korean or Vietnam wars, the last six United States presidents, or verifiable personal events, such as date of birth, marriage, or military discharge. Remote memory is regulated by the appropriate association cortex, but not the hippocampus, mammillary bodies, and the dorsal medial nuclei of the thalamus. Therefore, patients with substance-induced persisting amnestic disorder (such as Korsakoff syndrome) or early dementia of the Alzheimer's type still have intact remote memory, whereas in advanced Alzheimer's and Pick's disease and other frontotemporal dementia, remote memory becomes impaired due to cortical atrophy. Progressive dementias associated with abnormal movements, such as Parkinson's disease, Huntington's disease, and Creutzfeldt-Jakob disease, may interfere with remote memory at some stage.

Besides cognitive disorders, other psychiatric disorders—such as severe anxiety disorders, mood disorders with psychomotor retardation, agitation, or severe distractibility—can interfere with memory functions due to a lack of attention.

In dissociative disorders, such as dissociative fugue, dissociative amnesia, or dissociative identity disorder, retrograde amnesia occurs as a result of suppression or repression. This retrieval amnesia is not associated with anterograde (storage) amnesia; therefore, new learning occurs. These dissociative disorders may be reversible through hypnosis.

Patients with Ganser syndrome (dissociative disorder not otherwise specified [NOS]), as often seen in prison populations, also claim memory disturbances. They consistently give answers that come close to being correct:

I: How many legs does a horse have?
P: Five.
I: In which month is Christmas?
P: January.

4. ORIENTATION: CONFUSION

Ask the patient to state his name, time of day, day of the week, date, year, present location, address, and telephone number. Disorientation to time and place are less severe indicators of cognitive impairment than disorientation to person.

5. LANGUAGE: APHASIA

Whenever you notice that the patient is perplexed, has difficulties communi-
cating with you, or is indecisive in his goal-directed actions such as walking
to the chair or hanging up the coat, test him for deficiencies of comprehension and expression of language (aphasia), of recognition of complex sensations (agnosia), and of execution of routine acts (apraxia). Testing will
prevent you from misinterpreting aphasia as schizophrenic thought disorder, agnosia as psychomotor retardation, and apraxia as catatonia. *Phases* in
Greek means speech. Aphasia is a loss of the power of using speech.

Handedness

Before you test for aphasia, the patient's handedness should be determined.
Handedness and cerebral dominance are closely allied.

1. Ask whether he is right- or left-handed.
2. Assess with which hand he writes, holds a knife, throws a ball, or stirs his
   coffee.
3. Ask whether first-degree relatives are right- or left-handed (handedness
   is hereditarily influenced).
4. Observe the patient while writing. The natural right-handed person
   keeps his hand below, the forced right-handed person above the line of
   writing.

Right-handers have a left dominant hemisphere, left-handers sometimes
have a right dominant hemisphere. Footedness coincides 98% with hemispheric dominance while handedness coincides only 80–85%. (Note: Evaluate handedness prior to the administration of unilateral electroconvulsive
therapy [ECT], which should be given to the nondominant hemisphere).

Aphasic patients find it difficult to comprehend language (sensory or receptive aphasia) or express themselves verbally (motor or expressive aphasia). The aphasias also include reading and writing. The inability to read,
called alexia, represents a sensory (receptive) aphasia; the inability to write,
known as agraphia, represents a motor (expressive) aphasia.

Testing for sensory aphasia assesses whether the patient comprehends
the meaning of words, phrases, or sentences of increasing complexity by
listening or by reading (alexia).

Testing for expressive aphasia examines whether the patient can repeat
words or name objects of increasing complexity. Testing for agraphia inves-

tigates the ability of patients to write letters, words, and simple sentences. To screen for aphasia, start with a difficult task; if no deficiency is detected, move to the next test. If you spot problems, try simpler tasks to assess the severity of the disturbance.

Aphasias are further subdivided into four central and four pericentral types. Besides Broca's expressive and Wernicke's receptive aphasia, the central types include conduction and global aphasia. The pericentral types are transcortical sensory, anomic, transcortical motor, and isolation aphasia.

Central Aphasias

1. Broca's Expressive or Motor Aphasia

This is a result of a brain lesion of the prefrontal anterior speech area (Brodmann's area 44) (Fig. 5–3): the patient uses nouns and verbs without correct grammatical connection. Speech is nonfluent, dysarthric, and laborious, called *telegram-style* language.

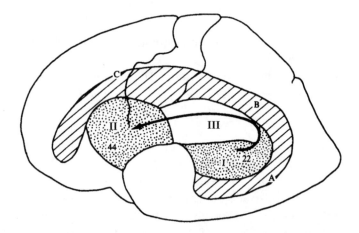

Figure 5–3. Location of cerebral lesion in different types of aphasias of the dominant hemisphere. *Roman numerals* refer to the lesions seen in central aphasias: *I* = Brodmann's area 22 in parietal lobe and posterior part of superior temporal lobe—comprehension (Wernicke's receptive aphasia); *II* = Brodmann's area 44 of prefrontal and frontal lobe of dominant hemisphere—fluency (Broca's expressive aphasia); *III* = connecting fibers between Wernicke's and Broca's speech areas—repetition (conduction aphasia). *Letters* refer to lesions seen in pericentral aphasias: *A* = border zone posterior to area 22—comprehension (transcortical sensory aphasia); *B* = connecting fibers from occipital lobe to limbic system in the second and third temporal gyri—naming (anomic aphasia); *C* = superior border zone to area 44—fluency (transcortical motor aphasia).

2. Wernicke's Receptive or Sensory Aphasia

This results from lesions of Brodmann's area 22 (Fig. 5–3) in the parietal lobe and in the posterior portion of the superior temporal gyrus. The patient has difficulty in auditory comprehension of your question. His language is characterized by fluent, effortless, well-articulated speech devoid of nouns. He may have push of speech. Since the patient often has no insight into his speech problem and has sometimes no apparent hemiparesis, sensory loss, or altered level of consciousness, his language disturbance may be misinterpreted as psychotic language (manic or schizophrenic).

3. Conduction Aphasia

This is due to a lesion of the arcuate fasciculus, that is, connecting fibers between the receptive and expressive speech center. Repetition of words and sentences is severely disturbed. The patient's speech is fluent but has pauses, because word finding is disturbed. Literal paraphasias are common.

"I like to drive my tar."

4. Global Aphasia

The patient can neither express his thoughts nor comprehend other people's speech. Only some syllables are uttered. This severe speech disorder is seen in extensive lesions of the dominant hemisphere with damage to both the expressive (Broca) and receptive (Wernicke) areas of speech.

Pericentral Aphasias

Pericentral aphasias are due to lesions surrounding the central sensory and motor speech areas of Wernicke and Broca.

1. Transcortical Sensory Aphasia

The patient repeats well, his spontaneous speech is fluent, but he does not comprehend what he hears or repeats. His speech is paraphasic. The deficit is caused by a posterior border zone lesion (Fig. 5–3, area A).

2. Anomic Aphasia

The patient speaks fluently, but with pauses to find words. He can repeat and comprehend well, but has difficulties in naming objects. He can neither name shown objects nor point to named objects. His word finding difficulties lead to paraphasias (Fig. 5–3, area *B*). The most severe anomias are found in lesions involving the second and third temporal gyri, which interrupt passageways from the occipital lobe to the limbic system. Higher lesions in the parietal temporal area are associated with substantial alexia and agraphia.

3. Transcortical Motor Aphasia

The patient can repeat and comprehend well, but does not have fluent speech (Fig. 5–3, area *C*).

4. Isolation Aphasia

The patient cannot name, or comprehend, and his speech is nonfluent. However, he can repeat and may have a tendency to repeat everything that is in hearing range, like a speech-trained parrot. This speech abnormality is called echolalia. The lesion involves the whole pericentral area (Fig. 5–3, areas *A, B,* and *C*).

Testing of Aphasias

Increasingly, psychiatrists, psychologists, and social workers encounter aphasias. It is less important to identify the subtype than to recognize its neurological origin. However, identification of a specific subtype may confirm an aphasia's neurological site. When you encounter a problem with speech in your patient, follow a simple sequence of tests to identify the type. Table 5–2 gives the performance profile for the aphasias. Figure 5–4 shows the decision tree for aphasia identification. If you suspect an aphasic syndrome, test at least writing, repetition, fluency, and comprehension.

1. Writing

All tests for aphasia show some degree of agraphia (writing difficulties); therefore writing ability should be tested first (Table 5–2). Screen for agraphia by giving the following instructions:

> "Write down, in one sentence, what the main problem is that brought you here."

If the patient fails this test, continue with systematic assessment. Testing of writing ability starts with dictation of letters and numbers. Next, the patient

Table 5–2. Performance profile of different types of aphasias

Aphasia type	Writing	Repetition	Fluency	Comprehension	Naming	Reading aloud with comprehension	Cerebral lesion (Fig. 5-3)
Central							
Receptive	–	–	+	–	+–	–	I
Conduction	–	–	+	+	+–	–+	III
Expressive	–	–	–	+	+–	–+	II
Global	–	–	–	–	–	–	I+II+III
Pericentral							
Transcortical sensory	–	+	+	–	–	–	A
Anomic	–	+	+	+	–	+–	B
Transcortical motor	–	+	–	+	–	–+	C
Isolation	–	+	–	–	–	–+	A+B+C

Note. + = intact. – = disturbed. +– = sometimes disturbed. –+ = frequently disturbed.
Source. Modified from Ross ED: "Disorders of Higher Cortical Functions: Diagnosis and Treatment." *Science and the Practice of Clinical Medicine: Neurology,* Vol. 6. Edited by Rosenberg RN, Dietschy JM. New York, Grune & Stratton, 1980.

should be asked to write down body parts or common objects. If he is successful with these tasks, he is asked to write a short sentence describing his family, the weather, or a picture on the wall. Agraphia should be diagnosed when basic language errors in spelling or substitution of letters, syllables, or words (paragraphias) not due to educational deficits are encountered. If the patient passes the writing task, she is probably not aphasic and you can stop your testing. (See decision tree, Fig. 5–4.) Agraphia can occur without aphasia, as in the cases of agraphia with alexia or with the Gerstmann syndrome (see Glossary). Agraphia cannot be excluded by asking the patient to write his name, because even in the presence of gross agraphia name writing may be preserved.

2. Repetition

The repetition of spoken language is only disturbed in the central aphasias, in which the central speech areas that bank the Sylvian fissure are lesioned. The pericentral aphasias are caused by lesions surrounding the central speech areas and thus have good repetition. Repetition can be affected by impaired auditory functions, disturbed speech production, or by disconnection between the receptive and expressive language areas.

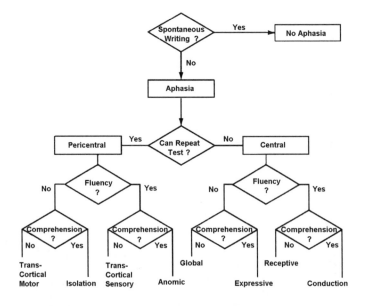

Figure 5–4.   Decision tree for eight different types of aphasias.

Test repetition by asking the patient to repeat words and sentences of increasing complexity. Ask the patient to repeat the material after you. Listen for errors in grammar, omissions, additions, paraphasias, and the inability to repeat the given material. For screening purposes, use the most difficult sentence (no. 10) first. If repetition is obviously disturbed, start with the easy tasks in order to establish a baseline for the extent of the disturbance.

1. Walk
2. School
3. Broadway
4. Dealership
5. Mississippi River
6. The woman went to the store.
7. Everybody left the house at the same time.
8. Let's go out to the park to walk the dog.
9. The tall blond policeman regulated the traffic downtown.
10. Every aspect of the problem needs more detailed discussion.

If the patient with agraphia passes the repetition test, she does not have a central but possibly a pericentral aphasia, that is, a lesion in areas *A, B,* or *C* (Fig. 5–3). If she fails this test, she has a central aphasia, that is, a lesion in area *I, II,* or *III* (Fig. 5–3). In any case, you have to test fluency next (Fig. 5–4).

3. Fluency

Observe it in the patient's spontaneous speech during the interview. Nonfluent speech is sparse, laborious, agrammatic, and filled with pauses for word finding. Nonfluent speech consists predominantly of nouns (telegram style). Nonfluent patients with central aphasia suffer from an expressive or a global aphasia. Nonfluent patients with pericentral aphasia suffer either from isolation (lesions in *A, B,* and *C* of Fig. 5–3) or transcortical motor aphasia (lesion in *C* of Fig. 5–3). Fluent patients with central aphasia suffer from a receptive (lesion in area *I* in Fig. 5–3) or conduction aphasia (lesion in area *III* of Fig. 5–3). Those with pericentral aphasia have either anomic (lesion in area *B* of Fig. 5–3) or transcortical sensory (lesion in area *A* of Fig. 5–3) aphasia (Fig. 5–4).

Fluent speech may also be quite unintelligible (jargon aphasia) or otherwise empty of content, full of abnormal words (paraphasias) and neologisms (self-invented words or phrases).

There are two types of neologisms: 1) the symbolic, repeatedly used neologism of patients with schizophrenia or other psychotic disorders, and 2) the paraphasic, newly invented, random, nonsymbolic, and rarely repeated neologism of aphasic patients with a lesion in the speech center. Neologisms indicate either pathological creativeness or inability to find the correct word. An example of the first is:

"The compterum that controls me and observes me,"

and of the second:

"The onlyness is how wellabit can I not take."

In milder forms, aphasic language contains abnormal words (paraphasias) that affect mainly verbs and nouns; it is filled with articles, conjunctions, and interjections. There is often pressure of speech, distinguished from mania by the fact that manic patients have neither paraphasic nor aphasic problems. Lack of fluency points to a cerebral prefrontal lesion, fluency with paraphasia to a postcentral upper posterior temporal lobe or parietal marginal gyrus lesion.

4. Comprehension

This should be tested in a fashion that does not require much expression, so that expressive aphasia is not misread as a comprehension disability. Ask the patient to point to his eye, leg, and nose. If he is successful, ask for sequences of increasing length, such as:

"First point to your nose, then to your right eye, then to your left ear, then to your right knee."

Patients with normal comprehension are usually able to point to four objects in sequence. A second method consists in asking six or more yes/no questions:

"Does Monday come before Wednesday?"
"Does the year have 13 months?"
"Is winter in Chicago warmer than summer?"
"Do you harvest potatoes in Iowa in December?"
"Is snow frozen water?"
"Do women wear athletic supporters?"
"Does the earth go around the sun?"

All questions should be answered correctly. If you have tested fluency and ability to repeat and comprehend, you can identify which of the eight subtypes of aphasia is present (Fig. 5–4). In other words, central lesions impair the ability to repeat, anterior lesions the ability to be fluent, and posterior lesions the ability to comprehend.

5. Naming and Word Finding

Ask the patient to name the objects that you point to. Repeat approximately 10 times. Use parts of the body, parts of a watch, and parts of clothing. Naming is usually more disturbed in the pericentral than in the central aphasias (Table 5–2). Thus this test can confirm your diagnosis of a central or pericentral aphasia, which you have established with your testing of repetition.

6. Reading Aloud and Comprehension

These skills are tested by having the patient read names of objects aloud and then asking him to point to them. A more difficult task is to have him read sentences aloud and then ask him yes/no questions about the content.

> "Two ladies played bingo in a nursing home."
> "Were the bingo players female?"
> "Was there more than one bingo player?"
> "Did they play bingo at the church?"

Usually, reading, comprehension, or both are disturbed in the aphasic patient.

You may encounter aphasias in your geriatric patients. Interpret aphasic language as part of a neurological syndrome and not as a schizophrenic thought disorder. A misdiagnosis can be fatal. If the aphasia is due to a tumor or abscess in the brain, surgical intervention, instead of long-term treatment with neuroleptics, may be needed. Also, you should be able to differentiate pseudodementia without aphasia in a depressed patient from true dementia with aphasia—aphasia being one of the four cognitive disturbances of all types of dementia (the other three being apraxia, agnosia, and disturbance in executive functions).

6. KNOWING: AGNOSIA

The parietal lobes of the cerebral cortex integrate sensory input; damage to these lobes causes deficits called *agnosias*. Agnosias are disorders of "knowing," the inability to recognize forms and the nature of objects or sensations. There are several types of agnosia, such as the inability to identify objects by touch, to recognize letters traced on the skin, or to recognize objects and pictures of faces (Table 5–3). Agnosias may include disorientation in space, the improper designation of body parts, right-left disorientation, as well as sensory inattention, or denial of illness or defect.

Test agnosias by asking the patient to identify objects (e.g., a key or coin) placed in their hand, or to identify numbers traced on the back of their forearm. Evaluate finger identification and right-left orientation simultaneously by asking the patient, for example, to lift up the ring finger of the left hand. In summary, agnosia is the inability to conceptualize complex sensations.

Criteria for expressive language disorder and mixed receptive-expressive language disorder are provided in DSM-IV-TR under "Communication Disorders" (American Psychiatric Association 2000, pp. 58–64).

7. PERFORMING: APRAXIA

Apraxias refer to the inability to execute purposeful actions and goal-oriented manipulations of objects. Apraxias are caused by damage to the premotor gyrus of the frontal cortex or the right parietal lobe. There are several types of apraxias, such as inability to carry out a movement, to determine what the movement should be, to organize the logical sequence of movements for acts such as dressing, or to construct simple forms or copy designs (Table 5–4).

Apraxias are assessed by having the patient perform some customary act (e.g., light a match), imitate an imaginary action (e.g., thread a needle), or construct a simple form (e.g., build a triangle from three pencils).

8. PATHOLOGICAL REFLEXES AND MOVEMENTS

Complement the testing of apraxias by testing the frontal lobe reflexes, which are abnormal when inhibitory pathways in the frontal lobe are interrupted.

Table 5–3. Agnosias and associated neuroanatomical lesions

Agnosia	Test	Lesion	Associated syndrome
Right-left	Pointing to right and left parts of own or examiner's body	Genetic or dominant parietotemporo-occipital region	
Finger	Lift, name, and point to individual fingers	Same as right-left	
Gerstmann syndrome	Finger and right-left identification, writing and calculation	Dominant parietal lobe	
Actual visual	Name presented object or describe its use without picking it up	Bilateral visual association cortex, areas 18 and 19	
Associative visual	Name objects after they were selected and their use described	Left occipital lobe and posterior corpus callosum	Alexia
Prosopagnosia	Recognize familiar faces without hearing their voices	Bilateral occipitotemporal and right inferior temporo-occipital	
Associative color	Name different colors	Disconnection of visual and language area	Alexia with agraphia
Actual color	Point to different colors	Bilateral inferior temporo-occipital	Prosopagnosia
Geographic	Find way to familiar environment; find cities on a map	Generalized right or left hemisphere	Right-left agnosia, spatial neglect

Table 5–4.   Apraxias and associated neuroanatomical lesions

Apraxia	Test	Lesion
I. Ideomotor		
Buccofacial	Blow out a candle, protrude tongue, blow a kiss	Any lesion in the following circuit leads to apraxia: 1. Verbal comprehension in dominant Wernicke area to 2. kinesthetic memories in supra-marginal gyrus to 3. transmission to dominant premotor area for activation of motor memory to 4. transmission to pyramidal neurons of motor strip for execution of action
Limb	Wave, wipe nose, swat a fly, scratch neck, snap fingers, ring a doorbell, use a foot pump	As above; isolated left limb apraxia is due to lesion of 5. pathway from dominant premotor to nondominant premotor area via anterior corpus callosum or 6. from this premotor area to motor strip
Whole body	Ride a bike, bowl, curtsey	Pyramidal and extrapyramidal motor system
II. Ideational	Complex tasks such as taking out a piece of gum, unwrapping the gum, sticking it in mouth, crumbling the wrapper, and throwing it in the trash; or complete dressing	Widespread bilateral cortex, especially both parietal lobes

Babinski reflex: Scratch the outside margin of the sole of the patient's foot longside. An upward motion of the patient's big toe is pathological.

Glabella reflex: Tap the forehead above the bridge of the nose. The eyes blink after the first few taps; if no extinction occurs (perseverative glabella reflex) the test is positive, which is an extrapyramidal sign observed in Parkinson's disease and neuroleptic-induced parkinsonism.

Grasp (forced grasping) reflex: The patient grasps the examiner's index finger when his palmar surface between thumb and index finger is stroked.

Palmomental reflex: Downward movement of the ipsilateral angle of the mouth appears when the inner surface of the hand is firmly scratched from the thenar to the hypothenar eminence.

Rooting: Scratch below one angle of the patient's mouth. A pulling down of the ipsilateral angle of the mouth is a positive response.

Snout reflex: Snout appears when the upper lip is tapped.

Sucking reflex: Sucking movement appears when the upper lip is lightly stroked.

Motor Functions

The patient carries out abnormal induced movements by demand, often regardless of the consequences.

Pathological obedience: Ask the patient to stick out his tongue. He will repetitively obey, even if he receives a pin prick in the tongue each time.

Waxy flexibility: Present when the patient remains in the body position you put him in.

Ambitendency: Ask the patient to sit down. The patient alternates between opposing movements, like bending down to sit down, but rising up instead and repeating this several times, until he finally stands up for the rest of the interview.

Cooperation (*Mitmachen*):   Instruct the patient to resist all movements. In spite of the instruction he can be pushed in all directions with a light touch of a finger. The opposite behavior is seen in opposition (*Gegenhalten*).

Opposition (*Gegenhalten*):   The patient, even though instructed to allow you to move his limbs, resists movements with a force proportionate to the applied force.

Echopraxia: The patient imitates actions, such as hand clapping or snapping, or copies complete actions of you and other people. Echopraxia is seen in transcortical motor aphasias and catatonia, and is normal in early childhood.

Forced grasping: The patient shakes hands whenever a hand is offered, even though you have instructed him not to do so.

Magnet reaction: You touch the patient's palm and withdraw your fingers slowly; the patient follows the examiner's fingers with his hand. Both forced grasping and magnet reaction can be seen in some dementias and catatonia.

Negativism: An accentuation of opposition in which the patient resists all movements of his limbs by the examiner (passive movement) or tries to do the opposite of what he is signaled to do.

Perseveration: The patient repeats a movement over and over after a command such as:

> "Open your mouth."

In compulsive perseveration he repeats the movement until he is asked to do another task. Most abnormal-induced movement can be observed in patients with schizophrenia, catatonic type, other psychotic disorders, and some dementias.

9. RANGE OF AFFECT

To differentiate disturbed affect due to right hemispheric cortical lesions from that of functional psychoses, Ross (1982) has proposed one test that measures a patient's ability to recognize and imitate affect. He asked patients with right cortical lesions to say, with as much expression as possible as if they were actors, emotionally charged sentences. Depending on the site or the lesion, these patients were not able to express affects or recognize them in others. We have used this approach with psychiatric patients. We have asked them to enact some of the nine basic transcultural innate affects (Izard et al. 1983; also compare Chapter 4) using the following phrases:

Negative affects:

> I'm angry. [anger]
> I'm disgusted. [disgust]
> I feel guilty. [shame]
> I'm sad. [sadness]
> I'm scared. [fear]

Positive affects:

I'm surprised. [surprise]
I feel safe. [content]
I'm happy. [joy]
I'm interested. [interest]

Rate each affect on a scale from 0 to 4. Give 1 point for each of the following four elements of affective expression: modulation in tone of voice, facial expression, gestures including body position, and rhythm of speech. Ask patients who score 0 or 1 for a particular affect to imitate you. Read each sentence that was rated 1 or less to the patient and demonstrate change in tone of voice, facial expression, body language, and rhythm of speech; that is, you attempt to express the sentence in a manner that would give you a rating of 4. Then have the patient repeat the test.

Guidelines for scoring each of the three elements are as follows.

Tone of voice: Patient changes loudness, pitch of voice, and melody of the sentence. If positive give one point.

Facial expression: Patient makes facial changes around mouth, forehead, and eyes. If yes, reward with one point.

Gestures and body position: A patient changes body position, stance, and gestures. If it clearly expresses affect, give one point.

Rhythm of speech: Patient changes rate of speech, length of vowels, and stress on syllables. Noticeable changes are rewarded with one point. There are no extra points for dramatic or accentuated changes.

This test is not validated for different psychiatric and neurological patient populations. Only a few clinical impressions have been collected. Patients with damage to the right frontal lobe and possibly disturbances of the limbic lobe have difficulty expressing their feelings (Ross 1982). Patients with conversion, somatization disorder, and mania may exceed a rating of 30. Low ratings often occur in patients with major depression, severe, with melancholic features.

For psychiatric patients, statements that reflect some of their genuine feelings appear to be more diagnostic. For instance, some anhedonic schizophrenic patients with flat affect become more lively when they express thought contents related to their delusions. Leonhard called these patients "affect laden paraphrenics." They have a better recovery rate than his "systematic schizophrenics" (Leonhard 1979). We have used some of these test questions on patients with major depressive disorder. These patients can express the negative affects of our scale but have difficulties with the positive affects. To measure the patient's ability to experience his affect over a long time period use an analogue rating scale: 0 indicating that the patient cannot feel this affect at all and 10 that he feels this affect frequently and intensely.

10. SUGGESTIBILITY: DISSOCIATION

Certain psychiatric symptoms and signs appear to be due to autosuggestion, such as conversion and dissociative symptoms that can be produced and removed under hypnosis. Therefore the ability to be hypnotizable or highly suggestible may be a necessary but not sufficient condition for the development of these symptoms. Hypnotizability may have a genetic component, since dissociative identity disorder runs in families.

Suggestibility is the patient's willingness 1) to imagine a feeling or picture such as:

"Let your head hang down so that it starts to feel heavy and pulls on your neck muscles,"

and 2) to comply voluntarily with a request such as:

"You start to breathe slower and slower."

High suggestibility (autosuggestion) may be associated with conversion, dissociative, or somatization disorder in some of these patients. Even if true, not suggestibility as such, but uncontrolled uncritical autosuggestion would be necessary to explain the symptoms in these disorders.

Testing Suggestibility

1. Sway test: Ask the patient to stand upright, keep both feet together, and close his eyes. Then ask him to imagine that he is standing on one end of a 6-foot-long board facing the other end. Let him imagine that somebody is slowly lifting the other end in front of him . . . that he is losing his balance . . . that he starts to sway more and more and is falling backward. Assure the patient that you will catch him if he falls. Repeat to him:

"If you can really imagine it, how the board is slowly lifted, you will fall backward. Imagine it . . . imagine it . . . now you are falling . . . falling . . . "

The test is positive when the patient sways markedly or falls back.

2. Tired eyelid test: Ask the patient to look up to your lifted index finger, a foot in front of and a foot up from his forehead, without lifting his head. Then ask him to imagine that his eyes are tired and the lids get heavy . . . that they will slowly close, while he is still looking at your finger. The test is positive when the patient's eyelids slowly close, while the eyes are still focused on your finger.

3. Finger-sticking test: Ask the patient to fold his hands and clasp his fingers tightly. Then ask him to imagine that the fingers stick together. That a force from above and below presses his fingers together. Tell him that he cannot pull them apart, no matter how hard he tries. Ask him to try, while he imagines the force. The test is positive when the patient does not pull his hands apart.

4. Pendulum test: A small object (like a ring) is fixed to a string in a pendulum fashion. The patient holds the pendulum between two fingers of his nonsupported arm and hand. Ask him to imagine that the pendulum starts to swing, first in a small circle and then in a larger and larger circle. The test is positive when the object starts to swing in a circle.

Do not put your authority on the line by suggesting that the patient will have a certain sensation, or make a certain movement. Always make it clear to him that it is his task:

"If you want to imagine that your arm feels heavy, you will start to feel the weight."

That way a failure is his and not yours.

11. ABSTRACT THINKING: CONCRETENESS

Abstract thinking is regulated by the language area of the dominant hemisphere. To test abstract thinking, ask the patient to listen to a proverb. Then ask for its meaning. For example:

"Don't cry over spilled milk."
"A stitch in time saves nine."

If the patient responds that one should not worry over past mishaps, or one is better off to fix a small problem before it becomes a big problem, he can abstract. But if he answers:

"If you cry over spilled milk you have not only lost milk, but also tears,"

or

"If you make one stitch you don't have to make another one,"

he shows concrete thinking.

Patients with schizophrenia sometimes may give awkward interpretations of proverbs:

"Milk is white and tears are clear. They don't mix."

The interpretation of proverbs unfamiliar to the patient may not always test concreteness.

Another drawback of the proverb test is that the patient who has experienced many psychiatric evaluations has learned the correct answer. Furthermore, proverb interpretation is not standardized and normative data are lacking. Some investigators have reported that only 25% of non-brain-damaged adults can interpret proverbs correctly (MacKinnon and Yudofsky 1986). Proverbs are culture-dependent and have therefore little diagnostic value (Taylor 1993). Concrete thinking appears to be a function of low intelligence rather than of schizophrenia (Payne and Hewlett 1960). You can observe it also in the dementias.

Completion test: Ask the patient to complete several conceptual series (e.g., 1, 3, 5, or A, 2, B 4, C, ?).

Similarity test: Ask the patient to find similarities:

"What do an apple and a banana have in common?"
"A car and a submarine?"
"Peace and justice?"

Problem solving: Test problem-solving ability by asking a patient to perform hidden calculations, for instance:

"If you have a total of 27 soda bottles, with twice as many in one refrigerator than another, how many bottles are in each refrigerator?"

or

"If you can get to work by bike in 45 minutes but drive there three times as fast by car, how long would it take you to drive?"

12. INTELLIGENCE: DEMENTIA, MENTAL RETARDATION

Intelligence functions can be crudely assessed with the Rapid Approximate Intelligence Test (RAIT; Wilson 1967), which consists of a multiplication task: 2×3; 2×6; 2×12; 2×24; 2×48, etc. The nonretarded patient should be able to multiply 2×24. Patients who cannot multiply 2×24 have an 85% probability of having a Wechsler Adult Intelligence Scale (WAIS) IQ score of less than 84 (Wilson 1967, Wechsler 1981).

A test that assesses verbal abilities and thinking more than calculation is the intelligence test by Grace H. Kent (Table 5–5). A quick procedure that will give you a score that reflects a patient's intelligence is the combined use of the Kent Test and the RAIT. Both are easy to remember.

We have reorganized the Kent Test into four problem-solving questions (1–4) and six knowledge questions (5–10). A patient who can solve the problems correctly has at least average intelligence (Table 5–6). We give such a patient credit for the first three knowledge questions because of their simplicity. Therefore such a patient has the following score of 26:

12 points credit for the simple knowledge questions (5–7).
14 points credit for the problem-solving questions (1–4).

The bright normal person (Table 5–6) or the person with superior intelligence can also correctly answer the last three knowledge questions (8–10). A patient who fails to correctly solve the four problem questions is then evaluated with the three simple knowledge questions. If he fails to answer these, he falls clearly in the defective range and may be diagnosed as mentally retarded if his school record also shows poor performance. Thus you need only four problem-solving questions and one multiplication task, i.e., 2×24, to exclude or establish the presence of subnormal intelligence (see test in Table 5–5).

Scores of both types of questions may be added up and used to esti-

Table 5–5.   Kent Test

	Maximal score
Problem solving	
1. "If the flag floats to the south from which direction is the wind?" Correct answer: North	3
2. "At what time of the day is your shadow the shortest?" Correct answer: Noon	3
3. "Why does the moon look larger than the stars?" Correct answers: Lower down = 2 points Nearer objects appear larger = 4 points	4
4. "If your shadow points to the northeast, where is the sun?" Correct answer: Southwest	4
Knowledge	
5. "What are houses made of?" One point for each material up to four points.	4
6. "Tell me the name of some fish." One point for each fish up to four points.	4
7. "Give me the names of some large cities." Excluded are small hometowns. One point for each city up to four points.	4
8. "What is sand used for?" One point for playing, two points for construction use, four points for glass.	4
9. "What metal is attracted by a magnet?" Two points for steel, four points for iron.	4
10. "How many stripes are in the United States flag?" Correct answer: Thirteen	2
Total score	36

Source.   Reprinted with permission. Copyright 1946, The Psychological Corp., San Antonio, TX.

mate the patient's intelligence. Table 5–6 provides a comparison of the two tests. A more refined and age-controlled test is the WAIS. Intelligence tests should be used by a qualified psychometrist or psychologist.

In mental retardation, the degree of retardation can be determined with appropriate intelligence tests (American Psychiatric Association 2000, pp. 41–42). Such testing allows the interviewer to determine four degrees of severity:

| 317 | Mild retardation | IQ 50–55 to approximately 70 |
| 318.0 | Moderate retardation | IQ 35–40 to 50–55 |

Table 5–6. Rapid assessment of intelligence

Intelligence range	Kent score	Wilson score	Approx. IQ
Defective	0–18	2 × 12	<70
Borderline	19–20	2 × 24	70–80
Dull normal	21–23	2 × 48	80–90
Average	24–31	2 × 96	90–110
Bright normal	32–33	2 × 192	110–120
Superior	34–35	2 × 384	120–130
Very superior	36	2 × ?	>130

Source. Wilson IC: "Wilson Rapid Approximate Intelligence Test." *American Journal of Psychiatry* 123:1289–1290, 1967; Kent GH: *E-G-Y Scales.* New York, Williams & Wilkins, The Psychological Corporation, 1946.

318.1	Severe retardation	IQ 20–25 to 35–40
318.2	Profound retardation	IQ below 20–25

In diagnosing mental retardation, pay attention to other commonly associated mental disorders, such as attention-deficit/hyperactivity disorder, mood disorders, pervasive developmental disorders, stereotypic movement disorder, and mental disorders due to a general medical condition such as head trauma. The specific etiological factor of dementia appears to combine with specific psychiatric disorders:

- Lesch-Nyhan syndrome with intractible self-injurious behavior
- Fragile X syndrome with attention-deficit/hyperactivity disorder and social phobia
- Prader-Willi syndrome with hyperphagia and compulsivity
- Williams syndrome with anxiety disorders and attention-deficit/hyperactivity disorder

You can find a brief review of predisposing factors for mental retardation in DSM-IV-TR (American Psychiatric Association 2000, pp. 45–46).

13. SERIAL TESTING OF SELECTED PSYCHOLOGICAL STATES

The multiaxial system of DSM-IV-TR assigns Axis V for the rating of general functioning ranging from 0 to 100. Besides this global rating, you may desire

to quantify the patient's state of functioning with a rating scale in a more focused, disorder-specific manner. Such a score can serve as a baseline for
follow-up evaluations and allows you to document, for instance, the progression of a dementing process or the efficacy of your treatment.

Several scales are used by clinicians. Most of these scales are routinely
used in efficacy and comparative studies of established and investigational
drugs that are presented to the FDA (Food and Drug Administration). The
measurement of a few selected states is described below (van Riezen and
Segal 1988).

Cognitive Impairment Disorders

In geriatric patients, look first for decline of executive functions (Royall et
al. 1992) as signs of beginning dementias that involve the frontal lobe. Second, assess for dementias with subcortical involvement. Third, assess for
dementias that affect memory and the overall cognitive state of functioning.
Three simple office procedures are available:

1. Executive Interview (EXIT)
2. Qualitative Evaluation of Dementia (QED)
3. Mini-Mental State Exam

The EXIT and QED are reproduced in the Appendix, and the Mini-Mental
State Exam is shown in Table 5–7.

The Mini-Mental State Exam is increasingly used to measure the cognitive state of functioning (Folstein et al. 1975). It is a simple procedure and
has been validated against anatomical findings characterizing dementia of
the Alzheimer type (Table 5–7). For the diagnosis of dementia, the
Mini-Mental State Exam is reproduced in Table 5–7.

The maximum score on the Mini-Mental State Exam is 30. Interpretation
of test scores is given below. Regarding retest reliability, retesting within 24
hours with the same examiner and with a different examiner yields a Pear-
son coefficient of .89 and .83, respectively, and within 28 days a product
moment correlation coefficient of .98. The validity mean score for elderly
normals is 27.6 (n = 63); for uncomplicated mood disorder, depressed 25.1
(n = 30); for depression with disturbances in orientation and memory that
occurred after the onset of the depression 19.0 (n = 10); and for dementia
9.7 (n = 29) (Folstein et al. 1975).

The three dementia scales (EXIT, QED, and Mini-Mental State Exam)
can be used to evaluate the decline of multiple areas of the brain in an over-

Table 5–7. Mini-Mental State Exam

Maximum Score	Item	Achieved Score
(5)	What is the . . . (year) (season) (date) (day) (month)? Give *1 point* for each correct answer.	/——/
(5)	Where are we now? (county) (state) (city) (hospital) (floor) or (address)? Give *1 point* for each correct answer.	/——/
(3)	Name three objects: *table, comb, tree*. One second to say each. Ask the patient to repeat them after you have said them. Give *1 point* for each correct answer on the *first* trial. Repeat the 3 words until the patient can say the 3 words. Number of trials: ———.	
(5)	Spell "world" backwards. Give *1 point* for each correct letter in *dlrow*.	/——/
(3)	What are those 3 words I said to you? Do not give clues. Give *1 point* for each correct word.	/——/
(2)	Show the patient a pencil and watch and ask the patient to name them. Give *1 point* for each correct word.	/——/
(1)	Please say what I say: "No, if's, and's, or but's." Give *1 point* if no error.	/——/
(3)	A 3-stage command: "Please listen. Take this paper (point) in your right hand; fold it in half and put it on the floor." Do not repeat. Give *1 point* for each correct act.	/——/
(1)	Show the patient the card with the sentence: *Close your eyes.* Ask the patient to read it and do what it said. Give *1 point* if the patient closes his eyes.	/——/
(1)	Say: Please write a sentence here (give the patient a pencil and piece of paper). Any sentence will do. Give *1 point* if a complete meaningful sentence is written.	/——/
(1)	Show the patient the card with a figure. Ask him to copy it. Give *1 point* if the drawing resembles the figure. Ignore small tremulous lines.	/——/
(30)	TOTAL SCORE	/——/——/

Source. Reprinted from Folstein MF, Folstein SE, McHugh PR: "Mini-Mental State: A Practical Method for Grading the Cognitive State of Patients for the Clinician." *Journal of Psychiatric Research* 12:189–198, 1975. With permission from Pergamon Press, Oxford, UK.

lapping fashion. Together with the Kent Intelligence Test and the Rapid Approximate Intelligence Test, you have available a test battery that allows you to measure the degree of decline of your patient's brain functions.

General Purpose Scale

A general purpose rating scale that has been widely used to measure thought content, organization of thinking, and disturbances of affect is the Brief Psychiatric Rating Scale (BPRS). This scale allows you to quickly obtain a profile of the state of mental functions, including hallucinations and delusions (Overall and Gorham 1962).

Mood Disorders

The severity of mood disorders is usually measured with the widely known Hamilton Psychiatric Rating Scale for Depression (HPRSD) (Hamilton 1960), or with the Montgomery-Asberg Depression Rating Scale (MADRS) (Snaith et al. 1986) and the Mania Rating Scale (MRS-11) (Young et al. 1978).

Anxiety Disorders

The Hamilton Anxiety Scale (HAMAS) measures the general state of anxiety (Hamilton 1959), the Sheehan Scale (Sheehan 1983) measures panic, and the Yale-Brown Obsessive Compulsive Scale (Y-BOCS) measures obsessions and compulsions (Goodman et al. 1989a,b) as different components of anxiety.

A wide array of disorder-specific, validated, and standardized rating scales is available and the number is increasing (van Riezen and Segal 1988). In our experience, a small set of repeatedly used scales is practical and sufficiently measures baseline state and its change.

Mental Status Findings as Support for Diagnosis: A Caveat

In Chapters 4 and 5 we have described the mental status examination. Clinical disorders have their typical mental state. The patient's behavior has an immediate diagnostic impact to the point that some interviewers claim they can "guesstimate" a diagnosis in the first 20 seconds. However, such reliance on the mental status may herald misdiagnosis, since the mental status can change dramatically within 24 hours.

Mental status assessment is only one of three essential elements of diagnosis, the other two being psychiatric history and family history (see Chapter 6). Mental status assessment complements the longitudinal aspect of the patient's psychopathology with cross-sectional data. Gauron and Dickinson

(1966a,b) found that the experienced clinician "depended less on the presence . . . [and] paid more attention to the clinical picture in relation to past history . . . " Let us focus on this point in the next chapter.

CHECKLIST

Chapter 5: Testing

This checklist is designed to help you scrutinize yourself. You fulfill minimum standards by testing orientation, memory, and intellectual functions. Give yourself a B if you supported your principal diagnosis by one focused test, such as testing for aphasia, apraxia, and/or agnosia in the patient with dementia, or testing hypnotizability in the patient with dissociative disorder. Give yourself an A if you used more than two focused tests for the principal diagnosis.

1. I selected appropriate tests to complete my diagnostic assessment.

2. The patient had problems with attention and concentration.
    If yes, I assessed attention and concentration by:
    digit span
    serial 7s (3s) backward
    naming the months backward
    spelling words backward

3. The patient showed signs of perseveration. If yes, I assessed perseveration by:
    copying of changing patterns
    repeating number-letter combinations
    tapping at certain letters

4. The patient had impaired memory. If yes, I assessed immediate memory by:
    word repetition
    figure drawing
    story repetition

5. I assessed short-term memory by:
    recall of four words after 10 minutes

6. I assessed long-term memory by:
    recall of the beginning of the interview description of last meal (verified)

7. I assessed remote memory by:
    recall of historic events
    personal, verifiable dates (birthday, marriage, etc.)

8. The patient was disoriented. If yes, orientation was assessed
    by asking for:
    his name
    place of the interview
    day of the week
    date
    time of day

9. I assessed handedness/footedness by:
    asking for it
    asking with which hand the patient
       writes
       holds a knife
       throws a ball
       stirs coffee
    observing hand position while writing
    asking with which foot the patient kicks a ball

10. The patient had a speech disorder. If yes, I assessed aphasia by:
    having him write down his chief complaint
    having him repeat sentences
    having him carry out commands
    observing his fluency

11. The patient had one of the following speech disturbances:
    central aphasia (inability to repeat)
    expressive aphasia (nonfluency)
    neologistic speech
    paraphasic speech

12. I tested the patient for agnosias by:
    writing letters on his hand
    having him identify coins by touch only
    having him name his fingers
    having him point to right and left body parts

13. I tested the patient for apraxias by asking him to perform imaginary
    actions such as:
    blow out a candle (buccofacial)

use a fly swatter (limb)
swing a tennis racket (body)
entire act of gum chewing (ideational)

14. I tested the following frontal lobe reflexes:
Babinski
glabella
grasp
palmomental
rooting
snout
sucking

15. I observed the following abnormal movements:
waxy flexibility
echopraxia
perseveration
forced grasping
magnet reaction
mitmachen
gegenhalten
negativism
ambitendency

16. The patient had a disturbance of affect. If yes, I tested it by the
9-affect test.

17. The patient seemed to have conversion/dissociative symptoms. I
tested his suggestibility by:
sway test
tired eyelid test
finger-sticking test
pendulum test

18. The patient showed intellectual impairment. I tested his ability to
think by:
proverbs
completion test
similarities
Kent Test
multiplication table 2×3, 2×6, 2×12, etc.

19. The patient showed an abnormal emotional or cognitive state.
    I established a baseline by a standardized scale:
    Brief Psychiatric Rating Scale (BPRS)
    Hamilton Psychiatric Rating Scale for Depression (HPRSD)
    Mania Rating Scale (MRS-11)
    Montgomery-Asberg Depression Rating Scale (MADRS)
    Hamilton Anxiety Scale (HAMAS)
    Sheehan Panic Scale
    Yale-Brown Obsessive Compulsive Scale (Y-BOCS)
    Executive Interview (EXIT)
    Qualitative Evaluation of Dementia (QED)
    Mini-Mental State Exam

CHAPTER SIX

FIVE STEPS TO MAKE A DIAGNOSIS

1. **Diagnostic Clues**
   Discomfort
   Chief Complaint
   Signs
   Expanding Versus Focusing
   Differential
2. **Diagnostic Criteria**
   Clinical Disorders (Axis I)
   Personality Disorders (Axis II)
   Psychosocial and Environmental Problems (Axis IV)
   Disorders Not Otherwise Specified (NOS)
   Checking for Unexplored Disorders
3. **Psychiatric History**
   Premorbid Personality
   Course of Clinical Disorders
   Course of Personality Disorders
   Treatment History
   Social History
   Medical History (Axis III)
   Family History
4. **Diagnosis**
   Assets and Strengths
   Diagnostic Formulation
   Multiaxial Diagnoses
       Axes I and II
       Axis III
       Axis IV
       Axis V
5. **Prognosis**

SUMMARY

Chapter 6 offers five steps to make a diagnosis: 1) collecting diagnostic clues, 2) checking diagnostic criteria, 3) assessment of the psychiatric history, 4) diagnosis with multiaxial assessment, and 5) prognosis.

▲ ▲ ▲ ▲ ▲

But where shall the wisdom be found?
And where is the place of understanding?

—The Holy Bible, King James Version,
Job 28:12

▼ ▼ ▼ ▼ ▼

INTRODUCTION

There is no single diagnostic approach that works optimally for all interviewers or all patients. There may not even be one style that is always beneficial or always harmful in every case. Many interview styles will lead you to a correct diagnosis but each involves gathering and analyzing information.

In the following we describe the work of two psychiatric residents whose interviewing styles reflect two extremes on a continuum.

Here is Ken Steiff's highly structured style. After one open-ended question at the beginning of the interview, Dr. Steiff presented the patient with a laundry list of psychiatric symptoms. For this purpose he had prepared about a dozen sheets, each with the symptoms of one psychiatric disorder. During the interview he would underline the symptoms that the patient endorsed. If the symptoms fulfilled diagnostic criteria for a disorder, he would mutter to himself:

"Wow!"

and

"That's it! Here we are!"

Then he told his patient: "You see you have somatization disorder; here is the proof. Look at all the symptoms you have."

How did the other residents who trained with Dr. Steiff respond to his interview approach? Even though they agreed with his diagnostic impressions, they found his interviewing style inappropriate. He did not use enough open-ended questions to become gradually more specific. He was not client-centered, that is, only slowly and cautiously introducing more directive techniques. Instead, he behaved like a computer programmed for symptom checking.

How did the patient respond to Dr. Steiff's approach?

"He really seems to know what he is talking about. I have been with a couple of therapists before, and all they did was beat around the bush. They did not seem to know what's going on with me at all. That's unlike Dr. Steiff. He really is on top of things."

This was not the only patient who appreciated Ken's style. He developed a following like the other residents. Maybe he had a lower return rate than others, but those who came back seemed to swear by him.

Here is the opposite, an unstructured diagnostic style. Dr. Rosa Dahl let her patients talk about what they wanted; she tolerated digressions, complaints, praises, gossip, and lengthy conversations. If a symptom surfaced, she did not follow up. It took her several visits to establish a diagnostic impression. Her long-term patients claimed that she was one of the best psychiatrists they had seen.

If the patient is considered the judge, we would have to conclude that for any interview style there will be patients for whom the approach works. Generally, the positive response is based on a match between the personalities of the patient and the interviewer.

If we use research results, both Ken's and Rosa's styles seem to be justified. Gauron and Dickinson (1966a,b) report that two major coordinate axes could be superimposed on the approaches to making a diagnosis. One involved the dimension structured versus unstructured. The other involved the dimension inductive-logical versus intuitive-alogical.

Mendel (1964) divided therapists into hedgehogs and foxes. The hedgehog is a problem solver with a probing, analytic, pragmatic mind depending on logic (a friend of DSM-IV-TR we may add), while the fox engages in scattered and diffuse thinking, waiting for experiences to take shape in his mind (a critic of DSM-IV-TR we may suspect). Interestingly, Gauron and Dickinson (1966a,b) found that the interviewer did not use the same approach in every case. Thus the hedgehog uses predominantly the left side and the fox predominantly the right side of his brain.

The ideal solution: use both approaches. Listen to the patient, follow the direction of his thought, see where it carries you (the intuitive method), then analyze your global impression, trace its origins, and test and verify the observations (the left-sided method). Conversely, in some patients start systematically with the chief complaint, include likely and exclude unlikely diagnostic options (left-sided method), and then ask yourself what your overall impression of the patient is, how your specific observations fit in (the right-sided approach). Have you missed the forest because of all the trees?

Like Ken and Rosa, interviewers may be successful despite a one-sided interviewing style if they communicate a genuine concern to their patient. What Ken's and Rosa's patients responded to was the genuine caring of these interviewers. It seems clear that rapport plays a central role in determining the extent to which the interviewer can collect diagnostically significant data.

How can you determine then which diagnostic approach is right for your patient? The best indication is feedback from the patient. If he opens up, is interested in the interview, contributes voluntarily, smiles, asks questions, and offers intimate details, you can consider your approach successful, at least in the short run. If the patient complies with your suggestions and treatment, returns for future appointments, and progresses in the solution of his problems, his behavior confirms that things have worked out in the long run. Whatever your personal style, if you follow five logical steps, you will be able to establish your diagnoses quickly and reliably.

1. Diagnostic Clues

As soon as the patient gets in contact with you, no matter what the setting, you like to establish rapport (see Chapter 2). This first step allows you to observe the patient for diagnostic clues in his behavior. You also get a feeling for his motivation to see you. All these observations may take place before you approach his chief complaint.

Starting with the first contact, assemble a running list of all possible diagnoses. From your observations and the patient's symptoms or disturbed behavior, hypothesize which major psychiatric or personality disorders are compatible with these clues. Thus you generate a list—we call it *list no. 1 of included psychiatric disorders.*

During the same screening process, you also make observations and obtain clues that exclude other psychiatric disorders. We call this *list no. 2 of excluded disorders.*

Besides lists nos. 1 and 2, you are left with the disorders that you have not covered yet. We call this *list no. 3 of unexplored disorders*.

You can conceptualize the diagnostic process as follows: from your long list no. 3 that consists of unexplored disorders, you derive a list no. 1 of included disorders, and a list no. 2 of excluded disorders. What is left is a dwindling list no. 3 of the unexplored disorders.

As you begin, screen the patient's report, chief complaint, and behavioral clues for the main diagnostic areas of psychiatric disorders: psychotic symptoms, mood disturbances, cognitive impairment, irrational anxiety (avoidance behavior or increased arousal), and physical complaints. Add psychosocial and environmental problems, and lifelong patterns of maladjustment to this catalog. Then organize this information into your diagnostic list no. 1, including a wide variety of major psychiatric and personality disorders or psychosocial and environmental problems. Use overinclusive questions for this step, questions that have high sensitivity but comparatively low specificity for psychiatric disorders. List no. 1 has all diagnostic options for the differential diagnosis; it grows during the first part of the interview, while list no. 3 of unexplored disorders and problems shrinks.

2. Diagnostic Criteria

After the patient has revealed his problems, scrutinize list no. 1. Determine the duration of essential psychiatric symptoms or syndromes. Assess their severity in terms of their impact on the patient's life. If you find more than one syndrome, assess their temporal and causal relationship to each other (see below). Check whether the reported symptoms and observed signs satisfy the criteria for one or more disorders—in other words: Test your diagnostic hypotheses!

DSM-IV-TR emphasizes in the introduction (American Psychiatric Association 2000, p. xxxii) that the diagnostic criteria should not be applied mechanically or in cookbook fashion but should be implemented using your clinical judgment. For instance, if the clinical presentation falls short of meeting the full criteria for a diagnosis, the exercise of your clinical judgment may still justify the diagnosis as long as the reported symptoms are persistent and severe. Thus, DSM-IV-TR criteria are meant "to serve as guidelines to be informed by clinical judgment" (p. xxxii).

Continue to examine one by one all major and personality disorders, and psychosocial and environmental problems in your list. During this second step use questions of high diagnostic specificity geared to identify all essential signs and symptoms of a disorder. The list of excluded disorders (no. 2) grows during this process at the expense of list no. 1, because now you exclude by detailed examination the previously included disorders. Go beyond the patient's chief complaint; now you don't ask him what he wants to tell but what you want to know. Thus you transform list no. 3 into list no. 1 or 2. At the end of the successful diagnostic interview, list no. 3 should be entirely eliminated.

3. Psychiatric History

If symptoms, signs, and problems pass the criteria test for a disorder, get more supportive evidence through premorbid history, the course of the disorder, and family history. Exclude medical disorders as the cause of the symptoms. If the problems fail the criteria test for a disorder, eliminate this disorder from list no. 1 and add it to list no. 2, the list of excluded disorders. Thus you shorten list no. 1 further in favor of list no. 2. Assess the impact of the disorder on the patient's life and obtain a measure of the level of severity.

4. Diagnosis

Organize your diagnostic impressions into DSM-IV diagnoses recorded on five axes. Run your diagnostic impressions through a decision tree to determine present, principal, and past diagnoses on Axes I and II. Complement this assessment by coding medical disorders, psychosocial and environmental problems, and global assessment of functioning on Axes III–V, respectively.

Summarize biological, psychological, and social factors that contribute to the patient's diagnosis. This so-called diagnostic formulation highlights precipitating and etiological factors of the patient's disorders.

5. Prognosis

Complete your multiaxial assessment with an explicit prognosis. Factor in the nature of the patient's clinical and/or personality disorders. Pay attention to how he handles the treatment contract and how he responds to it (see Chapter 7). It reveals his attitude toward his disorder and his willingness to comply with treatment. For practical purposes, the degree of compliance may outweigh the other factors in determining prognosis.

These five steps are not locksteps—they are not even necessarily consecutive steps, with the exception of step 1. These steps are logical steps, that is, at some time during the interview you have to elicit all pathology; at some time you have to determine duration, severity, and relationship of all pathology; at some time you have to get a history; and at some time you have to put it all together into a list of diagnostic impressions. The order in which you do it is often determined by what the patient wants to talk about. As long as his elaborations contribute to any of these diagnostic steps, you may want to follow his leads—a jumpy interview can still produce a complete list of diagnostic impressions.

Besides a stepwise approach, clinicians observe that "sometimes the diagnosis bursts into consciousness before one is aware of the reason why" (Sandifer 1972). Is this intuitive brilliance? Or is it simply a showy example of the interviewer's capacity to quickly ratchet through the steps in the diagnostic process? It may be both. To understand the nature and the importance of diagnosis, it is helpful to follow the steps involved in determining the major disorder, both to arrive at an appropriate diagnosis as well as to develop an organized treatment plan. Here is how to apply the five steps.

1. DIAGNOSTIC CLUES

Patients seek consultation for a number of reasons. Some come to you for administrative reasons, perhaps needing a certificate to return to work. Others are ordered by the court. Some need an evaluation requested by a third party, and others come for a second opinion, or advice. But most patients come because they know they need help and are desperate for intervention. Your initial goal is to help them express their problem.

How do you best proceed? It is risky to be too direct. The patient may freeze up. If you move too slowly, some patients will get impatient; therefore take a middle road: give the patient room and time until you have established rapport, until he trusts you and starts on his own to talk about himself and his problems (see Chapter 2).

Even if good rapport is established, some patients will persist with small talk; you may choose to converse until the patient expresses some change or dissatisfaction with his life, then summarize his difficulties for him.

Others may expect that you ask them directly for their chief complaint.

"You should find out what's wrong with me. Isn't that what you are paid for?"

Finally, there is a group of patients who overtly show disturbed behavior during the interview that you may take as an invitation to explore those signs closer.

Accordingly, you encounter three expressions of a problem: 1) discomfort, 2) chief complaint, and 3) signs.

Discomfort

A patient may appear tense and uncomfortable. He may refuse to talk to you at all, or he may start to talk about other people, about family members with psychiatric problems, or about movies in which a psychiatrist appeared. He may offer his opinions about health care, politics, art, or any topic unrelated to his problem. Or, he may talk about changes in his life, express feelings that "things are not right," but can only poorly describe what is going on. He may only slowly realize that his sleep, appetite, or sex drive have changed, that he avoids people, and that his mind is less sharp than a year ago.

You may choose to stay with an indirect conversational approach or probe further by asking him for his chief complaint, by confronting him with his behaviors, or reflecting his statements. As you talk to him, you may first get an idea about his present level of functioning before you find out if he has lifelong or recent problems, and he may be unable to adequately describe these changes.

With such a patient, it is your goal to eventually formulate—implicitly or explicitly—the chief complaint for him. If you meet such a patient who is not clear about his complaints, be careful not to increase his anxiety.

Chief Complaint

Most outpatients, especially those who come for treatment in a private practice setting, are cooperative. They may tell you spontaneously or expect you to ask them why they came to see you. Use phrases such as:

> "What kind of problems brought you here?"
> "How can I help you?"
> "Tell me what's troubling you."

Give them a chance to express their problems in their own words. Most patients give a chief complaint that involves about one or more of the following four problems:

Symptoms

They are either essential (also known as core) or associated symptoms of clinical disorders, such as:

> "I can't eat out anymore. Last time I went to a restaurant I thought I had a heart attack. In the emergency room they told me there is nothing wrong with my heart."

Patterns of Maladjusted Behavior

They reflect a lifelong pattern of maladjustment and problems in relating to other people, such as the following case shows. Here is Mr. Robert P., a white, 34-year-old car mechanic:

> "I always mess up just when I seem to establish myself. I'm so impulsive. I get so angry that I destroy what I accomplished. It happened again in the last few weeks."

Stressors

Stressors are generally outside events that have triggered or caused the person's current malaise. As the following example shows, Mr. Paul A. identified a business crisis as the precipitating factor:

> "I'm a farmer. Business is bad. I'm in debt and I have to work two jobs to get out from under. Now I got that heart attack and I worry. My doctor told me that I can't work the farm any more. I can't sleep because I don't know what to do."

Stressors may be single, multiple, recurrent, continuous, or specific developmental events, such as leaving home, getting married, or becoming a parent, being widowed, or facing death.

Interpersonal Conflicts

Conflicts with spouse, family members, boss, colleagues, or neighbors can be the major factor identified by the patient as the source of his problems.

> "Jim, my husband, does not know what intimate is,"

one patient complained.

> "He can't give me what I need and I probably can't give him what he needs. We've had no sex for the last 3 months. If we do it I have to initiate it. But I don't mean that he is not sexual, you know, we are just not intimate with each other. Now, I have met somebody else. I see him every week or every other week but I feel guilty because I'm still attached to Jim and I can't let go."

Signs

A patient may show behavioral disturbances during the first few minutes of the interview that point to a psychiatric problem. Such disturbances may represent signs and clues of a disorder, visible in his mental status. You may opt to start the diagnostic decision process by confronting the patient with it now, rather than exploring it later:

P: [talks in a very low voice when he first meets the interviewer in an outpatient clinic]
I: You talk so softly. Is there a special reason?
P: Yes, I'm afraid somebody from the waiting room is listening outside the door.

Register suspiciousness as a delusion occurring in all psychotic disorders, especially in schizophrenia, paranoid type, and delusional disorder, but also in psychotic disorder due to the dementias, substance-induced psychotic disorders, or major depressive disorder with psychotic features. In paranoid personality disorder, the suspiciousness does not reach the level of a delusion.

P: [insists on having his wife present at the interview]
I: You wanted your wife to be in here with us. Can you tell me how she can help us with the interview?
P: Yes, she can explain everything better. I have a hard time concentrating. That's why I brought her all the way from X [a town 150 miles away].

Register dependent behavior as seen in dementia, major depressive disorder, avoidant or dependent personality disorder.

P: [has rings on all her fingers]
I: You are wearing beautiful rings on each of your fingers.
P: You forgot my thumbs . . . I put them all on when I feel bad but have to go somewhere.

Register flamboyant behavior as seen in bipolar disorder or histrionic personality disorder, and also with intoxication.

These examples are characteristic of a group of psychiatric disorders. Follow up on observed signs if you feel they lead you to the patient's main problems. If the patient will not talk to you, you will have to find a way to confront him about the signs you observe. In most cases, this further questioning will yield his cooperation. If the patient consistently resists your efforts to elicit information, consult *The Clinical Interview Using DSM-IV-TR, Volume 2: The Difficult Patient* (Othmer and Othmer 2002).

Expanding Versus Focusing

After you have some idea of the patient's main problem(s), you can pursue one of two different avenues: expand and try to discover more problem areas, or focus on what you have already identified. Further screening of problem areas is useful because it may shed more light on the previous one. Zeroing in on the just explored area on hand may strike the iron while it is hot. Both are appropriate in different instances. Let the patient lead you.

Expanding

If you screen for more problems, use questions such as:

"Are there any other problems?"
"Is this your main and only problem?"

Screen the 13 diagnostic areas that often become the point of origin for a descriptive decision tree (also compare Table 6–1):

1. cognitive impairments
2. pattern of substance use
3. psychotic symptoms
4. mood disturbances
5. irrational anxiety, avoidance, increased arousal
6. physical complaints or anxiety about illness
7. factitious behavior
8. dissociative problems
9. sexual problems
10. eating disturbances
11. sleeping problems
12. problems with impulse control
13. adjustment problems

In addition, look for psychosocial or environmental problems, lifelong patterns of maladjustment, and periods of impaired functioning.

Broad, open-ended questions are useful here. Questions with high sensitivity help to spot unusual experiences such as extrasensory perception (psychosis) or feelings of being on an emotional roller coaster (mood swings). Diagnostic specificity of open-ended questions is—by design—low.

Focusing

If you decide to focus on a problem, ask the patient with open-ended questions to offer more details. Use techniques such as clarification and continuation to steer him back to his problem when he digresses. Encourage him to elaborate on three areas:

Table 6–1.   Essential symptoms of clinical disorders (Axis I)

Disorder	Essential symptoms
Cognitive disorders	
Deliria	Disturbed consciousness, inattention, perseveration, decreased alertness, memory impairment, disorientation, perceptual disturbances developing over a short period of time, hyperactivity or lethargy (or alternating between the two)
Dementias	Memory impairment, cognitive disturbances such as aphasia, apraxia, agnosia, and impairment of executive and social functioning
Amnestic disorders	Impairment of memory and learning with significant effect on social and occupational functioning (transient or chronic)
Substance-related disorders	
Dependence	Presence or history of tolerance, substance-specific withdrawal symptoms, consumption in larger amounts than intended, unsuccessful efforts to cut down, persistent use despite wasting of time, and negative social, occupational, psychological, and physical consequences
Abuse	Recurrent maladaptive use persistent over a 12-month period, leading to failures at work, school, or home, and to physically hazardous situations, legal problems, and negative social and interpersonal consequences
Intoxication	Reversible substance-specific syndrome due to recent ingestion with behavioral or psychological maladaption
Withdrawal	Substance-specific reaction to cessation of heavy and prolonged intake, causing significant impairment in important areas of functioning
Schizophrenia and other psychotic disorders	
Schizophrenia	Hallucinations, delusions, disorganized speech, grossly disorganized or catatonic behavior, negative symptoms for at least 1 month and with social and occupational dysfunction of 6 months' duration
Paranoid type	Delusions or frequent auditory hallucinations
Disorganized type	Disorganized speech and/or behavior, with inappropriate affect, no catatonia
Catatonic type	Immobility or excessive motor activity, mutism, posturing, stereotyped movements, echolalia, or echopraxia

Table 6–1.   Essential symptoms of clinical disorders (Axis I) *(continued)*

Disorder	Essential symptoms
Residual type	At least two negative symptoms or attenuated hallucinatory or delusional experiences
Schizophreniform disorder	Psychotic episode lasting at least 1 month but total episode <6 months
Schizoaffective disorder	Uninterrupted period including at least 1 month of psychotic episode with either major depressive or manic episode not due to substance abuse; in addition, delusions or hallucinations occurred for at least 2 weeks in the absence of prominent mood symptoms
Delusional disorder	Nonbizarre delusions without other psychotic symptoms not due to substance abuse for at least 1 month
Brief psychotic disorder	Duration of psychotic episode lasting more than 1 day but less than 1 month
Shared psychotic disorder	Similar delusion in two individuals in close relationship
Psychotic disorder due to general medical condition	Psychotic episode etiologically related to a general medical condition
Substance-induced psychotic disorder	Evidence of substance intoxication or withdrawal preceding by less than 1 month or concurring with a psychotic episode without the patient's insight; evidence of etiological relationship between substance use and psychotic disorder
Mood disorders	
Depressive disorder	Depressed most of day or diminished pleasure in normal activities for a continuous 2-week period
Bipolar I disorder, manic	Abnormally and persistently elevated expansive or irritable mood lasting at least 1 week
Bipolar II disorder	One or more major depressive episodes with at least one hypomanic episode
Cyclothymic disorder	Presence of hypomanic symptoms for at least 2 years
Substance-induced mood disorder	Presence of significantly depressed, elated, or irritable mood, starting within 1 month of substance intoxication or withdrawal; the mood disturbance appears to be etiologically related
Anxiety disorders	
Panic disorder	Panic attacks (unexpected)
Panic disorder without agoraphobia	Recent, unexpected panic attacks followed by 1 month or more of recurrence

(continued)

Table 6–1.   Essential symptoms of clinical disorders (Axis I) *(continued)*

Disorder	Essential symptoms
Anxiety disorders *(continued)*	
Panic disorder with agoraphobia	Same as above, with anxiety about being in places from which escape would be difficult or embarrassing
Agoraphobia without history of panic disorder	Anxiety about being in places from which escape would be difficult or embarrassing
Specific phobia	Excessive anxiety about specific situation or object
Social phobia	Excessive, persistent fear of social or performance situations with avoidance
Obsessive-compulsive disorder	Obsessions and/or compulsions
Posttraumatic stress disorder	Flashbacks and dreams about a traumatic event
Acute stress disorder	Exposure to a threat of death or serious injury
Generalized anxiety disorder	Excessive anxiety and worry occurring more days than not for at least 6 months
Substance-induced anxiety disorder	Predominant anxiety, panic attacks, obsessions or compulsions starting within 1 month; the anxiety disorder appears to be etiologically related to substance intoxication or withdrawal
Somatoform disorders	
Somatization	Many medically unexplained complaints beginning before age 30 and occurring over several years
Conversion disorder	Symptoms affecting voluntary motor or sensory functions, neurologically unexplained and not intentionally produced
Hypochondriasis	Preoccupation with fears of having a serious disease resistant to medical reassurance
Body dysmorphic disorder	Preoccupation with imagined defect in appearance, or exaggeration of a slight physical anomaly
Pain disorder	Severe pain associated with psychological factors
Factitious disorders	Physical and/or psychological symptoms intentionally produced or feigned to assume the sick role
Dissociative disorders	Amnesia, fugue, multiple personalities, depersonalization, derealization, trance

Table 6–1.   Essential symptoms of clinical disorders (Axis I) *(continued)*

Disorder	Essential symptoms
Sexual and gender identity disorders	
Sexual dysfunctions	Dysfunctions in desire, arousal, and orgasm; pain during intercourse
Substance-induced sexual dysfunctions	Dysfunctions starting within 1 month and appearing to be etiologically related to substance intoxication or withdrawal
Paraphilias	Over a period of 6 months recurrent episodes of intense sexual arousal concerning exhibitionism, fetishism, frotteurism, pedophilia, masochism, sadism, voyeurism, or transvestism
Gender identity disorder	Cross-gender identification, including treatment to change gender
Eating disorders	
Anorexia nervosa, restricting type	Willful starvation, distorted body image, amenorrhea (in females)
Bulimia nervosa, purging type	Recurrent episodes of binge eating followed by vomiting, excessive use of laxatives, or excessive exercise
Primary sleep disorders	
Dyssomnias	Insomnia, hypersomnia, narcolepsy, breathing-related sleep disorder, circadian rhythm sleep disorder
Parasomnias	Nightmares, night terrors, sleepwalking
Substance-induced sleep disorders	Significant distressful, attention-demanding sleep disturbance starting within 1 month and appearing to be etiologically related to substance intoxication or withdrawal
Impulse disorders	Uncontrolled impulses harmful to self and others, including intermittent explosive disorder, kleptomania, pyromania, pathological gambling, and trichotillomania
Adjustment disorders	Maladaptive reaction to a psychosocial stressor occurring within 3 months of onset of stressor and ceasing within 6 months of termination of the stressor
Mental retardation*	Pattern of general intellectual impairment starting before age 18

*Since this disorder also affects functioning and adjustment in adult life, it is included in this table.

Severity: Do his problems interfere objectively with his life and limit his social effectiveness and/or lead to (subjective) suffering?

Course: How long did he have the problems? Was the onset insidious or sudden? Did the disorder become worse or better with time? Was there any particular pattern?

Stressor: Does the patient believe that some outside event brought on his problems? Was there any physical abuse, sexual abuse, or a catastrophic trauma that contributed to the development of a psychiatric disorder?

After you have collected information about these three areas, decide whether it points to a clinical disorder, a personality disorder, or a psychosocial or environmental problem.

Clinical disorders, similar to physical disorders, are characterized by a syndrome of symptoms and signs, or a pattern, or, in some cases, a single symptom such as a chronic delusion, which follows a predictable course, and is often familial. Specific stressors may be associated with the development of a dissociative disorder, conversion disorder, posttraumatic stress disorder, or an adjustment disorder. In contrast, personality disorders are chronic, lifelong patterns of maladjusted behavior, often without clear onset.

Psychosocial and environmental problems may be the result of psychiatric disorders but can also occur in response to a complicated marriage, divorce, work, legal problems, or other stressful situations.

Differential

What do you do after you have determined the patient's chief problem? You may find yourself in one of two extreme situations: too little information (situation 1), or (mis)leading information (situation 2). Here are the reports of two candidates who took the National Boards of Psychiatry and Neurology. Their experiences illustrate the two situations.

Situation 1

After his oral boards in psychiatry and neurology, Dr. Tim R. complained that he must have failed the examination, because his patient did not say much. The patient did not give a chief complaint, answered questions with yes and no only, and used phrases such as:

"They told me to show up here today."
"I guess that's in my record."
"I don't know."
"I forgot."
"Can't remember."

When asked what the patient's differential was, the candidate responded with irritation:

"How could I give a differential? I couldn't tell whether this guy was mentally retarded, had Alzheimer's disease, or was severely depressed. I couldn't tell a thing."
"So your patient could have had any of the psychiatric disorders listed in DSM-IV-TR?"

he was asked.

"Sure," the candidate answered, "any or none."
"NONE? You would have had to prove that. But ANY? If you only came up with a list of any disorders—there is your differential! The less you know about the patient, the longer your list of differential diagnoses, the more disorders you may want to discuss with your examiners. Scant knowledge about the patient means that many disorders of adulthood listed on Axes I and II of DSM-IV-TR can be included in your list."

Situation 2

Dr. Susan F.:

"They gave me this 33-year-old fellow who had a lot of paranoid delusions. I caught that right away. His chief complaint was 'My neighbors are out to get me. They bought a satellite dish and directed it against my house. That makes me nervous.' I thought I lucked out—that's an easy case. What can be easier than a paranoid schizophrenic patient? So I told them what I thought. The examiners must have read the patient's chart. They asked me again and again what other diagnoses I would consider. I tried my best to convince them that in my book, the fellow has paranoid schizophrenia, but they must have thought that he has something else. I argued for quite a while, but I guess they were in the driver's seat."
"You probably would have passed your examination, if you had followed the rule of five."
"I never heard of such a rule,"

she said.

"The rule of five means that when you interview a patient, do not decide prematurely on one diagnosis. Challenge yourself, consider at least five diagnostic options."

The young lady looked puzzled.

"You mean I don't have to figure out what the right diagnosis is?"
"That's right; as long as you include the right diagnosis in your differential.
It's better to be overinclusive than overexclusive."
"How could I have found five diagnoses for my paranoid schizophrenic pa-
tient?"
"By looking for them. For instance, what kind of street drugs, if any, did your
patient take? Any amphetamines that could produce persecutory delusions?"
"I didn't ask that, because his delusions were so typically schizophrenic that
there was not any doubt in my mind."
"Did the fellow have a history of a head injury?"
"He was oriented alright; he could remember four objects after 10 minutes
and could do similarities fine. So I did not think that he had a cognitive im-
pairment."
"Are patients with delusional disorder due to a general medical condition al-
ways disoriented or unable to process information?"
"Hmm."
"How was his affect? Was there a history of depression or elated mood?"
"Why should a schizophrenic patient have elated mood or depressions? And
if he does, what's the difference?"
"That he might not be a paranoid schizophrenic patient after all."

This candidate had tried only to confirm her initial impression, and had
collected supportive evidence only for it, while ignoring other options. She
was pursuing her goal wearing blinders and elevated a symptom to a psychiatric disorder. Avoid this one-way-street trap.

The solution to the diagnostic dilemma of both candidates is the same.
Their information should be used to generate a list of all disorders that possibly could explain the patient's complaints and his mental state. On top of
that list should be the most severe and devastating disorders, followed by
the nonpsychotic and personality disorders, and finally the psychosocial
and environmental problems.

Here are three different types of cases you may encounter. If a patient
reports depressive symptoms, make a mental list of all disorders that fit this
account. Your catalogue could look like this:

- major depressive disorder
- bipolar I disorder, most recent episode depressed
- bipolar II disorder, most recent episode depressed
- dysthymic disorder
- adjustment disorder with depressed mood
- schizoaffective disorder, depressive type

- cyclothymic disorder
- substance-induced mood disorder
- mood disorder due to a general medical condition

If your initial impression suggests a stressor associated with anxious mood, your list may contain:

- adjustment disorder with anxious mood
- acute stress disorder
- posttraumatic stress disorder
- generalized anxiety disorder
- agoraphobia without history of panic disorder
- specific phobia
- social phobia
- panic disorder without agoraphobia
- panic disorder with agoraphobia
- avoidant personality disorder
- dependent personality disorder
- substance-induced anxiety disorder
- anxiety disorder due to a general medical condition
- delusional disorder

If your initial impression is a lifelong pattern of violent acts, generate a list such as:

- substance abuse
- substance dependence
- antisocial personality disorder
- intermittent explosive disorder
- impulse control disorder not otherwise specified (NOS)
- bipolar I disorder, most recent episode manic
- dissociative identity disorder

Work with an open mind in assembling these lists. Be overinclusive rather than overexclusive. Remember that the average patient fulfills criteria for two to three psychiatric disorders during his lifetime (Helzer et al. 1977; Othmer et al. 1981; Powell et al. 1982).

In summary, this step in diagnosis involves two approaches: including and excluding. Including supplies evidence to support a diagnosis, excluding provides evidence to eliminate a diagnosis. Thus, diagnosing generates three lists: list no. 1 consists of what to include, list no. 2 of what to exclude, and list no. 3 of what is still to be explored.

Both candidates neglected to develop these three lists. Otherwise, the first candidate would have realized that he had a long list of unexplored disorders to be discussed in light of his mental status observations, such as the patient's sex, age, demeanor, comprehension, speech, affect, orientation, and short-term memory, and then should have created list no. 1. Our second candidate was not aware that she had a long list no. 1 of disorders that share persecutory ideas.

This section taught you how to screen for psychopathology and problems, and how to make a differential. The next section helps you to verify some and exclude other disorders of your differential.

2. DIAGNOSTIC CRITERIA

At this point you have generated a list of preliminary diagnostic impressions in your mind. Review that list. You may face one of two extreme situations.

First, your list contains mainly disorders that belong to one of the 13 diagnostic areas described in DSM-IV-TR (see Table 6–1). For instance, your list contains mainly disorders that have in common psychotic symptoms or impaired reality testing, including two Axis II personality disorders:

- psychotic disorder due to a general medical condition
- substance-induced psychotic disorder
- schizophrenia
- schizophreniform disorder
- schizoaffective disorder
- delusional disorder
- bipolar disorder with psychotic features
- major depressive disorder with psychotic features
- brief psychotic disorder
- psychotic disorder NOS
- paranoid personality disorder
- schizotypal personality disorder

You could follow the diagnostic decision tree in Appendix A of DSM-IV-TR. You would then need to ask questions that allow you to make these decisions in proper order. DSM-IV-TR recommends excluding or verifying first a general medical condition when you encounter psychotic symptoms. Consequently, you would have to ask for any head injury or central nervous system disorder. In addition, you would have to examine the patient for the presence of disturbances usually associated with a cognitive disorder, such as fluctuations in alertness, distractibility, disorientation, amnesia, apraxias, agnosias, aphasias, or focal neurological signs and others as discussed in Chapters 4 and 5: Mental Status and Testing. If you cannot find a cognitive impairment due to a general medical condition, you would next have to exclude the direct physiological effect of a substance or toxin. Thereafter, ask for the duration of the psychotic symptoms. Did they last longer or shorter than a month? According to the answer, you will branch out to the next decision box until you end up at a "leaf," that is, a "point in the tree with no outgoing branches."

Such a diagnostic interview is, of course, possible, but it requires that you as interviewer take charge, direct the patient, and structure the diagnostic process: you ask the questions and the patient answers, preferably promptly and to the point. The problems with this approach are obvious. In your effort to follow your decision-making model, you will eliminate any spontaneity in the interview, suppress or possibly destroy rapport, and potentially lose valuable information. We therefore recommend that you postpone the decision making to the end of the interview. Let the patient move in different directions, let him elaborate here and there, and skip while you extract the descriptive features of his pathology.

Second, your list contains a wide variety of clinical, personality, adjustment, and mental disorders not otherwise specified (NOS; DSM-IV-TR), and psychosocial and environmental problems; a wide range of psychopathology—so to speak—without any focus on one of the 13 diagnostic areas. It is difficult to follow any single one of the proposed decision trees in DSM-IV-TR. An interviewer usually does what worked in the first situation (above). She scrutinizes her preliminary impressions by checking the descriptors of the collected symptoms and signs:

1. marking all symptoms and signs that are associated with a given disorder;
2. determining the duration of the symptoms and signs;
3. establishing the disabling nature of the symptoms;
4. listing preceding stressors; and
5. assessing the temporal relationship of the symptoms to each other.

For instance, if she finds hallucinations and delusions, she asks:

"What other symptoms emerged together with the hallucinations and delusions?"

"How long did they last? Did some last a shorter time than the others?"
"How much were you affected by these psychotic symptoms? Did you observe them with amusement, were they mainly present before sleep, or did they occupy all your time and energy?"
"Was there anything that brought them on abruptly, or did they sneak up on you slowly?"
"How did these hallucinations and delusions relate to your mood, your sleep and appetite disturbances, the guilt feelings and suicidal ruminations? Did they happen in a 2-week segment with a 6-month ordeal of mood disturbances, or did they dominate your life with depression occasionally fading in and out?"

Such an approach usually is comprehensive to the patient, memorable for the interviewer, and provides enough information to allow diagnostic decision making at a later stage.

In comparison to step 1, which was characterized by questions of high sensitivity, questions of step 2 usually have high specificity. Apply them to your preliminary diagnostic impressions formed at the end of step 1. They confirm or exclude certain diagnostic impressions.

With these descriptive features at hand, examine first the major psychiatric disorders of your diagnostic list, then the personality disorders. Finally, explore the psychosocial and environmental problems.

Clinical Disorders (Axis I)

How do you interview for clinical disorders?

During my psychiatric residency, one of our teachers impressed us with his interviewing style. He diagnosed a patient in a few minutes. "How does he do it?" I wondered. When I reconstructed his interviews after each session, I discovered he took advantage of the anatomy of the clinical disorders. First, he asked for the essential (core) symptoms and their severity. Then, he assessed associated, that is, less specific signs and symptoms only if the essential ones were present. When the essential symptoms were missing he would not waste time completing the catalog of symptoms for each disorder. He therefore avoided redundant exclusions.

Essential Symptoms

Table 6–1 lists essential symptoms for most clinical disorders. An essential symptom is a symptom that is necessary but not sufficient for the diagnosis of a disorder. For instance, you can diagnose alcohol abuse only when the patient drinks, or depression when your patient's mood is low.

Table 6–1 does not contain all DSM-IV-TR disorders and their sub-types—it is merely a demonstration guide. The essential symptoms for each disorder refer to the specific psychic functions that are disturbed in the respective disorder: level of consciousness, memory, and intelligence in the cognitive disorders; use of and control over substance intake in substance-related disorders; hallucinations, delusions, and grossly disorganized behavior in schizophrenia; territorial security in delusional disorder; mood, initiative, energy level, and risk taking in mood disorders; adaptation to threat in anxiety disorders; control over aggression, sexuality, and hygiene in obsessive-compulsive disorder; pain perception and somatic functioning in somatization disorder; amnesia and derealization in dissociative disorders; disturbances in sexual behavior and objects of desire, and cross-gender identification in sexual and gender-identity disorders; control over food intake in anorexia and bulimia nervosa; regulation of the sleep-wake cycle in sleep disorders; control of aggression in impulse control disorders; coping with stress in adjustment disorder; information processing in mental retardation. Most of the essential symptoms in Table 6–1 require associated significant impairment in social, occupational, or other important areas of functioning.

Questions to assess the essential symptoms of some of these disorders are listed below. Most have been validated (Othmer et al. 1989).

Cognitive disorders:

1. "What is your full name? I am going to say three words that I'd like you to remember. They are pencil, car, and watch. Would you say them? Good. I want you to remember the three words. It's very important. I am going to ask you to say them to me in a few minutes. Remember, the words are pencil, car, and watch."

2. "When were you born? What is the date of your birth?"

3. "What day of the week is today?"

4. "What month is it now?"

5. "What is today's date?"

6. "What year is this?"

7. "What is the name of this place we are in now?"

8. "What is the name of the city (or town, district, county) we are in now?"

9. "Would you tell me the names of two presidents of the United States?"

10." Now I am going to say a sentence. When I am through I want you to repeat exactly what I said. Ready? Listen."

a) "Next week I am going to take a drive in my green car."

b) "Tomorrow I am going to get some sugar and flour from the store."

11. "Would you tell me the three words I asked you to remember? What are the three words?"

12. "Now I am going to ask you to write a sentence: 'The sky is blue'."

Mental retardation:

"While you were in school, did anyone ever say that you were a very slow learner?"

If no:

"Did you ever have to go into a special education class when you were in school?"

Substance-related disorders:

1. "Has heavy drug or alcohol use ever caused you problems in your life?"

If yes:

"Has heavy drug use, or drinking, been a problem to you over the past year?"
2. "Have you ever used pot, speed, crack, heroin, ice, or any other drugs to make yourself feel good?"

If yes:

"Has anyone ever remarked on your use of drugs over the past year?"

Schizophrenia:

1. "Have you ever heard voices or seen things that no one else could hear or see?"
2. "Have you ever felt your mind or body was being secretly controlled, or controlled somehow against your will?"
3. "Have you ever felt others wanted to hurt you or really get you for some special reason, maybe because you had secrets or special powers of some sort?"
4. "Have you ever had any other strange, odd, or very peculiar things happen to you?"

If yes:

"Please tell me what they were."

If yes to any of the above:

5. "Did this happen even when you were not drinking or taking drugs?"

FIVE STEPS TO MAKE A DIAGNOSIS

Bipolar disorder, manic episode:

1. "Have there ever been times when you felt unusually high, charged up, excited, or restless for 1 week at a time?"
2. "Have there ever been times when other people said that you were too high, too charged up, too excited, or too talkative?"

If yes:

3. "How long do these mood changes usually last?"

If less than 1 week:

"What is the longest they have ever lasted?"

If still less than 1 week:

"Have these high, excitable moods ever stayed with you most of the time for at least 1 week?"

Major depressive disorder:

1. "Have there ever been times when you felt unusually depressed, empty, sad, or hopeless for several days or weeks at a time?"
2. "Have there ever been times when you felt very irritable or tired most of the time for hardly any reason at all?"

If yes on item 1 or 2:

3. "How long do these feelings usually last?"

If less than 2 weeks:

"What is the longest they ever lasted?"

If still less than 2 weeks:

"Have these feelings ever stayed with you most of the time for as long as 2 weeks?"

Panic disorder:

1. "Have you ever had sudden spells or attacks of nervousness, panic, or strong fear that just seem to come over you all of a sudden, out of the blue, for no particular reason?"

If yes on 1:

2. "Did you have these attacks even though a doctor said that there was nothing seriously wrong with your heart?"

If no:

"Tell me what the doctor said was wrong with your heart."

Phobic disorders:

1. "Have you ever been much more afraid of things the average person is not
afraid of? Like flying, heights, animals, needles, thunder, lightning, the sight
of blood, things like that?"

If yes:

"What were you afraid of?"
2. "Have you ever been so afraid to leave home by yourself that you wouldn't
go out, even though you knew it was really safe?"
3. "Have you ever been afraid to go into places like supermarkets, tunnels, or ·
elevators because you were afraid of not getting out?"
4. "Have you ever been so afraid of embarrassing yourself in public that you
would not do certain things most people do? Like eating in a restaurant, using a public restroom, or speaking out in a room full of people?"

If yes to any of the above:

"When your fears were the strongest, did you try to avoid or stay away from
(name feared stimulus) whenever you could?"

Obsessive-compulsive disorder:

1. "Have you ever been bothered by certain embarrassing, scary, or ridiculous thoughts that came into your mind over and over even though you tried
to ignore or stop them?"

If yes:

"Please describe them."
2. "Have you ever felt you had to repeat a certain act over and over even
though it didn't make much sense? Like checking or counting something
over and over or washing your hands over and over again though you knew
they were clean?"

Posttraumatic stress disorder:

"Have you ever experienced flashbacks, when you found yourself reliving some terrible experience over and over again?"

Generalized anxiety disorder:

1. "Have there ever been days at a time when you felt extremely nervous, anxious, or tense for no special reason?"

If yes:

"Have you sometimes felt this way even when you were at home with nothing special to do?"

If yes:

2. "Have these nervous or anxious feelings ever bothered you off and on for as long as 6 months or more at a time?"

Somatization disorder:

1. "Have you had a lot of physical problems in your life that forced you to see different doctors?"

If yes:

"Have doctors had trouble finding what caused these physical problems?"
2. "Did you start having any of these problems before you were 30 years old?"

Anorexia nervosa:

"Have you ever deliberately lost so much weight on a diet that people started to seriously worry about your health?"

If yes:

"Were you afraid of getting fat even when other people said you were thin enough?"

Bulimia nervosa:

1. "Did you ever have a problem with binge eating, when you would eat so much food so fast that it made you feel sick?"

If yes:

2. "When you were doing this, did you feel your eating binges were not really normal?"

If yes:

3. "Was the urge to binge sometimes so strong that you could not stop, even though you wanted to?"

If yes:

4. "After you had binged, did you often feel depressed, ashamed, and disgusted with yourself?"

If yes:

5. "Did you ever vomit after eating, use laxatives, or excessively exercise?"

Adjustment disorder:

1. "In the last 3 months have you been very worried or upset about something that happened to you? Like the death of a loved one, loss of a job, separation, divorce, an accident, serious illness, or that sort of thing?"

If yes:

2. "Do you feel that you had more trouble handling this situation than most people would have had?"

If you have identified an essential symptom of a psychiatric disorder, establish how long the symptom has been present. For example, has the patient been depressed, tense, and irritable for at least 2 weeks?

After you have identified essential symptoms and their duration, the next step is to assess severity. DSM-IV-TR considers as symptoms those complaints that cause "clinically significant distress or impairment in social, occupational, or other important areas of functioning." A patient who complains occasionally of feeling down but who fully functions at work and in his family and social life has a complaint, but it has not yet reached the intensity of a symptom. He may be mildly dysphoric but cannot be considered to have a psychiatric disorder. Zung (1972) reported on dysphoric mood in the general United States population: 48% were dysphoric under age 19, and 44% in the age bracket over 60 had abnormally high Zung Depression Scores. Data from a population of air traffic controllers also showed abnormally high depression scores (Barrett et al. 1978). These groups may not suffer from clinical depression, even though they admit to depressive feelings. Therefore, if you encounter a symptom, determine whether the symptom interfered with the patient's life; explore, for instance, whether he got into arguments, or abused his children, or was impatient with his customers, has missed work, was criticized by his spouse, lost a friend, needed outpatient treatment, or hospitalization.

Below are eight empirically tested questions to assess dysfunction by social interference. If the patient answers "yes" to one of the questions, in approximately 90% of the cases he will also fulfill the associated symptoms of that disorder (Othmer et al. 1989).

1. "Has [essential symptom, e.g., drinking, drug use, mood changes, etc.] ever interfered with your school, your work, or your job?"
2. "Has . . . ever caused you any problems with your family, or caused your family to worry about you?"
3. "Has . . . ever interfered with your social activities or friendships?"
4. "Have you ever gotten into trouble with the authorities because of your . . . ?"
5. "Has your health ever suffered from . . . ?"
6. "Have you ever received medication or treatment for your . . . ?"
7. "Were you ever hospitalized for . . . ?"
8. "When you had . . . were you able to live alone?"

When the patient has a psychiatric disorder, the effect on the patient is threefold: psychosocial impairment, interpersonal distress, and personal suffering. The patient may not understand that he is impaired psychosocially but he knows that he is suffering. Personal suffering frequently correlates with objective dysfunction.

Severity of the illness is reflected in a number of areas, including the family's reactions, social sanctions, impairment to general health, and the patient's general level of functioning. The response of the patient's family can be a key indicator. They may criticize, show disrespect, and ostracize the patient, or be supportive when the patient's suffering is clearly visible, as in the anxiety disorders.

Severity is also measured by the response of the public. Clearly, when law and order are violated through reckless driving, driving while intoxicated, or disturbance of the peace, the patient has a serious problem. Society also looks down on alcoholism and substance abuse, and may shun persons with other disturbing mental disorders, such as schizophrenia or bipolar disorder.

Severity can also be determined by the impairment to general health resulting from the disorder as, for instance, in alcoholism, substance abuse, and the cognitive disorders.

Severity is determined by the patient's general level of functioning. If you see a patient who has no clear chief complaint and you converse with him instead of exploring his problems, you may get an impression of his level of functioning before you know what factors impair it. DSM-IV-TR (American Psychiatric Association 2000) provides a Global Assessment of Functioning Scale (GAF Scale) that allows you to measure his level of functioning (see below section 3: Psychiatric History).

Associated Symptoms

After determining the essential symptoms, assess associated symptoms. An associated symptom is one that is frequently present in a disorder but not necessary for its diagnosis. For instance, insomnia is seen in depression, but also in many other disorders such as substance abuse, schizophrenia, bipolar disorder, and anxiety disorders. Associated symptoms are often vegetative, for example, anorexia, hyperphagia, or sexual dysfunction. They may also appear as unexplained pain in the lower back, abdomen, or head; as somatic perceptions such as dizziness, paresthesias, and weakness; or as general symptoms such as lethargy, tension, hopelessness, fear, and discouragement.

The number of associated symptoms for a disorder varies from patient to patient. A minimum number has to be present to fulfill diagnostic criteria for a disorder (see DSM-IV-TR). Assess them by asking open-ended questions such as:

> "What else have you noticed when you get depressed, you have your highs, your panic spells, and so forth?"

Most patients will list several symptoms. After such a patient-centered question use "disorder-centered" ones to confirm the diagnosis, such as:

"When you get depressed, how is your sleep . . . your appetite . . . your sex life, your concentration, your thoughts about the future, and your job performance?"

Make sure all associated symptoms concurred with the essential symptom(s) at the same time period. Find out which symptoms accompanied each other, and which occurred sporadically. The time reference is crucial to verify a past psychiatric disorder. Repeat the essential symptom or chief complaint when you ask for associated symptoms, or ask the patient whether the reported symptoms occurred together (see Q. 6 below):

1. I: What brought you here, Mrs. Holmes?
   P: I'm getting depressed again and cry very easily.
2. I: Can you tell me more about it?
   P: It seems to happen any time of the day, I get tearful and I start sobbing.
3. I: Have you had any other problems?
   P: Oh yes. I have bursting headaches and my sleep is not good.
4. I: Any problems with eating?
   P: Yes, how do you know? I had a raving appetite and gained close to 60 pounds.
5. I: Any other problems with eating?
   P: Maybe I should tell you about my vomiting. I thought I spit my heart out.
6. I: It is not clear to me whether all the problems happen at the same time.
   P: Oh, is that what you meant? Oh no. I had the problem with vomiting when I was pregnant.
7. I: What about the overeating?
   P: That was 3 years ago.
8. I: And with your sleep?
   P: That was the worst after I had the baby.
9. I: How is your sleep now?
   P: Oh it's fine. Maybe I sleep too long. I seem to be real exhausted.
10. I: And your appetite?
    P: Right now?
11. I: Yes.
    P: Too good. I even get up at night to get a snack. Can't stay away from that refrigerator.
12. I: Besides your crying spells and sobbing, what else has changed with you?
    P: I worry about my older daughter. She got herself pregnant and my husband is blaming me. I always had problems with my children and my husband.

If the interviewer had not clarified the temporal relationship of the symptoms, he could have mistaken them as associated symptoms of depression. However, the symptoms scattered over time suggested somatization disorder, a diagnosis that he later confirmed.

If your patient reports a sufficient number of associated symptoms to meet criteria for a major psychiatric disorder, you have established the inclusion criteria for that disorder. Now proceed in the same way for all other major disorders for which essential symptoms are positive.

Exclusion

If you have determined a patient's essential symptoms, their duration and severity, and have established the required number of associated symptoms, you now have sufficient information to diagnose the disorder. Yet you must await the results of your background exploration (see below section 3: Psychiatric History), since medical disorders can mimic psychiatric disorders. The presence of such a medical disorder may exclude the presence of a psychiatric disorder. In addition, in some cases, the symptoms of psychiatric disorders are also shared by some other psychiatric disorders (see below section 4: Diagnoses).

Sometimes you encounter essential symptoms of a clinical disorder but they do not interfere with the patient's life. For instance, a patient may notice chronic depressed mood, or anxiety, or anger, but none of these feelings interfere with his work, his family life, or leisure activities. He notices them but can overcome and control them. These feelings are subjectively noticed by the patient but do not impair him. In these cases, observe the patient but defer the diagnosis of a clinical disorder. Mild symptoms could herald the onset of the disorder.

Essential symptoms can also be too short in duration to meet criteria. If the symptoms are severe, it is best to make the diagnosis anyway, especially when the patient has to be hospitalized.

If essential symptoms are long and severe enough to meet criteria but are not accompanied by a sufficient number of associated symptoms, diagnose a not otherwise specified mental disorder (NOS). One study found such an incomplete manifestation of a disorder in 15%–20% of patients with positive essential symptoms (Othmer et al. 1989).

Personality Disorders (Axis II)

Like Axis I clinical disorders, personality disorders are defined categorically rather than dimensionally. If you try to verify a personality disorder, examine whether the patient fulfills the two sets of criteria typical for the anatomy of a personality disorder according to DSM-IV-TR:

1. Six general diagnostic criteria for a personality disorder (see DSM-IV-TR, A–F; American Psychiatric Association 2000, p. 689). These criteria de-

scribe a lifelong inflexible pattern of maladjustment in perceiving, feeling, relating, thinking, and impulse control in a wide range of social and
personal relationships causing significant functional impairment and
subjective distress.

2. The specific pattern of maladjustment that characterizes and defines
   each of the 10 personality disorders. This pattern can be viewed as a maladjusted pattern of response to general or specific triggers.

Patterned Lifelong Maladjustment

In a personality disorder, the pattern of maladjustment resurfaces throughout the patient's life. For instance, a patient displays symptoms of dysphoria, anxiety, and clinging whenever she anticipates or experiences a loss
of support. When you observe such a reaction, ask about a lifelong recurrent pattern, which is essential for a personality disorder.

Here is a case example that emerged in a conversation between a patient from Pakistan and the interviewer.

P: I'm crying day and night after I came here from Pakistan. I'm anxious, home-
    sick, and depressed and do not want to meet new friends. I lock myself in the
    bathroom. I cry and carry on and often keep the apartment complex awake by
    hollering and screaming at night. I can't adjust. I don't want my husband to
    leave.

I: Do you feel comfortable answering a few questions about yourself?

P: Sure, go ahead.

I: Tell me a little bit about your marriage. Was it prearranged by your parents?

P: Yes, it was.

I: When you got married, you moved in with your husband?

P: Yes, I did. Our wedding lasted 3 days and then I moved in with him.

I: Can you tell me how you felt when you moved in with him?

P: Oh, I cried for the first 2–3 weeks, was depressed, and called home all the time.

I: That sounds similar to the reaction you have now after you came to the States.

P: Hmm . . . I hadn't thought about that. You're right.

I: Do you know any other situations where you showed a similar response as
    when you got married and when you got to the United States?

P: When I moved away from Karachi, I had the same problem. I also had a hard
    time adjusting when I went to college. I felt like I couldn't survive without help.

I: You see? One so-called adjustment problem rarely comes alone. It seems to be
    hard for you to get away from your family and friends and adjust to a new envi-
    ronment.

P: Right, that's my feeling too. I seem to be very sensitive to loss of support.

I: Have you noticed that you got depressed or discouraged at any other times?
    Even when there is not a major change?

P: Let me see . . . Yes, I had a bad time when my parents could not come to visit
      me in college. I also cried at my sister's birthday when I could not go back
      home from college to be with her.

The stressor that triggered maladjusted behavior in the patient was the
loss of support and familiar environment. The maladjusted response is her
inability to overcome or restructure her need for support. This inability may
make her seek new dependencies rather than develop autonomy. Her repetitive maladjusted behavior shows a dramatic display of a childlike loss
reaction with depressive symptoms, which possibly qualifies her for the diagnosis of dependent personality disorder. However, the interviewer should
discuss with the husband whether her behavior is considered maladaptive
in her own culture.

Specific Pattern of Maladjustment

For a patient with dependent personality disorder, the loss of a close, supportive relationship is a trigger for her maladjustment. She perceives the loss
as a threat to her lifeline and herself as totally dependent upon this lost nurturing symbiosis. She responds to the loss with a host of depressive and
anxious symptoms and clinging behavior that, in contrast to major depression, remit with regaining of support and nurturing.

   Most patients with a personality disorder show patterns of maladjustment
with persons in three types of relationships or situations: intimate or sexual,
or familial; with organized social groups, at church or leisure activities; and
with colleagues at work. Therefore, ask the patient to describe her relationship to others. Explore whether your patient is callous, suspicious, or exploit-
ative, and whether she seems to fear, or be overly attached to, these groups.

   A more direct approach is to ask whether there are certain situations
that the patient has difficulties handling and may therefore dread and avoid.
She may describe the situations that trigger recurring maladjusted behaviors
and reveal a, to you, distorted perception of these situations.

   "Whenever I meet new people I prefer not to talk to them because I fear they
   may reject and criticize me. People are very critical. They seem to enjoy hurting you. Especially when they find out that you are weak, they take advantage of you. If you stay away from them, they are less likely to bother you."
   [avoidant personality]

   The interview itself is often a trigger situation for maladjusted responses. Observe if the patient relates to you during the interview in a pe-

culiar way. For instance, he is either blunt in his affect without being depressed or having hallucinations (schizoid personality); or dramatic, self-centered, and flirtatious (histrionic personality); or somewhat anxious, clinging, and asking for reassurance (dependent personality).

Find out what situations or stressors a patient is sensitive to. That will help you to identify the coping deficit and establish the diagnosis of a specific personality disorder. Most patients with a so-called "adjustment reaction" to a stressor also show a tendency for repetition, indicating a chronic coping deficit, in other words, a personality disorder. Thus the adjustment reaction may be the cross-sectional presentation of a personality disorder. A host of depressive and anxious symptoms accompany such a maladjusted reaction. These symptoms may occur at the mere anticipation of the trigger situation. Therefore whenever your patient reports a maladjustment, try to identify a possible stressor and screen her past for similar reactions to identify the underlying coping deficit. If the patient reports repetitive adjustment reactions, be alerted. Rigid, ingrained repetitiveness violates the essential criterion for an adjustment disorder.

Some patients do not describe a specific situation but a lifelong pattern of maladjustment, either symptoms or behaviors. Here is an example for lifelong symptoms:

"I'm shy and anxious and easily scared. I would like to be popular but I'm so afraid of being rejected. I'm inhibited and can't speak up for myself." [avoidant personality]

When the patient describes lifelong symptoms, link them to a clinical disorder. After remission, clinical disorders can leave some patients with a residual personality disorder (Winokur and Crowe 1975). Thus, personality disorders can sometimes be viewed as mild forms of the clinical disorders. They can also be precursors of the clinical disorders. Personality disorders show specific comorbidity and familial occurrence with clinical and other personality disorders. Thus, personality disorders and clinical disorders can be viewed as belonging to a spectrum that may have a genetic component (see Table 6–2). The studies for Table 6–2 have different reference points for Cluster A and B disorders (see next subsection, "Classification of Personality Disorders," for description of the three clusters of personality disorders specified in DSM-IV-TR). For Cluster A, the probands have the disorders listed under Familial Occurrence in column 3. For instance, probands with chronic schizophrenia or delusional disorder, paranoid type, have increased occurrence of paranoid personality disorder in their first-degree biological

Table 6–2. Personality disorders: comorbidity and familial occurrence

Personality disorder (prevalence in the general population)	Comorbid disorders	Familial occurrence (first-degree biological relatives)
Cluster A		
Paranoid (0.5%–2.5%)	Brief psychotic disorder Delusional disorder Schizophrenia Major depression Agoraphobia Obsessive-compulsive disorders Alcohol abuse Substance abuse Cluster A personality disorders Borderline personality disorder Narcissistic personality disorder Avoidant personality disorder	Probands with chronic schizophrenia or delusional disorder, persecutory type have increased occurrence of paranoid personality disorder
Schizoid (unknown)	Brief psychotic episodes Delusional disorder Schizophrenia Major depression Cluster A personality disorders Avoidant personality disorder	Probands with schizophrenia or schizotypal personality disorder have increased occurrence of schizoid personality disorder

		Schizophrenia (probands)
Schizotypal (3%)	Brief psychotic episodes	
	Schizophreniform disorder	
	Delusional disorder	
	Schizophrenia	
	Major depression	
	Cluster A personality disorders	
	Borderline personality disorder	
	Avoidant personality disorder	
Schizotypal (probands)		Schizophrenia and other psychotic disorders
Cluster B		
Antisocial (probands) (males: 3%; females: 1%)	Pathological gambling	Antisocial personality disorder
	Impulse-control disorder	Somatization disorder
	Substance-related disorders	Substance-related disorder
	Anxiety disorders	
	Depressive disorders	
	Somatization disorder	
	Other Cluster B disorders	
	Early-onset conduct disorder with ADHD	
Borderline (probands) (2%)	Substance-related disorders	Borderline personality disorder
	Bulimia nervosa	Antisocial personality disorder
	Posttraumatic stress disorder	Substance-related disorders
	Mood disorders	Mood disorders
	Attention-deficit/hyperactivity disorder	
	Other personality disorders	

(continued)

Table 6–2. Personality disorders: comorbidity and familial occurrence *(continued)*

Personality disorder (prevalence in the general population)	Comorbid disorders	Familial occurrence (first-degree biological relatives)
Histrionic (2%–3%)	Somatization disorder Conversion disorder Major depressive disorder Other Cluster B disorders Dependent personality disorder	No data
Narcissistic (<1%)	Dysthymic disorder Major depressive disorder Anorexia nervosa Substance-related disorders Other Cluster B disorders Paranoid personality disorder	No data
Cluster C		
Avoidant (0.5%–1%)	Mood disorders Anxiety disorders, especially social phobia Cluster A personality disorders Borderline personality disorder Dependent personality disorder	No data

Dependent (unknown)	Mood disorders Anxiety disorders Separation anxiety disorder Adjustment disorder Borderline personality disorder Avoidant personality disorder Histrionic personality disorder	No data
Obsessive-compulsive (1%)	Anxiety disorders (probands)	No data
Obsessive-compulsive (probands)	Mood disorders Eating disorders	

relatives. However, for schizotypal personality disorder probands, we also know the comorbidity in first-degree relatives. The family studies of Cluster B start out with the probands who have a personality disorder listed in column 1. For instance, probands with antisocial personality disorder have first-degree relatives with antisocial personality disorder, somatization disorder (in females), and substance-related disorders. For histrionic and narcissistic personality disorders (Cluster B) and all Cluster C disorders, no family studies are listed in DSM-IV-TR. Table 6–2 clarifies that probands with obsessive-compulsive personality disorder have as comorbidity mood and eating disorders rather than obsessive-compulsive disorder. However, patients with an anxiety disorder, including obsessive-compulsive disorder, may also have first-degree relatives with obsessive-compulsive personality disorder. For a psychodiagnostic interview, it is important to investigate such relationships.

Research on linkage among specific psychiatric disorders and personality disorders over recent years is incomplete and has produced complex and partly contradictory results (Fulton and Winokur 1993; Eppright et al. 1993; Lilienfeld et al. 1986; Gunderson and Sabo 1993; Thaker et al. 1993; Southwick et al. 1993). Several of these studies include family history data to decide whether specific Axis I psychiatric disorders congregate in the family of patients with certain personality disorders (Black et al. 1993). Paranoid personality, for example, may phenomenologically belong with a spectrum of schizophrenia, paranoid type, and delusional disorder. The strength of the genetic link awaits further study (Fulton and Winokur 1993). A review of the present literature is beyond the scope of this book.

Classification of Personality Disorders

Personality disorders can be classified by a maladjustment in social and interpersonal situations affecting two or more areas (Table 6–3):

1. Cognition
2. Interpersonal functioning
3. Affectivity
4. Impulse control

DSM-IV-TR groups personality disorders into three clusters. The first cluster, referred to as *Cluster A*, includes paranoid, schizoid, and schizotypal personality disorders. People with these disorders often appear odd or eccentric. The second cluster, referred to as *Cluster B*, includes antisocial, borderline, his-

Table 6–3. Personality disorders as maladjusted patterns of cognition, interpersonal functioning, and affectivity/impulse control

Personality disorder	Situation	Cognition	Interpersonal functioning	Affectivity/ impulse control
Cluster A				
Paranoid	Close interpersonal relations	"People sneak up on me and harm me."	Guarded distance, secretive, devious, scheming, counter-attacking	Suspicious, jealous, angry, hypervigilant
Schizoid	Close interpersonal relations	"People are meaningless to me."	Avoids social involvement	Cold, stiff, distant, aloof
Schizotypal	Close interpersonal relations	"Others have special magic intentions."	Imagines love or rejection without evidence	Inappropriate excitement, hostile aloofness
Cluster B				
Antisocial	Social standards and rules	"Rules limit me from fulfilling my needs."	Violation of social rules, standards, and law	Impulsively angry, hostile, cunning
Borderline	Personal goals, close relations	"Goals are good; no, they are not; people are great, no they are not."	Changing goals, ambivalent relations	Labile mood and affect
Histrionic	Heterosexual relations	"I have to show intense emotions to impress."	Flirts, shows exaggerated, nongenuine emotions	Excited by positive, dysphoric by negative response
Narcissistic	Evaluation of self	"I'm the only person that counts."	Self-centeredness, expects recognition without contributions	Labile, grandiose, deflated feelings

(continued)

Table 6–3. Personality disorders as maladjusted patterns of cognition, interpersonal functioning, and affectivity/impulse control *(continued)*

Personality disorder	Situation	Cognition	Interpersonal functioning	Affectivity/ impulse control
Cluster C				
Avoidant	Close interpersonal relations, public appearance	"People reject and criticize me."	Escapes and avoids social appearances	Anxious, withdrawn
Dependent	Self-reliance, being alone	"I hate to be alone."	Giving up own goals to cling to others (parents)	Anxious, panicky
Obsessive-compulsive	Close relationships, unstructured situations, authority	"My rules must prevail, uncertainty is frightening; feelings interfere with thinking.	Emotional restriction, rigid, angry if his rules are broken; defiance of authority	Anxious, angry, resentful
Personality disorders not otherwise specified (NOS)				
Depressive	Self-image, attitude toward others	"I am inadequate and worthless. Others are not helpful either."	Self-derogatory, critical and judgmental of others	Gloomy, remorseful
Passive-aggressive (negativistic)	Deadlines, demands to perform	"They impose on my freedom, but it is dangerous to resist openly."	Procrastination, broken commitments	Anxious, angry, resentful
Sadistic	Weak, dependent persons	"I have to show them who is boss; I can make them eat shit."	Cruel, restrictive acts against defenseless people	Pleasure derived from the suffering of others
Self-defeating	Situations and relationships difficult to master	"I have to endure hardship to prove myself worthwhile."	Enters or creates situations that promise hardship	Indulges in suffering

trionic, and narcissistic personality disorders. The third cluster, referred to as *Cluster C*, includes avoidant, dependent, and obsessive-compulsive personality disorders. When you diagnose a personality disorder, decide which cluster best fits the patient's behavior by using Table 6–3 and answering the following three questions:

1. Does the patient tend to be isolated because of socially cold, suspicious, or strange behavior?
2. Does he impose on others; is he dramatic and self-centered?
3. Is he afraid of others, anxious, submissive, or restricted?

Cluster A: During the interview the patient appears suspicious, blunted, odd, or eccentric. He may tell you that others think he is a loner, inaccessible, hard to get to know, and easy to overlook and ignore. He may be described as untrustworthy, strange, and "nutty."

During the interview, ask the patient who shows paranoid perceptions whether he has friends he can trust, or whether it is easy for him to open up to others. He may answer that he cannot trust anybody, thus concurring with your impression of a paranoid personality.

Ask the patient who appears blunt and disinterested whether he is usually unemotional, or disinterested in other people's feelings. He may answer that he feels as much as the computer he plays games with, thus qualifying for the diagnosis of schizoid personality disorder.

Ask the patient with out-of-body experiences, superstitious beliefs, oddities in dressing, or peculiarities in responding whether he has experienced extrasensory perception. His vividly described experiences will help you to establish the diagnosis of a schizotypal personality disorder.

Cluster B: Such a patient appears emotionally labile, or shows excessive emotional responses during the interview. He may report that he is flying off the handle easily, and that others call him unstable and erratic. He may say he cannot establish stable relationships. Check the chronicity of these behaviors. You may ask:

"You seem to be a very emotional person."
"It appears to me that you have stronger feelings than others."
"Do you think that being more emotional has affected your relationship to others?"

Most patients with a Cluster B personality disorder will agree with your perceptions. After you have established hyperemotionality, assess characteristics that differentiate the disorders of this cluster.

Illegal or violent actions that started in the teenage years point to the diagnosis of antisocial personality. This disorder is more common in males. Rapid mood swings (with or without a history of bipolar disorder), self-mutilation, suicide attempts, or even brief psychotic-like experiences occurring during stress may indicate a borderline personality. Exaggerated, multiple unexplained somatic symptoms are more often reported by females than males. They involve menstruation, sexual activity, and the abdomen. Such complaints may suggest the diagnosis of histrionic personality.

Egocentric and grandiose behavior, with little regard for others, may portend the diagnosis of narcissistic personality. Similarities in the symptom profiles of these personality disorders with somatization disorder and rapidly cycling bipolar disorder have been observed.

Cluster C: A patient in Cluster C appears anxious, dysphoric, phobic, or obsessive during the interview. To differentiate the disorders in this cluster, look for the following characteristics:

- If he is shy, weighs his words, asks for reassurance, or speaks up reluctantly, consider avoidant personality.
- If he is clinging, too dependent, always requiring care, or inviting aggression, consider dependent personality.
- If he appears perfectionistic, tries to be precise, is annoyed by unstructured situations, consider obsessive-compulsive personality disorder.

Personality disorders not otherwise specified (NOS): Sometimes a patient shows a variety of pathological responses, depending on the social situation. He may show dependent behavior toward authority figures, obsessive demanding behavior toward subordinates, and passive-aggressive tendencies toward colleagues. This is where diagnosing becomes complex. DSM-IV-TR allows you to assign more than one personality disorder. This rule transforms the typological into a multidimensional approach.

Table 10–1 in Chapter 10 lists DSM-IV-TR criteria for 10 personality disorders. It can also be used in identifying features of personality disorders, including those personality disorders that have characteristics of more than one specific personality disorder.

Personality disorder NOS can also be used for personality disorders that in DSM-IV-TR need further study, such as depressive and passive-aggressive (negativistic) personality disorders. Furthermore, DSM-IV (American Psychiatric Association 1994) considered sadistic and self-defeating personality disorders as possible entities. These four personality disorders are listed in Table 6–3.

Psychosocial and Environmental Problems (Axis IV)

The chief complaint may reflect a psychosocial problem. Louise is a 48-year-old, stay-at-home mother of three children. She complains about difficulties dealing with her husband. He is too demanding, pushes her too hard, and has no understanding for her feelings. Until a few months ago she could keep up with his demands, but lately they have overwhelmed her. She also reports that she does not love her children anymore because they are so rebellious.

Such an interpersonal conflict may be a clinical disorder, a personality disorder, an adjustment reaction, or a psychosocial problem. Check all four possibilities.

First, examine whether the interpersonal conflict is the expression of a clinical disorder. Attempt to translate the conflict into symptoms by temporarily ignoring the content of the complaint and instead focusing on the disturbed psychic functions. Probe for symptoms such as irritability, low energy, decreased sex drive, and social withdrawal. Then search for essential features that are associated with these symptoms. For instance, ask about recent substance abuse, or depressed feelings expressed in crying spells, bouts of hopelessness, guilt, and disturbances in appetite and sleep. Find out whether the patient may have obsessive thoughts or compulsions that make her too rigid in dealing with her family, or somatic symptoms that draw her attention to her physical problems and deprive her of the patience necessary to handle her family. If you can translate the patient's psychosocial problems into essential symptoms of a clinical disorder, pursue that disorder rather than an adjustment disorder.

Explore whether the psychosocial problem is caused by a personality disorder. If the problem has recurred throughout her life, find out whether it arose from a coping deficit in handling certain situations such as living independently, making and keeping contact with people, or establishing and maintaining stable relationships. A lifelong recurrent coping deficit points to a personality disorder.

Consider an adjustment disorder if you find a onetime stressor followed by some psychiatric symptoms, provided you can first exclude clinical disorders and personality disorders. Indeed, the prevalence of adjustment disorders is strongly related to environmental factors. In the general population, it is

2%–8%. In a hospital inpatient consultation service, it is 12%. In a mental health outpatient setting, it is 10%–30%. In populations of patients who have experienced a specific stressor such as cardiac surgery, it is 50%. The prognosis of this disorder is worsened in patients, especially younger ones who have a comorbid condition such as attention-deficit/hyperactivity disorder. In these patients, the adjustment disorder may progress to a more severe mental disorder.

If the interpersonal conflict cannot be explained by a clinical disorder, a personality disorder, or an adjustment disorder, consider a psychosocial problem without a psychiatric disorder, a condition that becomes the focus of treatment due to its life-disrupting qualities:

- academic problems
- adult antisocial behavior
- bereavement
- borderline intellectual functioning
- childhood or adolescent antisocial behavior
- malingering
- noncompliance with treatment
- occupational problems
- other conditions that may be the focus of clinical attention
- other interpersonal problem
- other specified family circumstances
- parent-child problem
- phase-of-life problem

DSM-IV-TR proposes nine categories for psychosocial and environmental problems. These problems can have dramatic effects on patients in a number of different ways. They may affect the diagnosis, the treatment, or the prognosis of Axis I and Axis II disorders. Some examples of psychosocial and environmental problems include: family problems, death of a significant other or a child, sexual or child abuse, difficulty with acculturation, illiteracy, extreme poverty, problems at work or unemployment in general, and legal problems (either as perpetrator or victim). These can be called "problems of living" or "outside stressors." Acute and severe stressors are often reported as chief complaints:

> "My son committed suicide, and after that happened I cried all the time, neglected my daughter, and became quite irritable with my husband."

Also, patients focus on the stressor, rather than on their reaction to it, when the impact of the stressor is expected to strike in the future:

"My husband told me he wants a divorce."
"My daughter has a boyfriend and I'm afraid they will get married soon. He is a military man, and expects to go to Germany. Since she is my only child and I'm a widow, there will be nothing left for me but my pet canary."

If a patient talks about a stressor as the cause of his psychiatric problems, then it is important to investigate the relationship between the stressor and the disorder (Zimmerman et al. 1985). In this instance the Axis IV psychosocial and environmental problems may give rise to an adjustment disorder of Axis I, thus showing a cause-and-effect relationship.

A psychosocial or environmental problem (stressor) may be related to a psychiatric disorder in five different ways: 1) as a time marker, 2) as a magnifier of psychiatric symptoms, 3) as a consequence of a psychiatric disorder, 4) as a trigger, or 5) as a cause of a psychiatric disorder.

If a patient claims a stressor is the source of his distress, the most conservative assumption is to doubt this explanation and assume that the stressor is just a memorable event that coincides somewhat with the onset of a psychiatric disorder; in other words, such a stressor is a *time marker*.

To accept a stressor as more than that, you have to go beyond description. To accept a stressor as cause is an interpretation that cannot be proven with certainty. Here is what you can do: Exclude the possibility that the named stressor is merely a result of the psychiatric disorder rather than its cause as, for instance, a magnifier of the impact, or a consequence of the disorder. You also want to exclude a life stressor as a mere trigger before you accept the stressor as a true cause (compare in the Glossary, **stressor**).

Maladaptive Reaction

After you have explored the nature of the stressor, evaluate the maladaptive reaction. It may manifest itself in two ways, behaviorally and symptomatically. Behaviorally, the patient may show a decline in occupational functioning, social activities, or in his relationships to others. Symptomatically, the patient may report symptoms and show signs in excess of what you would normally expect as a reaction to stress.

DSM-IV-TR lists six maladaptive reactions as part of an adjustment disorder as follows: with anxiety, with depressed mood, with disturbance of conduct, with mixed disturbance of emotions and conduct, with mixed anxiety and depressed mood, and NOS. Mixtures among them may also occur. The reaction should be time limited and not persist beyond 6 months; otherwise, a diagnosis different from adjustment reaction should be made.

Adjustment disorders are associated with suicide attempts, suicide, substance abuse, and somatic complaints. They may cause decreased compliance with the treatment of a general medical condition.

Three-Month Rule

DSM-IV-TR requires that you demonstrate a temporal relationship but not a causality between stressor and response. The maladaptive reaction has to occur within 3 months of the stressor and not persist for more than 6 months. This arbitrary rule excludes psychiatric disorders that follow a stressor by a year (anniversary reaction) or more.

Exclusion of Clinical Disorders

Symptoms of adjustment reactions resemble those of major depressive disorder, anxiety disorders, or antisocial personality disorder, respectively. The patient's and family's history and the mental status will distinguish them. Exclude as adjustment reactions psychiatric disorders that fulfill criteria for any other DSM-IV-TR Axis I or Axis II disorders. The patient's perception of psychological causality between stressor and response then becomes irrelevant for the diagnosis, but—of course—not for the treatment of the disorder.

Accepting an insufficient number of depressive symptoms as part of an adjustment reaction rather than major depressive disorder NOS becomes plausible when the patient has neither a personal nor family history of mood disorder and when the symptom profile is distinct from a mood disorder; for instance, if the patient is distractible, and depressed only when reminded of the stressor, has no vegetative symptoms (such as anorexia or early morning awakening), and is tearful and requests assurance rather than being emotionally withdrawn.

A patient with a personality disorder may develop symptoms under stress. Make sure that the maladaptive response is not just an activation of his preexisting personality disorder. For instance, a patient with antisocial personality disorder may under stress commit unlawful acts, or neglect work and family; a patient with dependent personality disorder (which may be more common in females) may become dysphoric when deserted; and a patient with avoidant personality disorder may become anxious when asked to appear in public. Such responses are exacerbations of the underlying personality disorder but not indications of an adjustment disorder.

Disorders Not Otherwise Specified (NOS)

When a patient reports a single symptom, try to link it to an essential symptom of a clinical disorder. An effective way is to ask:

"When you have symptom X, what other problems do you notice?"

He may respond with:

"When I have my low back pain, I wake up too early and feel rotten all day. I just sit around and don't want to do anything, and I hope that nobody will bother me. Wouldn't you feel the same way if you had that kind of pain?"

This answer shows how a patient frequently forms an opinion about his illness, explains a set of symptoms by the presence of others, and reports only the "causative" symptom. This patient may have an affective disorder in which the back pain becomes the thought content. If you can pair the reported symptom with an essential symptom you have identified it as a possible associated symptom for a clinical disorder.

If you cannot elicit any other associated symptoms, investigate the *severity* of the symptom; does he have to think about it continuously, avoid other people because of it, or is he affected in his marriage? If so, pursue the symptom further.

Isolated signs and symptoms are often physical, such as medically unexplained headache, dizziness, and back pain. There are isolated compulsions such as handwashing, counting, not stepping on cracks; monosymptomatic delusions such as a bad odor (often genital), protruding evil eyes, skin infestation by unidentifiable organisms, or being secretly loved by an important person (erytromania); and isolated mood disturbances such as constant complaining, chronic dysphoria, or silliness.

Here is an example of an isolated delusion.

Mrs. Turner is a 49-year-old, white, married woman who accompanies her husband with bipolar disorder to the clinic. She asks to see his physician alone.

I: Mrs. Turner, you wanted to talk to me about your husband's treatment.
P: That's right. I want to impress on you the terrible things that you've done to him.
I: Let me hear about it.
P: Ever since my husband started on lithium, he sweats terribly. The lithium salt must be in his sweat, because it destroys my linen.
I: That's interesting. I've never heard anything like that before. Tell me more about it.
P: I'm also allergic to the lithium. I can't get close to him because of it. We haven't had sex since he started on it.
I: Have you noticed any other changes in you since then?
P: No, not really. Nothing that I can think of . . .

I: Any changes in your sleep, appetite, or general well-being?
P: Oh no. None whatsoever.
I: How are you coming along with your work?
P: Just fine. I have a job that I enjoy and I get my housework done. My husband tells me what a good housekeeper I am.
I: Can you tell me about your social life?
P: We belong to a church group, we play bridge regularly with friends, I have a girlfriend, and my husband has his own friends who come to see us.
I: What have you done about that problem with your husband's medication?
P: I had my own lithium level checked. I have also sent the bedsheets to a lab for analysis, and I've talked to several drug companies that make lithium.
I: Any results?
P: The typical response. Nobody seems to want to make a commitment. My own level was 0.0025.
I: Do you feel people want to mislead you?
P: Oh no, they just don't seem to know. By the way, the real reason I wanted to talk to you is to ask you to stop the lithium. I have heard you are running an experimental program with a new drug. I want you to enroll my husband in this program so that we can have a normal life again.

A diagnostic interview with Mrs. Turner produced no psychopathology other than her monosymptomatic delusion—she had no other delusions or hallucinations, and no history of substance abuse, or conversion symptoms. Her affect was appropriate and normal in range. She had normal eye contact, and memory and intellectual functions were intact.

For the diagnosis of an isolated sign or symptom, determine first whether it is indeed isolated; second, whether it represents a disturbance of thinking, mood, or somatic function; third, which code classifies it the best as an atypical disorder (NOS): psychotic, mood, anxiety, somatoform, or dissociative disorder.

Checking for Unexplored Disorders

After you have verified some initial diagnostic impressions and excluded others, you are left with a list of psychiatric disorders that are unexplored—list no. 3. Remember, a chief complaint reflects only what the patient chooses to talk about. Therefore, to be comprehensive you have to reach beyond the boundaries of the chief complaint and what the patient volunteers. Use a disorder-oriented approach and explore essential symptoms that the patient does not offer. You may be surprised by what you find.

> Rachel, a 27-year-old African-American female presented with depressed affect.

P: I'm 5 months pregnant. While I save for our baby, my husband spends all his money at the races. I just can't take it anymore.

I: You must really feel let down.

P: You better believe it. I cry for hours.

I: How long has that been going on?

P: My husband has always worked long hours, but since I got pregnant with our second child, it's gotten worse. Now he even stays out overnight.

I: You seem to feel stuck.

P: Stuck and desperate. I can't sleep, I lost my appetite, I don't feel like talking to anybody.

The interviewer felt quite empathic and protective of the patient, and in the remainder of the interview stayed within the limits of her spontaneous complaints. His list of diagnostic possibilities included: adjustment disorder, with depressed mood; major depressive disorder; and bipolar disorder, most recent episode depressed.

Two days after this interview, the patient's aunt called. She complained:

"My niece is still drinking like a hole. She drives her husband out of the house. This poor fellow has tolerated her drinking for the last three years. Isn't there anything you can do about it?"

Rachel had never mentioned her drinking or other substance abuse during the interview. When the interviewer confronted Rachel with the aunt's concern, Rachel reluctantly admitted to her drinking but claimed that her husband was exaggerating it. Nevertheless, the interviewer had made the mistake of restricting himself to the patient's initial chief complaint. He never generated a list no. 3, let alone assessed it.

Screen for hidden clinical disorders by asking for their essential symptoms (Table 6–1), especially for memory problems, substance use, physical problems, "spells," and avoidance behavior. To screen for personality disorders, ask your patient whether he had a rough life and got into situations that were difficult to handle.

3. PSYCHIATRIC HISTORY

Premorbid Personality

The assessment of the premorbid personality serves three functions in the clinical interview:

1. It is the baseline for the patient's present functioning. Ask the patient and relatives to what extent the patient deviates from his "normal self."
2. It supports the diagnosis, since some psychiatric disorders are associated with specific premorbid features. For instance, patients with bipolar disorder may show cyclothymic traits, while patients with schizophrenia often show odd behavior and are socially isolated prior to the onset of the disorder. If diagnosis and premorbid personality do not match, reconsider your diagnosis.
3. It sets the therapeutic goal beyond which treatment is less likely to produce improvement.

The technique to assess the course of a psychiatric disorder, that is, onset, duration, and severity, differs whether you deal with a clinical or a personality disorder.

Course of Clinical Disorders

When you probe for the onset of clinical disorders, start with questions such as:

"When did you first experience your present problems?"
"When was the first time in your life that you had problems like this?"
"Do you remember when you experienced this for the first time?"

Check whether the present disorder may have occurred in a different form. The patient who has a current depressive disorder may have started with manic symptoms, the one with schizoaffective disorder may only have had depressed or irritable mood, and the patient with schizophrenia may have shown predominantly catatonic or paranoid symptoms. A patient may not consider these different manifestations as part of his present disorder. If so, educate him about the connection of past and present problems to facilitate communication.

Along with the assessment of onset, ask questions such as:

"Up to what age were you free of any problems?"

A discrepancy between reported age of onset of a disorder and the age up to which the patient felt healthy may occur in disorders with an insidious onset or a prodromal state.

Mr. Steve M., a 27-year-old, white, single clerk in a grocery store, demonstrates such a gap between the end of mental well-being and the onset of illness.

I: When did all these problems start?
P: Oh, when I was about 21 years old. I became very depressed, heard voices, and was afraid of women.
I: Hmm.
P: And from then on it seemed to always get worse.
I: Up to what age do you think you were completely well and had none of these problems?
P: Until I was 17.
I: 17?
P: Yes, I remember I enjoyed going out and was even pretty successful with the girls. They seemed to like me then.
I: So what happened between 17 and 21?
P: I don't know . . . something . . . I noticed it first at work.
I: What do you mean?
P: I think people at work didn't really like me.
I: How could you tell?
P: They were talking behind my back. I always had the feeling they were laughing about me.
I: What were they talking about?
P: I don't know, but I thought they were thinking I'm queer or something. I heard them say something about "another of those homosexuals." I pretended that I did not notice it. But I did not really feel comfortable going out with them. I always had the feeling I had to pretend.
I: Did you hear voices at that time?
P: No, I don't think so. But I sure picked up the remarks these guys made.

This interview exemplifies how the duplicate question of:

"When did your illness start?"
"When was the last time that you were healthy?"

uncovers the period between end of health and onset of illness. This approach will help you decide whether the onset was insidious or acute. Explore to what extent a clinical disorder interferes with the patient's psychosocial functioning as shown above.

The duration of a clinical disorder may vary from several weeks to a lifetime, and the severity of symptoms (course of illness) may be either chronic stationary, chronic progressive (frequently with exacerbations), episodic, or vacillating. Remissions may be complete or not, leaving the patient with a residual symptomatology or functional deficit (Fig. 6–1). For instance, 1 year after onset, 40% of patients with major depression are still depressed, 40% have recovered, and 20% have some depressive symptoms. Risk factors for a poorer prognosis include preexisting dysthymic disorder, severity of initial major depressive episode, comorbidity with a chronic general medi-

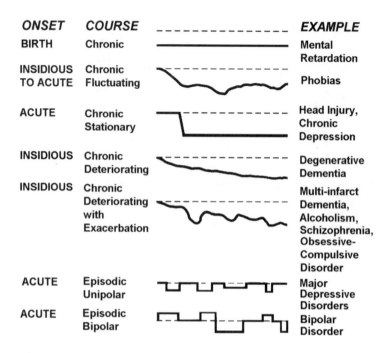

ONSET	COURSE		EXAMPLE
BIRTH	Chronic		Mental Retardation
INSIDIOUS TO ACUTE	Chronic Fluctuating		Phobias
ACUTE	Chronic Stationary		Head Injury, Chronic Depression
INSIDIOUS	Chronic Deteriorating		Degenerative Dementia
INSIDIOUS	Chronic Deteriorating with Exacerbation		Multi-infarct Dementia, Alcoholism, Schizophrenia, Obsessive-Compulsive Disorder
ACUTE	Episodic Unipolar		Major Depressive Disorders
ACUTE	Episodic Bipolar		Bipolar Disorder

Figure 6–1.   Natural course of various psychiatric disorders. *Dashed line* = normal.

cal condition, and substance dependence, especially alcohol and cocaine dependence. Symptoms of some cognitive disorders, some substance-related disorders, and schizophrenia may show a characteristic worsening. Symptoms of antisocial personality disorder may show gradual improvement over a lifetime due to a "burnout" effect. Symptoms of panic disorder, somatization disorder, and obsessive-compulsive disorder, especially if untreated, show a chronic course with exacerbations.

Help a patient who cannot focus on his condition by a graphic approach. Draw a horizontal time line and ask him:

> "If this line represents your life and the beginning represents your birth and the end your present age, where on this line do you think you were first bothered by others and their sneakiness?"

Put each complaint in relationship to the patient's present age and plot them along this time axis (see "Course" section in DSM-IV-TR for each disorder).

Course of Personality Disorders

To obtain information about the onset and duration of a personality disorder you need to modify your approach. Personality disorders are lifelong patterns of maladjusted behaviors that are often ego-syntonic. They first become noticeable during the teenage years. You can assess onset and duration by focusing on either recurring interpersonal conflicts or maladaptive personality features. Track back a conflict that the patient has volunteered such as:

"I have trouble with my husband,"

and identify the part that the personality disorder plays in that conflict. Personality disorders do not always have a poor prognosis. In particular, two Cluster B disorders, antisocial and borderline personality disorders, improve during the third and fourth decade of life in up to 50% of patients. In borderline personality disorder, diagnostic criteria are no longer fulfilled at 10-year follow-up. Similar improvement with age may be seen in avoidant personality disorder.

A Personality Trait

Some patients with a personality disorder recognize their maladaptive personality trait such as shyness, perfectionism, or emotionality. Use this awareness to ask for the onset of the personality trait:

"When did you first notice that you were shy, perfectionistic, or overexcitable?"

Expect an answer such as:

"As long as I can remember."

Realize that personality features and social conflicts are two sides of one coin: recurring conflicts may express a pathological personality trait and, in turn, pathological personality traits cause recurrent interpersonal conflicts.

Focus on the following key areas to assess *severity:* friends, sexual relationships, family life, work life, bonds in the community, and leisure-time activities. A severe personality disorder affects three areas: work, love, and leisure, while a milder form may have less impact. Another measure of severity is the number of similar conflicts a patient has within a year.

Treatment History

Psychiatric disorders show some evidence of specificity of response to certain drug treatments. Therefore, a detailed history of treatments and treatment responses can serve at least three purposes:

1. It can help to reconstruct what type of diagnoses another psychiatrist may have entertained if records are not available and the patient does not remember his symptoms. For instance, a patient may report that he received twelve electroconvulsive treatments and that he was able to return to work after he was discharged from the hospital. Such a report suggests that the patient's therapist diagnosed a mood disorder.
2. It may help to identify responsiveness to certain treatment modalities. For instance, Keith reports:

   "I took Wellbutrin for 3 months, and then Serzone for 4 months, and I didn't get any better. My mother went to Dr. J., who switched her from Serzone to Paxil when she didn't respond. Paxil really helped her."

   Not only disorders but also response to medication may be partly genetically determined. Entertain a treatment attempt with a specific serotonergic reuptake inhibitor such as paroxetine (Paxil) for a patient like Keith.

3. It may help to confirm your own diagnosis. For instance, your patient shows a confusing picture of chronic maladjustment but you are impressed by periods of increased activity and energy followed by social withdrawal and suspiciousness. The patient does not fulfill criteria for bipolar disorder but at best has a combination of a personality disorder and mood disorder NOS. You decide to treat this patient with lithium. Two months later, the patient reports that the fights with his wife and children have stopped, that he got a promotion at work, and that everybody comments on his calmness. He also tells you that the appearance of his desk at work has changed.

   "It's not cluttered up any more. All of a sudden I take care of things as they come, I file them, or throw them away. Four years of psychotherapy and many hours reading books on how to manage time have not accomplished what these little lithium capsules do for me. Amazing."

Such a response, even though not treatment specific, may for practical purposes confirm your impression that the patient had a bipolar disorder NOS. For these reasons, a personal and family history of treatment response is important. Treatments with some specificity for certain disorders are summarized in Table 6–4.

Social History

Divide the social history into its premorbid and morbid part. From the premorbid history assess the developmental milestones and the highest degree of psychosocial functioning. Milestones such as psychomotor and speech development, toilet training, and school performance are especially important when learning disability or mental retardation are complicating factors. Address six areas of school performance:

1. Slow learning, as expressed by repetition of the first grade, and need for special classes or schools, indicates mental retardation or mental dysfunctioning persisting into adulthood. Check for circumscribed deficits such as dyslexia or acalculia.
2. Disciplinary problems, such as lying, stealing, cheating, running away from home, and violent behavior toward superiors, peers, or animals

Table 6–4. Psychotropic agents and their specificity for the treatment of clinical disorders

Clinical disorder	Psychotropic agents
Alcohol use	Disulfiram, naltrexone
Opioid use	Methadone, naltrexone
Psychotic disorders	Neuroleptics, including atypicals; clozapine
Bipolar disorders	Lithium, valproate, carbamazepine, gabapentin, lamotrigine, topiramate, atypical neuroleptics
Major depressive disorder	SSRIs, venlafaxine, nefazodone, tricyclics, mono-, tetra-, and heterocyclics, MAOIs, ECT
Panic disorder with and without agoraphobia	SSRIs, tricyclics, MAOIs, alprazolam, propranolol
Obsessive-compulsive disorder	SSRIs, clomipramine
Generalized anxiety disorder	Benzodiazepines, buspirone, SSRIs

Note. ECT = electroconvulsive therapy. MAOI = monoamine oxidase inhibitor. SSRI = selective serotonin reuptake inhibitor.

suggest conduct and antisocial personality disorders. Oppositional defi-
ant disorder frequently precedes the childhood-onset type of conduct
disorder (American Psychiatric Association 2000, p. 97).

3. Hyperactive behavior, which may explain impulsivity and performance
   failure in adulthood. It may be related to a personality disorder.
4. Phobias, obsessive and compulsive symptoms, or depressive symptoms
   often start in childhood or adolescence. Obsessive-compulsive symptoms start later in females than in males. During puberty, the prevalence
   of depression among females is twice that among males. These symptoms often reach the threshold for disorder before adulthood.
5. Sporadic school attendance, social withdrawal, anger outbursts, and decline in hygiene may precede adult schizophrenia.
6. Arguing with teachers and objecting to rules paired with temper tan-
   trums, resentfulness, and vindictiveness may point to oppositional defi-
   ant disorder.

Use the patient's work record to gauge whether his past employment
corresponds with his intelligence and educational background. Explore and
analyze the social interaction with colleagues, superiors, and subordinates.
Screen the military record (if applicable) for discipline problems, substance
abuse, promotion, demotion, and type of discharge.

Compare the patient's highest premorbid functioning in work and family life with his functioning during morbidity. The distance between the two
indicates the impact of the disorder on the patient's life, while premorbid
functioning sets the treatment goal. Thus, recovery is freedom from symptoms
and also return to premorbid functioning. A measure to quantify premorbid,
morbid, and present functioning is the Global Assessment of Functioning
Scale (GAF Scale, DSM-IV-TR). It allows you to rate global functioning from
1 to 100, 100 being the highest level of functioning. A score of 0 reflects inadequate information. The GAF Scale has two components: 1) the presence
of symptoms, including their severity (i.e., mild to severe) and their duration
(i.e., transient to chronic); and 2) the level of functioning in a wide range of
activities; social effectiveness; satisfaction with life; and mastery of problems.
A GAF score assigned to pivotal points of the patient's life quantifies the impact of mental disorders on your patient's functioning at a specific point in
time, such as current highest level in past year or at discharge from the hospital. Your final rating is *not* an average of symptom level and level of functioning, but must reflect the *worse* of the two. DSM-IV-TR provides a four-
step approach for this scale (American Psychiatric Association 2000, p. 33).
Frequently used, the scale may quantify the natural course of the disorder.

Social history can be used as a detection device for a psychiatric disorder in patients who try to conceal mental problems. For instance, a patient is evaluated for a heart transplant and wishes to get a high priority for the operation. He believes that his past antisocial history and substance abuse, including alcohol, may deny him this privilege. He therefore denies all such symptoms. If you suspect a rewriting of his past, ask for a thorough, year-by-year, or even month-by-month social history. Divorces, job losses, arrests, convictions, jail sentences, driving while intoxicated citations, and hospitalizations for injuries in fights are hard to hide. At least, discrepancies and contradictions will emerge, which will then lead you to the concealed psychiatric conditions.

Medical History (Axis III)

Physical disorders may complicate or mimic psychiatric disorders. This knowledge can help you avoid a misdiagnosis in two ways.

1. *Medical Disorders as Cause of Psychiatric Symptoms*

When you take a medical history, and encounter neurological, endocrinological, metabolic, collagenic, cardiovascular, or other medical disorders in addition to psychiatric symptoms, examine whether these disorders or their treatment with pharmacological agents could possibly be responsible for the psychiatric symptoms. For instance, a patient has been diagnosed as having lupus erythematosus. Subsequently, she develops a multitude of anxious and depressive symptoms. Her psychiatric personal or family history is negative. Entertain the possibility that these symptoms are due to the lupus and that they may respond to different medications than a mood disorder, for instance to neuroleptics rather than to antidepressants. If you feel that the general medical condition is responsible for the psychiatric symptoms, you should make the diagnosis of anxiety disorder due to a general medical condition or mood disorder due to a general medical condition, respectively, rather than generalized anxiety disorder or major depressive disorder.

Table 6–5 shows which physical conditions (left column) are frequently associated with psychiatric symptoms and therefore the cause of a delusion, hallucination, mood disorder, anxiety disorder, or personality change due to a general medical symptom. Consider the relationship especially when you work on consultation service and are called to diagnose and treat psychiatric symptoms in medical patients.

Neurological disorders may present with psychiatric symptoms. Focal neurological deficits, such as anesthesia and paralysis, or the essential symp-

Table 6–5.   Psychiatric symptoms associated with Axis III conditions: physical disorders

Physical disorders	Panic	Anxiety	Depres-sion	Episodic	Delu-sions	Dereali-zation
Neurological disorders						
Transient cerebral ischemia	+					
Cerebral ischemia	+	+				
Multiple sclerosis	+	+	+			
Posterolateral sclerosis	+					
Wilson's disease	+	+			+	
Huntington's chorea	+	+				
Polyneuritis	+					
Niemann-Pick					+	
Homocystinuria					+	
Brain tumor			+			
Marchiafava-Bignami					+	
Encephalitis					+	+
Herpes simplex encephalitis				+		
Creutzfeldt-Jakob			+			
Normal pressure hydrocephalus					+	
Granulomatous meningitis					+	
Alzheimer's and Pick's diseases			+		+	
Brain abscess					+	
Temporal lobe epilepsy					+	+
Ménière's disease	+	+				
Head injuries		+				
Endocrinopathies						
Thyroid, parathyroid, adrenal, insulin	+	+	+		+	
Pheochromocytoma	+			+		
Electrolyte imbalance						
Na, K, Ca, Mg, HCO			+		+	
Collagen vascular disorders						
Lupus erythematosus		+	+	+	+	+
Others		+	+			

(continued)

Table 6–5. Psychiatric symptoms associated with Axis III conditions: physical disorders *(continued)*

Physical disorders	Panic	Anxiety	Depression	Episodic	Delusions	Derealization
Circulatory disorders						
Paradoxical atrial tachycardia	+					
Coronary insufficiency	+					
Anemia		+				
Congestive heart failure					+	
Hypertensive encephalopathy					+	
Infections						
Tuberculosis, brucellosis	+	+				
Toxoplasmosis					+	
Malaria (cerebral)	+	+			+	
Viral: hepatitis, pneumonia mononucleosis	+	+				
Subacute bacterial endocarditis					+	
Carcinoma						
Oat-cell (lung)	+	+				
Leukemia			+			
Pancreatic cancer			+			
Lymphoma			+			
Vitamin deficiencies						
B$_1$, B$_6$, B$_{12}$, niacin, folic acid		+	+		+	
Systemic disorders						
Nephritis		+				
Uremia			+			
Early cirrhosis			+			
Psoriasis			+			
Gout			+			
Amyloidosis			+			
Regional enteritis			+			
Ulcerative colitis			+			
Acute intermittent porphyria				+		
Pancreatitis				+		

Note. + = present.
Source. This table was constructed with the help of information contained in Hall RCW, ed: *Psychiatric Presentations of Medical Illness. Somatopsychic Disorders.* New York and London, Spectrum, 1980. Permission granted to quote and abstract from this book.

toms of a cognitive disorder such as lethargy, confusion, disorientation, amnesia, or intellectual deterioration give them away. These indicators, however, are missing in the early stages or in mild manifestations of some neurological disorders. A high index of suspicion is then needed to lead you in the right direction.

Endocrine disorders are as often a cause for misdiagnosis as the neurological disorders. Hypo- or hyperfunction of the thyroid, parathyroid, adrenal cortex, or insulin-producing Langhans cells are responsible for the emergence of psychiatric symptoms.

Electrolyte imbalance, usually a depletion of sodium, potassium, calcium, or magnesium, causes psychiatric symptoms and so can high potassium levels. Serum bicarbonate levels outside of the normal range may also mimic symptoms of depression.

Collagenic disease of the vascular system, such as lupus erythematosus, rheumatoid arthritis, periarteritis nodosa, and temporal arteritis can be associated with symptoms of anxiety and depression. Systemic lupus erythematosus can virtually mimic all psychiatric symptoms, including delusions and derealization.

Cardiovascular disorders, especially paroxysmal atrial tachycardia and coronary insufficiencies, can mimic panic disorder, while congestive heart failure and hypertensive encephalopathy may induce delusions. The remaining physical disorders listed in Table 6–5, such as chronic infections, some carcinomas, some vitamin deficiencies, and some systemic disorders, may occasionally present with symptoms of depression and anxiety but only rarely with delusions.

Usually, a physical disorder is not mistaken for a psychiatric disorder. Occasionally, however, the medical presentation may be preceded by panic, anxiety, or depression. Or the episodic course of some physical disorders suggests a mood disorder (where an episodic course is typical). Here are eight such disorders:

- multiple sclerosis
- herpes simplex encephalitis
- pheochromocytoma
- systemic lupus erythematosus
- acute intermittent porphyria
- pancreatitis
- systemic mastocytosis
- chronic Epstein-Barr viral syndrome

Often, interviewers associate delusions and derealization so strongly with a psychiatric disorder that they overlook a general medical condition.

2. Psychiatric Symptoms as Indicators of Undetected Medical Disorders

Avoid misdiagnosis when you encounter psychiatric symptoms in older patients with a negative personal and family psychiatric history; when the symptoms occur in an unusual combination; when they show an unexpected course; or when they present at an age for which the onset of the respective psychiatric disorder is rare. For instance, Ronald, a high school teacher in his late fifties, shows symptoms of depression and persecutory delusions for the first time after an episode of indecent exposure at the school's gym. Consider early manifestations of Pick's disease, if you can exclude by laboratory tests or history other medical disorders. Table 6–5 can help you consider and exclude, or verify physical conditions as possible causes of psychiatric symptoms. For instance, the patient has one of the following psychiatric symptoms: panic attacks, generalized anxiety symptoms, depressive symptoms, episodic symptoms, delusions, or derealizations. Find this symptom as one of the headings in Table 6–5. Identify all the medical disorders that can cause this symptom. Then check whether the patient may have one of these disorders. If yes, consider that the patient has a psychiatric disorder due to a general medical condition.

Your work setting often determines the likelihood of a patient having psychiatric symptoms due to a general medical condition. Consultation psychiatrists, family practitioners, and psychiatrists in rural areas may more frequently encounter physical and pharmacological causes for psychiatric symptoms than those professionals in multidisciplinary settings such as a university outpatient clinic, where mental health professionals often work in a tertiary care function and where those patients with general medical conditions are filtered out.

The side effects of pharmacological agents (Table 6–6) may be mistaken for symptoms of a psychiatric disorder. Table 6–6 shows most of these agents grouped according to their therapeutic use with a residual category. These agents are not considered psychotropic except for the stimulants, the autonomous nervous system agents, the antihistamines, and some vitamins, especially vitamin B_6, which facilitates the metabolism of some monoamine neurotransmitters (Hall 1980).

Psychiatric symptoms due to these agents are not limited to toxic effects or interference with brain metabolism such as delirium, confusion, disorien-

Table 6-6. Psychiatric symptoms associated with side effects of nonpsychiatric medications

Drug category	Psychiatric symptoms															
	D	S	I	R	IN	A	E	H	DL	P	DR	C	DS	L	T	AT
Anti-infectious agents																
Sulfonamides	+		+	+						+						
Sulfones			+		+					+						
Anthelmintics										+		+				+
Antituberculars	+						(+)			+		+				
Antimalarials			+							+				+		
Trichomonacides	+		+		+							+				
Antihypertensives																
Rauwolfia alkaloids	+	+													+	
Ganglionic blockers											+	+			+	
Beta-blockers	+			+									+			
Autonomous nervous system drugs																
Sympatholytics	+									+					+	
Sympathomimetics				+	+					+					+	
Anticholinergics				+				+		+	+	+	+			
Stimulants																
Amphetamines	+							+	+	+			+			
Phenylphenidate			+	+	+				+	+						

Psychiatric symptoms

Drug category	D	S	I	R	IN	A	E	H	DL	P	DR	C	DS	L	T	AT
Analgesics																
Salicylates			+	+								+				
Acetaminophen, phenacetin			+	+					+			+				
Propoxyphene	+						+					+				
Analgesics, other	+		+	+						+		+				
Hormones																
Insulin			+		+					+		+				+
Oral antidiabetics												+				
Thyroid drugs			+	+	+											+
Adrenocorticosteroids			+		+		+			+						
Estrogens	+		+	+	+	+										
Estrogen + progestins								+								
Diuretics																
Carbonic anhydrase inhibitors			+										+			
Xanthines			+	+	+						+					
Diuretics, other						+						+				
Others																
Antineoplastics	(+)	(+)	(+)		(+)		(+)			(+)	(+)	+	(+)			
Cardiac glycosides	+							+	+			+	+			

(continued)

Table 6–6. Psychiatric symptoms associated with side effects of nonpsychiatric medications *(continued)*

Drug category	Psychiatric symptoms															
	D	S	I	R	IN	A	E	H	DL	P	DR	C	DS	L	T	AT
Antihistamines	+			+	+		+	(+)			+				+	+
Vitamin B complex		+	+	+	+							+				
Antitussives			+					+	+							
Diphenoxylate	+						+									
Diphenidol								+		+		+	+			
L-Dopa	+	+				+		+		+		+				
Vascular muscle relaxants	+					+							+			+
Antiarrhythmics	+			+	+		+	+								
Nicotinic acid			+	(+)		+										
Hydantoins								+	+						+	
Succinimides	+		+				+					+		+		
Narcotics	+			+	+		+	+					+			
Narcotic antagonists	+							+			+					

Note. D = depression. S = suicidal. I = irritability. R = restlessness. IN = insomnia. A = anxiety. E = euphoria. H = hallucinations. DL = delusions. P = psychosis. DR = delirium. C = confusion. DS = disorientation. L = lethargy. T = tremor. AT = ataxia. + = present. (+) = possibly present.
Source. This table was abstracted from information contained in Hall RCW, ed: *Psychiatric Presentations of Medical Illness. Somatopsychic Disorders.* New York and London, Spectrum, 1980.

tation, lethargy, tremor, and ataxia. Therefore, you may overlook a drug induction unless you ask the patient to bring in all medications he has been taking for the last 2 months. Ask especially the elderly, for whom drugs have a prolonged half-life of excretion. Note that the average geriatric patient takes nine agents daily, which may lead to drug interaction and potentiation.

Include in your medical history a list of all hospitalizations and disorders the patient was treated for in his lifetime. Assess the patient's compliance with his past medical treatment and his response to the various agents. Both help to predict compliance and therapeutic response to your anticipated treatment.

Use Table 6–6 in two ways:

1. Examine whether a patient who takes any of the medications listed in Table 6–6 may have had psychiatric symptoms that coincided with the beginning of that drug treatment.
2. Examine whether psychiatric symptoms that occur in patients without a personal or family psychiatric history, in an atypical form, or at an unusual age are due to medications taken for a physical ailment. With Axis III, DSM-IV-TR offers a way to code the general medical condition or conditions for which the medication is taken. Tables 6–5 and 6–6 can help you with Axis III diagnoses. On Axis I you code the medication-induced psychiatric disorder.

Family History

Studies suggest most major psychiatric disorders are familial. Monozygotic twin studies and adoption studies favor the interpretation that the disposition to psychiatric disorders is genetically transmitted, even though the mode of transmission is unknown (Goodwin and Guze 1989; Wender et al. 1986).

Family history can be used to confirm a psychiatric diagnosis and to predict course and treatment response in young patients with their first affliction, especially when making the differential diagnosis of psychotic depression versus schizophrenia, or bipolar disorder NOS versus schizophrenia. For instance, if your patient has had several depressive episodes but first-degree relatives suffered from bipolar disorder, suspect bipolar disorder in your patient also. Such knowledge may caution you against the use of antidepressants that could precipitate a manic or hypomanic episode, but suggest a combined use with a mood stabilizer. But if first-degree relatives of a patient with major depressive disorder have documented chronic schizophrenia, scrutinize your patient's course for evidence of social decline to exclude schizophrenia.

Family studies on personality disorders are in progress. Since some personality disorders appear to be somewhat associated with major psychiatric disorders, and since the latter are familial, it is not surprising that personality disorders may also be familial (see Table 6–2). Therefore, ask your patient whether any of his first-degree relatives could be described as: 1) loner, odd, or eccentric; 2) in social trouble (the "black sheep" of the family); or 3) dependent, abused, rigid, or resentful. Such questions may puzzle your patient initially. He may not know, only to return later with ample information after he talked to parents and other relatives who had concealed some family secret. Such awareness helps *you* to predict his course and outcome and *him* to understand the nature of his disorder. It reduces his guilt and his unjustified blaming of his parents for their alleged sins committed in his upbringing.

4. DIAGNOSIS

Coming up with a diagnosis makes sense out of madness. It labels the disorder, not the patient; it condenses a multitude of data into one term; it serves communication, and allows prediction of treatment response and outcome.

The diagnostic assessment expresses your judgment and your conclusions about the patient. For inpatients, it should contain the following standards:

1. the patient's assets and strengths,
2. the diagnostic formulation including biological, psychological, and social factors, and
3. a multiaxial diagnosis.

Assets and Strengths

The need to gather this information is partly dictated by federal agencies in the United States, such as Medicare and Champus. At this time, Medicare requires the determination of the patient's assets and strengths, and of a diagnosis.

The standards used by HCFA (Health Care Financing Administration 482.61 b[7]) determine that an inventory of the patient's assets in descriptive terms is included in the psychiatric evaluation. The interpretive guidelines list as strengths the following: knowledge, interests, skills, aptitude, experience, education, and employment status. All of these may be useful in motivating the patient to actively participate in the interview process and in treatment.

Assessment of the patient's assets and strengths reflects in a positive way the abilities that remain after the psychiatric disorders have taken their toll on him. They will play a major role when you determine his treatment plan and prognosis.

Diagnostic Formulation

The American Board of Psychiatry and Neurology now requires that a candidate be able to discuss the diagnostic formulation, that is, a summary of the biological, psychological, and social factors that contribute to a patient's disorder. Since such assessment aids treatment planning, it is useful even after the board examination is over.

Biological Factors

The biological formulation summarizes the biological factors that contribute to a patient's psychiatric disorder. This includes:

1. psychiatric disorders in first-degree relatives as an indicator of genetic predisposition;
2. prenatal history as an indicator of damage to the fetus by mother's infections, other medical disorders, or substance use;
3. early development as indicator of the influence of general medical conditions that possibly retarded the child's development;
4. history of general medical conditions including seizure disorders and their treatment as indicators for the influence of these conditions on the patient's psychiatric history.

Psychological Factors

The psychological formulation includes an estimate of the impact that child-rearing techniques had on the patient's development of interpersonal skills and defense mechanisms. These effects may surface during the interview in the form of transference to the interviewer and defenses observed while the patient presents his problems. Interviewers with a psychodynamic orientation may include a structural summary of the patient's ego, id, and superego forces; a topological analysis of conscious and unconscious behaviors; and a history of psychosexual development, as proposed by Erikson (1969). Cognitive therapists may want to characterize the patient's irrational beliefs and self-defeating self-talk that may slow down her improvement and make her noncompliant with the treatment plan.

From a behavioral point of view, learned maladjusted behaviors should be described, such as avoidance behaviors in response to certain stimuli; pathological means of weight control, as seen in eating disorders; and substance abuse in response to environmental problems, to name just a few.

Social Factors

Describe the support systems that may have a positive or negative impact on the patient's psychiatric history. These include:

1. *Family.* May potentially harm the patient by the following situations: loss of parental figures through separation, divorce, or death; and physical, sexual, and emotional abuse. A history of abuse is often present in patients with dissociative disorders. Older patients may experience support or neglect from their children that may influence the outcome of their psychiatric condition.
2. *Religious institutions.* May have helped to develop the patient's spiritual strength or subjected her to brainwashing or coercion.
3. *Neighborhood.* May have helped to develop social standards or posed a threat to the patient's safety.
4. *School.* May have helped to develop academic skills, ambition, and positive role models, or was perceived as a place of failure, rejection, and punishment.
5. *Military.* A source to develop self-esteem or foster dependence and despair. It may be the source for trauma that may have contributed to the development of a posttraumatic stress disorder.
6. *Job or career.* May provide financial security or be the source of continuous stress and failure.
7. *Marriage.* May offer source of strength and support, or of persisting problems.

Multiaxial Diagnoses

Axes I and II

DSM-IV-TR encourages multiple psychiatric diagnoses on Axes I and II reflecting clinical and personality disorders. These diagnoses can be specified by terms such as principal diagnosis, provisional diagnosis, or "in remission" (see below). In many diagnostic systems, including DSM-IV-TR, a hierarchical principle is used to exclude certain psychiatric diagnoses to the benefit of others. Usually, the more pervasive disorder receives priority over the less pervasive disorder.

The absolute exclusion of one psychiatric disorder by another is limited to two situations:

1. If a psychiatric disorder is felt to be due to a general medical condition, then the additional diagnosis of the psychiatric disorder is not made. For instance, if a patient has major depressive disorder after chronic treatment with reserpine, he will receive the diagnosis of medication-induced depressive disorder and not the additional diagnosis of major depressive disorder.
2. The defining symptoms of one disorder are at the same time associated features of another disorder. For instance, a patient has schizophrenia and also reports some depressive symptoms. He will receive only the diagnosis of schizophrenia but not the additional diagnosis of dysthymia since dysthymia is thought to be part of schizophrenia.

In contrast, if a patient has obsessive and compulsive symptoms in addition to schizophrenia, he will receive the diagnosis of obsessive-compulsive disorder in addition to schizophrenia, since obsessions and compulsions are not thought to be associated features of schizophrenia (see DSM-IV-TR). The same applies to disorders that have a high comorbidity with schizophrenia, such as nicotine dependence (in 80%–90% of individuals), panic disorder, and some preexisting personality disorders, such as schizotypal, schizoid, and paranoid types, which are coded on Axis II with the specifier premorbid.

Principal diagnosis: Assign the principal diagnosis to the disorder that clinically most reliably and comprehensively explains symptoms present and that are the focus of attention or treatment (DSM-IV-TR). For instance, if a patient is presently alcohol dependent but also reports symptoms suggestive of dysthymia, the diagnosis of alcohol dependence is undoubtedly reliable and the major focus of treatment, while the dysthymic symptoms may be due to patterns of alcohol intoxication and withdrawal and are therefore less reliable. Therefore, the principal diagnosis is alcohol abuse or dependence and not dysthymia.

A patient may have more than one principal diagnosis. For instance, he may have experienced obsessions and compulsions for several years that significantly impaired his functioning. For the last 4 weeks, he became increasingly depressed and for the last 2 weeks, fulfills all criteria for major depressive disorder. This "new" disorder made him consult a psychiatrist in addition to his psychologist who was treating him with behavior modification for his obsessive thoughts and compulsions. Clearly, both disorders are additive in the impairment of the patient's functioning. They justify two principal diagnoses.

Provisional diagnosis: It happens that the interviewer can assess some symptoms of a psychiatric disorder but the patient's lack of cooperation does not allow him to investigate the full syndrome. The interviewer has the impression that the patient has all symptoms necessary to make the diagnosis but he lacks documentation. Rather than assigning a not otherwise specified diagnosis (NOS), the interviewer may choose to express the level of uncertainty by using a provisional diagnosis.

Past psychiatric diagnoses: DSM-IV-TR does not use the term "past psychiatric disorder." However, it uses the terms *in partial remission, in full - remission,* and *residual state* to indicate the status of previously experienced psychiatric disorders.

Diagnostic profile: If a patient has more than one psychiatric disorder, it is helpful to plot onset and end of each disorder on a time line. The zero point signifies the patient's birth, the units of the time line are the years of his life, and the end is his present age. The disorders are indicated with bars above it. On top of the graph are the disorders due to general medical conditions, followed by substance-use disorders, psychotic disorders, mood, anxiety, somatoform disorders, and so on, as they are listed in DSM-IV-TR. Such a display of a patient's diagnostic profile allows you to visualize the temporal relationship of all disorders. It presents the most succinct diagnostic summary.

Axis III

You report current medical conditions on Axis III. The separation of medical conditions from psychiatric disorders does not imply that the medical conditions differ from psychiatric disorders nor that they are less affected by behavioral or psychosocial factors. If a medical condition causes a mental disorder, it is listed on Axes I and III: on Axis I as a mental disorder due to a general medical condition and on Axis III as the general medical condition itself. If more than one Axis III condition is present, all should be reported. Especially include pregnancy and sexually transmitted disorders on this axis.

Axis IV

You report psychosocial and environmental problems on Axis IV. The DSM-IV-TR manual lists a host of V codes that refer to problems a patient might have with the primary support group, social environment, education, occupation, housing, economic situation, access to health-care services, interaction with the legal system, and other psychosocial problems. Relational problems with a parent, child, partner, or sibling are included here, as well as problems related to abuse or neglect. These problems constitute stressors that the patient has to deal with. These stressors can also include positive experiences, such as the birth of a child, if they bring on or exacerbate a mental disorder.

Axis V

You report global assessment of functioning on Axis V. The Global Assessment of Functioning Scale (GAF) quantifies the clinician's judgment of the severity of symptoms and level of functioning. The worst of the two components must be used for the final score. The authors of DSM-IV-TR propose the inclusion of three further scales. They are: the Social and Occupational Functioning Assessment Scale (SOFAS), the Global Assessment of Relational Functioning Scale (GARF), and the Defensive Styles Rating Scale (DSRS). The GAF rating summarizes the clinician's evaluation of only psychological, social, and occupational functioning. The DSM-IV-TR GAF Scale ranges from 1 to 100. One can conceptualize this scale as representing five levels of functioning:

1. Range 1–20 represents the patient who is persistently (1–10) or sometimes dangerous (11–20) and poses a threat to others or to himself, who has severe (1–10) self-neglect or commits serious suicidal acts, or who has gross impairment in communication (11–20). Such a patient needs to be committed to a mental institution if voluntary hospitalization cannot be achieved.

2. Range 21–40 represents the patient whose reality testing is severely impaired by delusions or hallucinations (21–30) or shows major impairments in all (21–30) or several areas such as work, school, family, or

impaired judgment, thinking, or mood (31–40). Such a patient cannot function without continuous supervision and a continuous support system. He should be treated as a psychiatric inpatient.

3. Range 41–60 represents a patient who has serious, nonpsychotic symptoms that interfere with his time management, such as obsessional rituals; lead to severe avoidance behavior and panic attacks; and impair (41–50) or interfere (51–60) with social, occupational, or school functioning. Patients with this rating usually need continuous pharmacotherapy and psychotherapy in a partial hospitalization or outpatient setting.

4. Range 61–80 represents a patient who has some mild (61–70) or transient symptoms (71–80), which cause difficulties in social, occupational, or school functioning. If they are transient and expectable reactions to stressors, the higher rating (71–80) is used. These are patients who may require occasional counseling and psychotherapy.

5. Range 81–100 represents a person who shows good functioning in all areas with a wide range of interests and activities and level of social effectiveness. Symptoms are absent or present in everyday occurrences such as examination anxiety (81–90). The highest rating is reserved for the person who manages all life problems successfully and is sought out by others for his positive qualities. Such a person requires no type of counseling.

This scale provides a convenient way to measure the patient's psychosocial competence and rounds off the diagnostic assessment.

5. PROGNOSIS

During the interview, we recommend that you share your diagnostic considerations and decisions with the patient in the form of diagnostic feedback. A good way to introduce this topic is with statements such as:

> "Let me wrap up for you what I found that you have suffered from. And let's see whether you agree with me."

Usually, patients appreciate being included in this process. They are anxious to know what you think about them; they also may feel rewarded after they have answered your questions. If you do this, patients may tell you how much they appreciate the feedback. Presenting the diagnostic impression to the patient easily sets the stage for the next step—the discussion of the treatment options. We will discuss this at greater length in Chapter 7.

The patient's response to your treatment suggestions clearly shows from a diagnostic point of view his attitude toward his disorder. It gives you an inkling of his degree of compliance. Together with the nature of his major psychiatric and/or personality disorder, his attitude toward his disorder and the treatment options contributes significantly to his prognosis.

Share this outlook with the patient. Tell him whether you think he has an excellent chance for full recovery, or express your concern about his low-level interest in his treatment and your sense that a lack of compliance may lead to a prolonged course of illness and future relapse. These issues may be expressed as concerns and not used as threats to enforce compliance (see Chapter 7). The prognostic feedback rounds off the diagnostic process.

Now you are ready to integrate what was taken apart: rapport, techniques, mental status examination, and diagnosing. You will understand how they interact and develop throughout the five phases of the interview.

CHECKLIST

Chapter 6: Five Steps to Make a Diagnosis

This checklist is designed to test your diagnostic skills. Complete this list after an interview.

1. What was the chief complaint?
2. List all psychiatric signs and abnormal behaviors (clues), if any, that you observed during the initial minutes of the interview.
3. List the differential diagnostic options (at least five) that these signs and behaviors suggested to you.
4. Did you address any signs or clues?
5. Give reasons why you treated clues the way you did.
6. Did the observed behavior or the chief complaint suggest a psychiatric symptom, a long-term maladjusted behavior, a psychosocial or environmental problem?
7. How did you follow up on the chief pathology?
8. How soon after the start of the interview did you have a list of five diagnostic options?
9. If the patient reported psychiatric symptoms as chief complaint, list all disorders for which these symptoms are:

    a. essential,

    b. associated.

10. Did you screen for essential symptoms?

11. Did you screen for a lifelong maladjustment?

12. If the patient reported lifelong maladjustment:

    a. describe the situations he is sensitive to,

    b. list the personality disorders that are associated with your patient's pathology,

    c. list the clinical disorders that could explain his maladjusted behavior.

13. Did you screen for a psychosocial or environmental problem?

14. If the patient named a stressor, determine how the stressor is related to the disorder: cause, trigger, time marker, magnifier, or consequence.

15. If the patient described a social conflict, discuss whether this conflict was the expression of:

    a. a clinical disorder,

    b. a personality disorder,

    c. an adjustment disorder,

    d. a psychosocial or environmental problem.

16. List all psychiatric disorders that the chief complaint could:

    a. include,

    b. exclude,

    c. be neutral to.

    Separate the disorders into clinical or personality disorders. Make sure you have included at least five disorders.

17. Did you get a description of the premorbid state?

18. List evidence for slow learning, learning disability, social isolation, disciplinary problems, phobias, obsessions.

19. In what way did the disorder interfere with the patient's intimate relationships, work, and hobbies?

20. Did you check for unexplored disorders? What type of disorders did you detect? List them!

21. When was the onset of the disorder? Was it sudden or insidious?

22. Was the course chronic, episodic, chronic progressive? Did it leave a deficit?

23. What is the impact of the disorder on the patient?

24. What was his response to previous treatment(s)?

25. List the medical disorders that could mimic the patient's symptoms.

26. List pharmacological agents the patient is taking that can mimic his psychiatric symptoms.

27. List the psychiatric disorders that occurred in the patient's first-degree relatives.
28. Did any blood relatives commit suicide?
29. Did any of the patient's first-degree relatives have the same psychiatric disorder as the patient?
30. What was the natural history of the patient's disorder in his first-degree relatives?
31. Which psychotropic drug(s) worked and did not work in the first-degree relatives who had a psychiatric disorder similar to your patient's?
32. List all psychiatric disorders for which the patient fulfills DSM-IV-TR criteria.
33. What is the patient's principal diagnosis?

CHAPTER SEVEN

FIVE PHASES AND THE FOUR COMPONENTS: HOW TO PUT IT ALL TOGETHER

SUMMARY

Chapter 7 shows how to synthesize the four components described in Chapters 2 through 6. It demonstrates how to conduct an interview by simultaneously establishing and maintaining rapport, selecting the most effective interviewing techniques, monitoring the mental status, and progressing in a flexible yet orderly manner in the diagnostic evaluation through the different phases of the interview.

Chapter 7 analyzes an interview with a cooperative patient, making use of the four components outlined in Chapters 2–6. The interview is short and shows the five phases. This chapter offers a bridge from the psychodiagnostic strategies to their applications to real-life interview situations.

▲ ▲ ▲ ▲ ▲

Healing is a matter of time, but it is sometimes also a matter of opportunity.

—Hippocrates, Precepts 6, ch. 1, ca. 460–400 B.C.

▼ ▼ ▼ ▼ ▼

Following Hippocrates, create that opportunity.

The four tasks of the interviewer are to establish and maintain rapport, to apply the appropriate interviewing techniques, to monitor the mental status, and to propel the diagnostic process. Several shifts in goal and topic occur during the course of the interview that subdivide it into five phases: 1) warm-up and screening of the problem, 2) follow-up of preliminary impressions, 3) history and database, 4) diagnosis and feedback, and 5) prognosis and treatment contract. Since the five diagnostic steps (Chapter 6) set the goal for each of the five phases of the interview, these five phases coincide somewhat with the steps. However, the five phases encompass more than the diagnostic steps. Each phase also includes rapport, techniques, and mental status.

This chapter will show how to use these four components in each phase of the interview. You will see the ebb and flow of the interviewer's work, and how she can maintain rapport, apply effective techniques, monitor mental status, continue to refine her diagnostic understandings, and arrive at an accurate diagnosis and efficient treatment plan. In this chapter, we offer you a succinct guide to the goals of each phase and an accessible, shorthand version of the integration of the different elements explored in this book.

The interplay of the four components and the five phases is summarized in Table 7–1. This table suggests guidelines and not strict procedures. It is intended to raise your awareness of tasks to be completed in an interview. The order of completion is often determined by the connections the patient makes and not necessarily by the order in Table 7–1. For instance, if the patient describes as his chief complaint severe symptoms of depression (phase 1 of the interview) and then makes the connection to his mother's depression and describes her disabilities, you may temporarily shift into assessing his entire family history (phase 3 assessment). This order follows the patient's needs. If this topic is exhausted you may then return to phase 1 and pursue assessment of further symptoms of depression, their severity,

Table 7–1. Five phases of the interview and the four components

Phase	Rapport	Technique	Mental status	Diagnosis
1. Warm-up and screening of problem	Put patient at ease, set limits, empathize with suffering, become a compassionate listener	Select productive and broad screening questions	Observe appearance, psychomotor functions, speech, thinking, affect, orientation, memory, and explore mood, insight, memory, judgment	Note clues, classify the chief complaint; assess symptoms, severity, course, stressors; list differential diagnoses
2. Follow-up of preliminary impressions	Become an ally, make shifts in topics clear	Shift topics, progress from open- to closed-ended questions	Assess thinking, thought content, suicidality	Verify or exclude diagnoses
3. History and database	Show expertise, interest, thoroughness, leadership and motivate for testing	Shift topics, handle defenses, fill in gaps, follow up clues, reconcile inconsistencies	Evaluate judgment, memory, test specific mental status functions and IQ	Assess course of disorders; impact on social life; family and medical history
4. Diagnosis and feedback	Secure acceptance of diagnosis	Explain disorders and treatment options	Discuss mental status findings, explore compliance	Establish diagnoses on five axes
5. Prognosis and treatment-contract	Assume the leadership role and assure compliance	Discuss treatment contract	Make inferences about insight, judgment, and compliance	Give prognosis; predict treatment effects

course, and the preceding psychosocial and environmental problems. Thus, you strike a balance between the opportunities that the patient offers and the overall organized interviewing process taught in these pages.

1. PHASE 1:
WARM-UP AND SCREENING OF THE PROBLEM

Goal: Find a relaxed tone and comfort the patient. Control aggressive, in-trusive, or delirious behavior. Show empathy. Elicit essential symptoms and signs of psychiatric disorders.

Rapport: Give the patient time to become familiar with you and the sur-roundings. Involve him in small talk so he can get used to your voice and the way you talk. Address his apprehension and show concern for his well-being. Put him at ease.

If your patient is aggressive or belligerent, as in the emergency room, set limits. Help him to recognize what you expect from him and what is ac-ceptable to you. Make him aware that cooperation is to his own advantage. Medicate the very excited or delirious patient. After he is sedated, conduct a modified diagnostic interview (see Chapter 9, section 3: Irritable Hyperac-tivity in Bipolar Disorder).

Sense the patient's suffering. Thus, you place your "visitor" in the pa-tient's role. Help him now to express his suffering and respond with empa-thy. Your compassion as listener deepens rapport. Be tactful and aware that you are dealing with mental pain—not with pieces of a puzzle, or a charac-ter in a novel. Interviewing is not just playing detective, or choosing—like a computer—the most efficient algorithms of a decision tree for the patient's problems. The focus of this early phase is the patient's mental anguish and not the interviewer's diagnostic curiosity.

Technique: During the initial period of small talk, test what type of ques-tions are most productive. Do open-ended questions work? Do they elicit detailed elaborations or rambling? Or short answers like:

> "I don't know."
> "You tell me."

Open this phase in one of two ways. Either follow up on a lead, such as disorientation, affect, hallucinations, delusions, or a thought disorder; or ask a variation of the question:

"How can I help you?"
"What kind of problems bring you here?"
"Where shall we start?"
"What's going on in your life?"

These questions will assess the chief complaint. Focusing on the chief complaint initiates the diagnostic process. What vocabulary does the patient prefer? Visual, abstract, or auditory? Can he comprehend long questions, understand their abstract meaning, and talk about familiar subjects without difficulties?

If your patient responds well to open-ended, nonstructured questions, use them and then switch to more structured and closed-ended questions when you need to pinpoint a symptom. If your patient is reluctant to talk about certain topics, or distorts the facts, recognize his resistance and underlying defense mechanisms and deal with them.

Mental status: Observe mental status functions such as appearance, psychomotor activity, speech, and affect during the warm-up. Anxiety (anticipatory and phobic) surfaces frequently here. As time goes on, the anxious patient may gain control over his affect. Therefore, register this initial anxiety for later follow-up. Similarly, look for signs of suspiciousness.

The themes of the small talk in the warm-up phase are not arbitrary. Choose topics that allow you to examine uncensored the patient's mental functioning. Is he oriented? Can he memorize well enough so that history taking will be reliable? Questions such as:

"When did you contact this office first?"
"Where did you park your car?"
"How easy was it for you to find the office?"

are nonconspicuous ways to test his recent memory.

The question for the chief complaint changes the character of the interview from *conversation* to *exploration*. This switch confronts you with the patient's degree of insight and understanding of his problem. This is very important to establish because insight determines how to approach his psychopathology (Chapter 2). Adopt the patient's view of his problems to help determine mental status functions, as well as increase rapport. This approach will yield better results than remaining an outside observer.

As an example, think of the patient with a drinking problem who continues to drive inebriated in spite of several arrests and two severe accidents, one nearly fatal. The family judges these acts as irresponsible and criminal. However, without a few drinks, the patient feels unable to overcome his agoraphobic feelings and panic attacks in order to go to work. If you adopt the patient's view of his drinking rather than that of his family (or society), you use his insight to interview him, which will help your rapport, mental status, and diagnostic assessment.

Diagnosis: Pick up clues of disturbed mental functions. They can be more productive in starting the diagnostic process than asking for the chief complaint. Regardless whether you pursue the clue or not, start forming diagnostic options for your list no. 1 (see Chapter 6).

The length of the warm-up period depends on the patient's cooperation. If he is reluctant or hesitant to talk to you, it will take longer to establish rapport than when he volunteers all information. When you both feel comfortable with each other, you are ready to screen the problem by assessing the chief complaint. This moves the patient's disorder into the center of the interview. The chief complaint confronts you with symptoms, patterns of disturbed behavior, reactions to stressors, and problems of living. Base your initial diagnostic impressions on these reports. Construct and keep track of the three lists (Chapter 6):

1. list no. 1 of likely disorders—be overinclusive
2. list no. 2 of excluded disorders
3. list no. 3 of disorders not yet checked

List the disorders according to the hierarchy as outlined in Chapter 6, that is, start with the major psychiatric disorders, followed by personality disorders, and psychosocial and environmental problems.

The four components of the interview interlock: while you ask for symptoms and problems, you observe at the same time the patient's mental status for emerging signs of disturbed behavior. Their follow-up by confrontation, for instance, fuels the diagnostic process. If these interventions disrupt rapport, identify the mental status functions responsible for the stalling—persecutory ideas or anger, for instance. Then change your technique to revive rapport and reengage the patient in the diagnostic process.

Monitor how the patient formulates, how he thinks, and how he processes information. Analyze what type of questions help him to open up and talk about his problems, and which questions distract and confuse him. Adjust your technique accordingly. Redirect when he digresses from discussing his own problems. What can you conclude from these observations for mental status and the differential diagnosis?

2. PHASE 2:
FOLLOW-UP OF PRELIMINARY IMPRESSIONS

Goal: To make diagnostic decisions and verify the probable and exclude the unlikely diagnoses.

Rapport: Phase 2 is the most taxing for the patient because he has to give you very specific information that allows you to make diagnostic decisions. While the previous phase was patient-centered, allowing the patient to select the topic and describe his pain and suffering, this phase becomes task-centered. The patient has to answer detailed questions, which sometimes are difficult and not always purposeful for him. Furthermore, your questions may seem to jump erratically from one topic to another. Recognize when the patient becomes puzzled, and explain the rationale for your topic selection and sequencing. This far into the interview, the patient should be convinced "that you know what you are doing," that you are not only a compassionate listener but also an expert.

Technique: Since during this phase you seek information that allows you to make specific diagnostic decisions, you use a variety of steering techniques: redirecting when the patient becomes too detailed about a topic, or accentuated or abrupt transitions when you need to cover different topics and to check out your diagnostic options. Since you are more active during this phase than in the previous one, you may encounter resistance and defense mechanisms that you have to handle.

Mental status: During phase 2 you request detailed and precise information from the patient. Thus, you become aware of selected mental status functions, such as thought content, remote memory (symptoms that occurred in the far past), and recent memory, insight, concept of words, goal directedness in thinking, tightness of associations, and speed of thinking. Since you may switch topics quickly, you can also judge the ease with which the patient can shift sets.

Diagnosis: Check out the disorders on list no. 1. Verify or exclude them. Decide whether the patient's complaints fit best a clinical, a personality, or an adjustment disorder. Frequently, you find a combination of one or more clinical disorders with a personality disorder. Try to separate them and follow up on each of them. This process shortens and solidifies list no. 1, the likely disorders; it lengthens list no. 2, the excluded disorders.

As in phase 1, there is no diagnostic progress without maintaining rapport, without continuous monitoring of the patient's mental status, and fine-tuning of assessment techniques. If the interviewer neglects any of these four components, he may miss information to support his diagnoses. Or he may not be able to make one at all. Insensitivity to mental status and rapport may put the whole interview in jeopardy; the result may be premature termination.

3. PHASE 3: HISTORY AND DATABASE

Goal: To get the history, the course of the disorder, the premorbid personality, the psychiatric family history, the medical and social history to confirm the diagnosis, to fill in gaps in history and the mental status assessment, and to follow up on clues and inconsistencies.

Rapport: Through assessing and understanding the patient's history your expertise will show. This thoroughness and interest in your patient's problems will intensify rapport.

In this phase, you cover territory known to the patient. He has given a history to health professionals before. However, there are obstacles to rapport in this phase: embarrassing topics—being fired from a job, imprisonment, drug abuse, venereal disease, unfaithful behavior. Beware of judgmental behavior. Your goal is to understand the patient, not judge his actions.

Master two rapport-related tasks during this phase:

1. Motivate the patient to take some tests. Testing taxes rapport because it may activate performance anxiety. It reminds him of a student role. If rapport is fragile, he may refuse testing (like Ms. M. in Chapter 9). To ensure cooperation, explain the purpose of each test carefully. Emphasize that there is no failing of the test; it serves to help and not to grade him. Provide him with immediate feedback about the results and how they relate to a possible diagnosis.
2. In the case of inconsistencies in the patient's story, ask the patient to help clarify what were to you confusing aspects of his story. If you confront the patient, you may arouse anxiety, suspicion, or anger. Therefore emphasize that you did not understand, that you are confused, rather than implying that he misinformed you.

Technique: Your goal during this phase is to keep the patient animated to give you a detailed history of his psychiatric disorders. Find new angles to help him explore his past. Generate new insights. Sudden transitions in topics revive the interview. Pay attention to his reality distortions and his resistance to give certain information. Identify his defense mechanisms, and handle them cautiously if they obstruct the diagnostic process. If this is your first contact with him, you may bypass them (see Chapter 3).

If you found inconsistencies, tell the patient that you don't have a clear picture about some events in his past, or that you need some help to reconcile A and B. If you have some clues, follow up on them by making the patient aware of your observations. Don't threaten him, but communicate that it is in *his* best interest that you understand the background of these inconsistencies or of these clues.

Mental status: Phase 3 gives ample opportunity to test the patient's remote memory. His past actions reveal his social responsibility. Extend the social history by exploring his future plans, which will give you a feeling for his judgment.

You may spot some gaps; you may have a vague notion about the patient's concentration, recent memory, and intelligence from the interview, but you feel you need quantitative data to clearly support your preliminary impression. Now is the time to test, just before the "feedback" phase (phase 4). Testing would have interrupted the flow of information earlier.

Diagnosis: Determine the duration of the patient's problems and their course. Was the course episodic, chronic, or deteriorating? Major psychiatric disorders may be associated with specific personality disorders; be aware of this relationship. Schizophrenia, for instance, may be preceded by a schizoid or schizotypal personality disorder. The patient's social history shows the impact of the illness on the patient's life.

The medical history may contribute to the psychiatric diagnosis. For instance, multiple unsuccessful surgeries point to somatization disorder; endocrinological disturbances may have triggered or complicated a mood disorder. Seizures or head injuries may have predisposed the patient to an amnestic disorder.

Finally, screen his first-degree relatives for evidence of psychiatric disorders. Bipolar disorder, schizophrenia, alcohol use disorders, panic, or obsessive-compulsive disorder in one or both parents or in siblings may increase your diagnostic certainty and may give you a glimpse of the patient's future.

Phase 3 solidifies the diagnostic impressions on list no. 1. When you review premorbid personality and history, and find a chronic course where you had expected remissions, you may detect a previously overlooked personality disorder. Add it to list no. 1 and scrutinize it.

Phase 3 completes the collection of evidence for your diagnostic impressions, your list no. 1. This phase also offers a chance to go beyond the chief pathology and screen for any other unexplored disorders, list no. 3. Screen especially for alcohol and substance abuse, which can imitate—during intoxication and withdrawal—a host of psychiatric symptoms. Thus, you reduce list no. 3 in favor of lists no. 1 or 2.

Clues not yet explored may be dealt with now. For instance, perhaps the patient looked at his watch repeatedly and polished his glasses eight times during the interview. Or perhaps he used the same phrase over and over such as:

"Typical for the government,"

or

"And then the usual thing happened again."

Now you may clarify inconsistencies between the patient's psychiatric history, your diagnostic impression, and previous treatment. For instance, explore whether the depressed or anxious patient who was treated with neuroleptics ever heard voices or had delusions that would justify such treatment. Or explore a mismatch of an event and his age, or of his schooling and his occupation.

Again, during this phase, the four components of the interview are interrelated. Your diagnostic impression will help you to decide which mental status tests to select, which gaps in history to close, which behavioral clues to follow, and which inconsistencies to reconcile. Your rapport and mental status findings will guide you in your technical approach.

Phase 3 is not rigidly separated from the preceding phases. Historical data may emerge earlier and aid your diagnosis. Favor a natural flow of information over a rigidly systematic approach. As long as the patient gives you pertinent information, let him lead you through his past; give him the chance to explain his history to you like an experienced museum guide.

4. PHASE 4: DIAGNOSIS AND FEEDBACK

Goal: To explain to the patient what is wrong with him.

Rapport: Your feedback should have two effects:

1. to give the patient confidence in your understanding of his problems, and make him accept you as an expert, and
2. to give the patient confidence in your treatment recommendation, and make him accept your guidance.

Your roles as expert and leader intensify rapport and may bring out his personality traits. The dependent patient may glorify you, while the narcissistic personality may try to dismantle you of your authority. To stay in control, recognize his personality traits. Register changes in attitude. If a negative interplay develops, address, discuss, and interpret it.

Technique: Open the diagnosis and feedback phase by telling the patient something like:

> "I have asked you a lot of questions and we have discussed many points. Is there anything you would like to ask me?"

After you have answered him, tell him what you have learned about his problems. Tell him how and why you think he is suffering. Link his suffering and his symptoms with the nature of his illness. Discuss in lay terms your working diagnosis. However, delay the disclosure of your diagnosis if it may affect him negatively. Explain what can be done to alleviate his suffering and to control his disorder, aiming at full remission.

Mental status: The patient's response to your feedback highlights three mental status functions: cooperativeness, insight, and judgment. They reflect how serious he is about seeking help. Lack of interest in treatment may be a clue for noncompliance. Patients who have concealed their suicidal tendencies throughout the interview may admit their hopelessness if you address their disinterest in help at this point. You should then consider hospitalization.

Diagnosis: Integrate all observations about rapport, mental status, and history. You should have a working diagnosis after 30 to 45 minutes of interviewing. Share some of the results of this integrative process with the patient. The patient may comply better with your treatment if you give him feedback. Feedback enhances the patient's understanding of his condition. You learn how well he accepts his disorder and the treatment options. His acceptance of them improves his prognosis.

5. PHASE 5: PROGNOSIS AND TREATMENT CONTRACT

Goal: To give a prognosis, select a treatment plan and agree on a treatment contract.

Rapport: Your guidance is essential during this phase. The more the patient recognizes your competence during the interview, the easier he will accept and follow your treatment recommendations, especially a patient who is dependent or enjoys gratification. The more he feels that he gets from you, the more likely he may bond and comply with the treatment. Present your prognosis in terms of treatment compliance. Give the patient your estimation about the outcome of his problems for both scenarios: his compliance or noncompliance with your treatment plan.

Technique: Discuss in- or outpatient care; the pros and cons of different modes of therapy available, such as types of psychotherapy, pharmacotherapy, or a combination thereof, or electroconvulsive therapy; cost; time involvement; and outcome measures. Point out that the treatment plan will be tailored to his needs. Tell him that at follow-up visits, you will ask him when he desires to come back and that you will consider his wish in scheduling. For outpatient care, indicate how often and how long he may have to be seen.

If you recommend pharmacological treatment, discuss type of medication, dose, timing, efficacy, and side effect profile. Be detailed about major possible adverse effects so the patient feels completely informed. Tell him what to do if they surface. Only then discuss the beneficial treatment effects. Ask the patient to always use the same pharmacy so that all prescribed medications are known to the pharmacist and possible interactions can be checked. Furthermore, ask the patient to read the patient information sheets from the pharmacy.

Avoid raising false expectations about treatment success. Prepare him for possible changes in the treatment plan. If and when he accepts your treatment plan and promises to comply with the details, you know that (for now) he may have accepted your guidance.

After the discussion of an individualized treatment plan, the patient may assume that you will be his therapist. In spite of this assumption, discuss this point explicitly. If you feel competent and are willing to treat him, tell him so; otherwise recommend a referral. Even if you want to work with the patient, he should be given the option to have you as his therapist or to request a referral. Some patients, for example, may feel that a therapist of a different gender may be more acceptable, or a therapist who lives closer to home. Your fees may be too high; he may want to use a mental health center. Before you initiate treatment, be sure that the patient fully accepts you as his therapist and that he made this choice in the presence of alternate options.

Currently, there are a multitude of health plans that channel the patient's choice, penalize him if goes outside the plan, and reduce or even exclude his benefits. Make the patient aware of these factors so that he checks with his insurance plan. If he chooses to see you, make sure both you and he understand clearly the limits of his benefits. Make him aware that he will be responsible for any additional expenditure. If free choice is important to him, and his plan is very restrictive, you might recommend other plans available through his employer. Emphasize the patient's right to choose.

After the patient has understood and agreed to the treatment plan and has accepted you as his therapist, close the treatment contract. Take details seriously and let him agree to all terms: how often and how long you will see him; how much you will charge for regular and broken but uncanceled appointments; who will cover for you when you are out of town; how he can reach you after hours. Tell him under which circumstances you expect him to call. The more explicitly he agrees to all terms, the more he will feel obliged to keep his part of the contract.

Mental status: The patient's comprehension of your prognosis and treatment plan and his insight into his problems become apparent. What may surprise you is the confidence that some patients express in their future and in their ability to comply with the treatment. Patients who are very confident and grandiose often intensely follow the treatment for a short period but when they experience setbacks—which they regularly seem to do—they drop out. For instance, a patient who abuses alcohol may tell you in glowing terms that Sunday was the last day he had a drop of it. No more from now on! He will empty all his liquor bottles, dump his drinking buddies, and start a new life with milk and honey. Without dampening the patient's enthusiasm, inform him that relapse should not be viewed as failure. Help him understand that relapse is part of the illness and that your goal is to help him recognize that the process of recovery takes time.

At the very end of the interview you may want to ask the patient how he felt at the beginning of the interview and how he feels now. Indicate to him that you are looking forward to seeing him again. Express a justifiable degree of optimism about the future visits and the anticipated progress.

6.   INTERVIEW WITH A COOPERATIVE PATIENT

Most psychiatric patients are cooperative. They answer questions to the point and engage in the interview either spontaneously, or at least after a brief warm-up period.

We have reproduced a typical interview with a hospitalized, 29-year-old, white female. We edited it by numbering all questions and adding some questions (Q.) and answers (A.) to illustrate what we discussed in Chapters 1–6. We also divided it into five phases to show how each phase contributes to rapport, mental status, techniques, and diagnosis. Important questions are italicized.

Phase 1: Warm-Up and Screening of the Problem

In an intensive medical care unit, the patient is sitting up in her bed in a hospital gown. Her ash-blond hair is unkempt, showing half an inch of new brown growth at the roots. She wears no makeup and her skin is pale and gray.

She glances at the psychiatrist when he approaches her area, which is separated from the neighboring beds by a partly drawn curtain. She licks her dry lips; her lower lip is bruised and swollen, presumably from the intubation 2 days ago. She looks older than her stated age. She swallows when the interviewer is ready to address her.

1. I: Hello, Mrs. Goodman, my name is Dr. O. Has Dr. M. told you that he wanted me to see you?
   P: Yes, he told me that.
2. I: Do you feel comfortable talking to a psychiatrist?
   P: Well . . . I don't know what good it can do . . . just asking a bunch of stupid questions isn't going to help me a bit. But I guess you do what you want to anyway, no matter what . . . [speaks hesitantly].
3. I: If you talk to me we may be able to understand what got you here.
   P: I know that anyway. I don't need you for that [slumps back into her pillow and turns to the side away from her interviewer].
4. I: Gee, you must really feel pissed that you bite my head off before I have even started to talk to you.
   P: Darn right.
5. I: Being that pissed . . . you sound as if you've gone through hell.
   P: [slowly she turns around and looks at the psychiatrist] I'm sorry . . . if I sound rude . . . I just can't help it, I'm so keyed up . . . any little thing makes me fly off.
6. I: Maybe you can get some things off your chest and, of course, if you feel too bad and if you can't take it just say so and we can continue later.
   P: Hmm . . .

7. I: How have you been treated here?
 P: Oh, I can think of a better place.
8. I: How long have you been in the intensive care unit?
 P: For the last 2 days. I came here Saturday night.
9. I: Can I do anything for you before we start . . . [waiting] like getting you something to drink?
 P: A glass of ice water would be fine [the interviewer goes to the nursing station to get it].
10. I: [after he returns from the station with a glass of water] What got you here in the first place?
 P: I had problems with my husband—we were arguing and fighting—and the kids got on my nerves. And so I couldn't sleep. On Saturday, I took some pills.
11. I: Took some pills?
 P: Well, I took all the prescription pills that we had in the house . . .
12. I: Hmm.
 P: Because I was tired . . .
13. I: [just looking at her]
 P: I just wanted to lay down and go to sleep.
14. I: [still looking at the patient]
 P: . . . and . . . and not wake up.
15. I: Hmm. You must have really felt awful . . . not wanting to wake up.
 P: Yeah I guess . . . I really had it. I felt all worn out.
16. I: So bad that you were ready to die?
 P: I wasn't thinking about it that way . . . at the time. I was . . . just tired of everything—like I said, I just wanted to lay down and go to sleep and forget everything . . . I didn't think about it as killing myself.
17. I: Just to get rid of all those feelings?
 P: Yeah. That's right. To kill all those feelings.
18. I: Do you still feel that way?
 P: Hmm . . . I don't know . . . I guess . . . at times.

Severity

19. I: What happens to you when you are that down?
 P: I don't want to move [pulls up her cover, turning away to the side]. I don't want to see anybody . . . I want to be left alone . . . just have peace and quiet [the patient closes her eyes].
20. I: Hmm . . . [the interviewer puts his hand on the patient's shoulder, which is covered by the blanket].
 P: . . . Not answer anything.
21. I: Ah . . . hmm, do you feel like this right now?
 P: Hmm . . . now . . . ? [turns to the interviewer and opens her eyes] Earlier I guess. Everybody gets on my nerves . . . I want to be left alone, everything is an effort.
22. I: I see . . . It must really bother you to talk to me now.
 P: Yeah . . . Hmm . . . eh . . . it's all right, I guess. You seem to understand; that makes it easier.

23. I: I see . . . so . . . you still feel down?
    P: Yeah, pretty much.
24. I: I'm so sorry that you have such a rough time. Were you so much down that you felt like out of it?
    P: Yeah, like losing my mind.
25. I: Like losing your mind? Like even hearing things?
    P: Yeah . . . I just would . . . like maybe . . . be in a room by myself . . . and I'd think . . . I heard somebody . . . heard somebody call me . . . call my name or something, but I didn't see anybody talking . . . and there wasn't anybody.
26. I: Yes, that happens to people when they feel really depressed . . . tell me more about it.
    P: Just my name . . . maybe two or three times . . . like I was aware of it . . . maybe not like a voice.
27. I: When you felt like this . . . could you get anything done . . . like your regular work?
    P: Oh no . . . everything was too much . . . I couldn't even go to the grocery store—it made me so nervous.

Course

28. I: When did it all start?
    P: I have had those feelings off and on. But it really got worse over the last 6 weeks.
29. I: Off and on . . . ?
    P: Yes. They hit me out of the blue.
30. I: And you could not go to the grocery store then either?
    P: Oh no . . . That was just in the last few weeks. Before that I was just crabby and bitchy . . . terrible with my kids and with Al [the patient's husband].
31. I: You could work back then?
    P: Yes, I could but I was draggy . . . just not worth a shit. But I guess I looked all right . . . from the outside. And it didn't really last that long.
32. I: And now?
    P: Now? Now that's different. It really hit me for a loop. I haven't had anything like this before.

Stressor

33. I: So it really hit you this time. Tell me what happened, what brought it on?
    P: Hmm . . . I felt pressured. It just seemed everybody was making demands on me . . . more than I could stand. And I felt . . . like I was trapped.
34. I: Trapped?
    P: Yeah, at work. We had a girl at work . . . she was going into surgery . . . and then we had another one going on vacation, and I was taking over both their jobs and mine . . . and I kept forgetting and misfiling things . . .
35. I: Ah, let's look at your concentration and memory a little later . . . Anyway, you said you felt pressured.

P: Pressured . . . yeah . . . I felt like closed in and trapped. I had to get things done and I couldn't. The more I tried the worse it got. I got all tangled up. That pulled me down.

36. I: [frowns] You felt overworked?

P: [irritated] Yeah, didn't I just tell you?

37. I: Being overworked pulled you down?

P: Yeah, at my job and at home . . . must have been . . . there wasn't anything else going on . . .

38. I: [raising his eyebrows] Hmm . . .

P: Don't you believe me?

39. I: [with emphasis] Of course, I believe you. It must seem that way to you.

P: What do you mean?

40. I: I mean you felt more pressure because there was more pressure . . . or maybe because you could take *less* pressure.

P: [annoyed] You're playing with words.

41. I: Maybe I play with how one can look at it.

P: [shakes her head] You confuse me.

42. I: I'm sorry . . . but let me ask you, has that happened before, that somebody was on vacation?

P: Oh yeah, it happens every year once or twice, for the last 5 years.

43. I: And then it gets to you?

P: Hmm . . . hmm . . . no . . . last year I just went to the supervisor. I just told him we were falling behind and he better send somebody else down . . . but Ron [the supervisor] couldn't do that, really. He had a girl answer some of the mail that I thought was important. The rest, he said, just had to wait.

44. I: Hmm . . . and this time?

P: This time was different. I didn't feel up to it. I felt I had to handle it . . . by myself. I couldn't face him and tell him that I couldn't pick up Rosie's work. So I just drudged along.

45. I: You could not face him?

P: Oh, it just didn't feel right. I just thought I'm letting her down if I complain behind her back. I couldn't do that.

46. I: So you felt you couldn't let her down?

P: Yeah, tattle on her.

47. I: How did you feel otherwise?

P: Crabby . . . down in the dumps, I guess.

48. I: So this time you feel different . . . different to begin with?

P: You mean because I was down I felt that way?

49. I: Yes, that's right.

P: But what else should have pulled me down?

50. I: Sometimes people feel down without a reason, we'll talk about that later.

P: But that's crazy . . .

Rapport: The patient rebuffs the interviewer's opening remarks. Right away, he addresses her despondent attitude toward him and shows sensitivity for her discomfort. He overcomes her territorial defense ("the patient turns away") with strong language to match her affect and to get her attention. He activates her guilt feelings when he confronts her with her hostility. When she shows regret, he quickly responds to her verbal signal ("keyed up") with empathy.

She puts him in the role of overwhelming authority (A. 2). He mollifies her by telling her that he can continue the interview later if she so desires (Q. 6). But he takes care not to encourage her to escape the interview, thus maintaining guidance. He shows concern for her well-being and tries to put her at ease by getting her something to drink.

Since the interviewer has some difficulties in establishing rapport initially, he delays the question for the chief complaint (Q. 10). And since rapport remains destabilized, he screens the patient's behavior for signs of resistance such as hostile posture, avoidance of eye contact, evasive or short yes/no-type answers.

He assumes a role as empathic listener (Q. 15, 22, 24, 26, 33). He exercises patience, waiting for her answers without pushing, to keep her in a spontaneous talking mode rather than in a reactive answering mode, where answers have to be extracted like teeth. He neutralizes her admission of a possibly embarrassing symptom (a hallucination, A. 25) as an experience typical of depression to put her at ease and to encourage her to elaborate on other psychotic symptoms.

A. 33–36 show that the patient interprets her dysphoric feelings as the result of stress rather than as a spontaneous shift in mood, showing that she has only partial insight. The interviewer attempts to challenge her perspective, but she maintains that her disturbed feelings are due to outside stress (Q. 38–41).

Technique: Initially, the distractible and hostile patient resists talking and is unwilling to cooperate with the interviewer. In this case, the patient shows unprovoked hostility, and he answers in kind by using slang to get her attention. Even though he is aware that this confrontational approach may provoke more hostility, he feels it is important to quickly put her in a responding mode. As soon as he has her attention—because she answers him, to the point—he attempts to replace the hostile interchange by an empathic approach. This works because it activates her guilt feelings. A. 9 concludes the warm-up phase; the patient appears to be at ease; she accepts a glass of water from him.

Q. 10 is broad and open-ended to allow the patient to select her topic. This question for the chief complaint (Q. 10) is introduced by an accentuated transition, which is viable here since the patient does not seem to be anxious or suspicious. The interviewer follows up on the clue ("I took some pills") by echoing (Q. 11), continuation (Q. 12–14), specifying (Q. 16), and summarizing (Q. 17) techniques. With Q. 18 he shifts to the present to probe for persisting depressive symptoms and suicidal ideation as mental status functions.

The smooth transition (Q. 19) aims at the severity of her depressions. Q. 33 introduces as a new topic the precipitating event using another smooth transition. In a subtle way, this question asks for her interpretation. He echoes her interpretation (Q. 34) but starts to question its accuracy, mainly by frowning (Q. 36) and eyebrow raising (Q. 38). The patient notices his doubts and responds with irritation (A. 36, 38, 40, 41). Starting with Q. 39, he suggests by his questions an alternate interpretation, namely that her problems may be due to a decrease in coping ability rather than to an increase in stress (Q. 39–50).

Mental status: *Observation* yields an alert, slightly disheveled female who looks older than her stated age. Her ethnic background appears to be Anglo-American. She does not maintain eye contact; she shows some evidence of psychomotor retardation. Her affect appears sad, irritable, despondent, and depressed; she does not smile when the interviewer walks in. She shows reactivity in her affect when he evokes guilt feelings.

Conversation reveals that the patient is alert and comprehends the questions. Her speech is goal-oriented and fluent but slow, with increased latency of response. She elaborates on the closed-ended Q. 1 and 2 rather than limiting herself to yes/no answers. She is oriented to place, person, and time; her short-term memory is grossly intact (she remembers correctly the time of admission).

During *exploration* the patient reports psychomotor slowing, suicidal ideation, and a fleeting auditory hallucination. She gives detailed responses indicating her cooperation. Her vocabulary expresses at least average intelligence. She interprets her symptoms as a reaction to outside pressure, which she feels she should have been able to handle. Her interpretation of her disorder seems to show limited insight, which is not easily corrected. Her attitude toward work and colleagues reflects a lack of assertiveness but presence of guilt feelings, and low self-esteem. She tries to overcome her inadequacy by obsessive work habits and increased effort, rather than by asking for assistance. Therefore, her approach shows impaired social judgment.

The interviewer prepares the patient for later testing of memory in phase 3 (Q. 124).

Diagnosis: The interviewer opens with a question for the chief complaint rather than following up on behavioral clues noticed during warm-up. The patient lists associated symptoms for depression: suicidal tendencies (A. 10), irritability, and social withdrawal (A. 19, 21). Q. 11–17 clarify the suicidal remarks as an intent to kill her depressed feelings rather than herself. Such suicidal gestures may express one or more of the following:

1. the wish to communicate severe suffering (cry for help);
2. frustration and anger against oneself;
3. an attempt to induce guilt in others;
4. an attempt to get rid of depressed feelings.

In contrast, hanging, shooting, and jumping from high places are generally more serious and often mostly successful suicide methods.

Q. 24–26 assess psychotic symptoms, hallucinations, and delusions, that is, severity of the illness. The patient experienced an auditory hallucination of having her name called. She explained this brief auditory experience as due to her nervous condition rather than as the effect of a magical event. Because of her insight, this hallucination is considered a pseudohallucination.

Q. 28: The switch from cross-sectional to longitudinal symptom assessment examines whether diagnostic criteria for depression are met, that is, duration of more than 2 weeks, which helps to distinguish depression from adjustment disorder with depressed mood, since depression has diagnostic priority over adjustment disorder (DSM-IV-TR). The patient fulfills diagnostic criteria for major depressive disorder.

Q. 33–50 assess as a precipitating event the increased work load, which the patient attempted to handle, rather than negotiating with her supervisors for a better work distribution. Guilt feelings and obsessive-compulsive tendencies may have contributed to such a behavior. It is unclear whether her guilt and obsessiveness are personality traits magnified by depression, or symptoms of a depressive episode.

From the patient's response, which indicates that she could handle similar situations in the past, we can conclude that the increased work load is not a cause for her depression—it is unlikely that it has triggered the depressive episode. The most plausible interpretation is that the patient was depressed to begin with and that her failure to adjust to the increased work load magnifies her decreased coping ability during her depression.

At the end of phase 1, the warm-up and screening phase, list no. 1 of possible diagnostic options includes:

- alcohol use disorders
- substance use disorders
- bipolar disorder, depressed
- major depressive disorder
- cyclothymic disorder
- dysthymic disorder
- somatization disorder
- histrionic personality disorder
- borderline personality disorder
- obsessive-compulsive personality disorder
- dependent personality disorder

All these disorders should ideally be scrutinized in phase 3. This list is not written in stone. As clues evolve during the interview, other disorders may be added (see below, panic and obsessive-compulsive disorder). List no. 2 excluded psychiatric disorders, such as adjustment disorder with depressed mood, and cognitive disorders. All disorders of DSM-IV-TR not mentioned in list no. 1 or list no. 2 remain in list no. 3, the unchecked psychiatric disorders.

Phase 2: Follow-Up of Preliminary Impressions

51. I: Hmm. Let's talk about it.
    P: You know I wasn't sleeping well. That's probably why. I just felt like I had to get out and away from everybody . . . I started to lose my appetite, and you know . . . just evasive things.
52. I: Evasive things?
    P: I don't want to talk about them . . . not now.
53. I: Evasive things . . . [looks at the patient but she does not answer] Sounds like you try to push them out of your mind?
    P: Yeah.
54. I: They must still bother you.
    P: It's so crazy . . . well, let's just forget about it now.
55. I: Must be difficult to talk about it.
    P: Yeah, I don't want to think about it any more. I really felt bad.
56. I: Yeah, you felt so bad that it even affected your sleep.
    P: Yeah, it was lousy.
57. I: What kind of sleeping problems?
    P: Oh, I'd stay up till 11:00 P.M. or 12:00 midnight, and I'd be up through the night . . . and I'd get up around 5:30 or 6:00 A.M. . . . and just go all day.
58. I: And your appetite?
    P: [does not answer]

59. I: Did you lose any weight?
    P: Yes, about 30 pounds . . . my clothes were falling off me. Everything looked too big.
60. I: What's your weight now?
    P: [laughs] I don't want to answer that [the patient weighs 176 pounds at the interview].
61. I: Did you want to lose that much?
    P: Yeah . . . but I also did not have any appetite.

Manic Episodes

62. I: You say: You feel crabby and down in the dumps now. Have you ever felt the opposite: Were you ever really up, so people would say: "My goodness, you are high, are you taking coke or something?"
    P: Yeah, like "What happened? Where did you get all that pep to do things, what's going on?" And the next day I'd be so low, you know.
63. I: How long did your longest high last?
    P: About 3 weeks.
64. I: For 3 weeks!
    P: Yeah, at least.
65. I: What kind of things did you do during that time?
    P: What do you mean?
66. I: Did you ever do something . . . that you regret now . . . like spending a lot of money, getting involved with something or someone?
    P: No, no, nothing like that.
67. I: What about your energy then?
    P: Oh, that was fine. I just felt contented—and I was pleased with everything around me.
68. I: How was your sleep during that time?
    P: Well, I stayed up late and got up early, but I slept through the night at least. I needed less sleep.
69. I: How was your speech?
    P: I might have talked faster.
70. I: Faster?
    P: Rattling—yeah [laughs, embarrassed].
71. I: Did others comment on that?
    P: Well, my husband would tell me to shut up once in a while [laughs again and blushes].
72. I: Does he usually do that?
    P: No, it's just when I got to rattling.
73. I: How often did you have that rattling period?
    P: I don't know. Not real often to that point, to that degree.
74. I: Did you start a lot of projects then?
    P: Well, I liked to be busy.
75. I: Did you get it all done what you started?
    P: Oh sure, it all fell right into place.

Substance and Alcohol Use

76. I: Did you ever take any street drugs to feel that good?
    P: [gives an empty stare] No . . .
77. I: Or for any other reason?
    P: No, never.
78. I: What about drinking?
    P: Liquor . . . ? No, I don't like any of it.
79. I: Do you take any pills . . . pain pills? If we looked in your medicine cabinet at home, what would we find?
    P: Nothing now.
80. I: And before that?
    P: Aspirins.
81. I: Often?
    P: When I got headaches, I would. But mostly my husband would take them.

Obsessive-Compulsive Disorder

82. I: Besides these depressive feelings—you described them really well—did you have any other concerns, anything else unusual?
    P: Like what?
83. I: For instance, thinking about the same things over and over again, not being able to push a thought out of your mind?
    P: Yeah, I've had that. I've been struggling with that over the last few weeks.
84. I: What kind of thoughts were those?
    P: Well, about two months ago for one thing, I kept having dreams that my little girl was dying . . . One Sunday morning in church I looked up in front and I could see her playing in her coffin up there, you know. For several days after that, all I could think about was seeing her laying up there. I got kind of panicky to the point where I hated to let her out of my sight. I was afraid something would happen to her.
85. I: Did you ever have the feeling that you yourself would harm her . . . accidentally . . . or even intentionally?
    P: No, like I said, when I could feel myself getting angry, I would send the kids out, because I knew I could get carried away spanking them. But no, I didn't ever really think I'd ever hurt her.
86. I: Did you have other thoughts that forced themselves into your mind?
    P: Yeah, but I don't want to talk about them.
87. I: You don't want to discuss them now . . . [after a pause]. Were these types of thoughts only there when you were depressed or were they present all the time?
    P: They were there quite a lot of the time . . . because that's what used to bring me down, you know. I'd be okay, and then I'd start thinking on things and then I would start feeling myself getting down . . . really getting depressed. And then when I was depressed, it was much worse to where it kept me there.
88. I: When did they first start?

P: Two or three months ago, I think.

89. I: Were these thoughts like visions that would come up in your mind . . . like with the coffin?

P: Yeah. Like that . . . like visions . . . but sometimes just thoughts.

90. I: Is there anything that you did about it? Any ritual or any kind of procedure to prevent those things from happening? You said, you did not let your daughter out of sight. Did you do any more than that?

P: No, there was nothing else to do.

91. I: Did you do things like checking . . .

P: [looks puzzled and frowns]

92. I: Like checking the locks . . . or the fireplace or the gas?

P: I didn't check anything.

93. I: Did you feel these visions or thoughts were really silly?

P: Hmm . . . One scared me. You know, I always felt like I wasn't going to have her until she was grown, from the time she was born, you know. But some of the other ones have been silly.

94. I: Can you tell me a few silly ones?

P: No.

95. I: You must feel quite embarrassed about them that you feel so strongly about hiding them—any reason?

P: Many reasons, but I won't discuss them either—you seem to know a lot about them anyway.

Panic Disorder

96. I: Okay. You say some of these thoughts scared you. Have you ever felt so scared that you had a spell of panic?

P: Yeah, that morning when I saw her up front in the coffin, I had to leave. I was shaking and crying [little laugh], you know, kind of on the verge of hysterical, I guess.

97. I: Did you have to fight for your breath?

P: No.

98. I: Just describe what happened to you when you had that spell.

P: I was scared, uptight, my hands were clammy.

99. I: Clammy? Also tingling?

P: No, there was no tingling.

100. I: And your vision?

P: My vision? There was nothing wrong with it, nothing.

101. I: And your heart?

P: Nothing wrong with my heart, just the same.

102. I: Any pounding?

P: No, nothing like that.

103. I: How often did you have these types of spells?

P: Not more than two or three times. It's just really started coming. This was just a couple of days ago.

Rapport: Mrs. Goodman gives a coherent history and elaborates spontaneously, all signs of good rapport. Therefore, further empathic remarks are not necessary. The interviewer continues to challenge her explanation for her depression. However, when she explains her depression as being due to inadequate sleep, he adopts her perspective; he forms an alliance with her without attempting further to correct her level of insight, thus preserving rapport.

She refuses to discuss obsessive thoughts (A. 51–54, 86, 94–95). This refusal may be due to an anxiety of being overwhelmed when discussing them, or fear to be considered "crazy" or "silly." Since her refusal is limited to symptoms not essential for a working diagnosis and immediate management, the interviewer, after repeated confrontation, expresses empathy with her refusal, and decides to abstain from further pressuring her and to bypass her resistance in order not to endanger rapport. She acknowledges his expertise (A. 95), which seems to justify his approach.

Technique: Q. 56–61 are specifications of symptoms mentioned in A. 51 using the techniques of specification (Q. 57) and checking for symptoms (Q. 58–61).

Q. 62–75: The interviewer approaches manic symptoms with a smooth transition. He contrasts her present depressive state with its opposite. After she admits to elation but denies unrestrained buying sprees (A. 66), he checks for other manic symptoms (Q. 67–69, 74, 75) with circumscribed open- and closed-ended questions. After a smooth transition (Q. 76), he screens for substance and alcohol abuse and excludes it.

Q. 82–95: He checks obsessive-compulsive disorder with a standard strategy: with broad questions (Q. 82, 83) he screens for the presence of essential symptoms of the disorder. Since the patient refuses to describe her obsessive thoughts, he confronts her with her resistance in Q. 87 and 95. When the patient refuses to discuss the reason for the resistance, he starts to discuss other pathology.

Q. 96–101: With a smooth transition he links the obsessions to panic disorder by picking up on the patient's clue "scared" (A. 93) and continues with open- and closed-ended, symptom-oriented questions.

Mental status: The remark about her colleague whom she could not let down represents nearly unrealistic if not delusional guilt. The patient also shows suppression of her possible obsessive thought content, which she seems to experience not as ego-dystonic but as threatening to her integrity. She experiences her aggressive impulses as difficult to control and sends her children outside. This also reflects a need for social withdrawal, which she acted out when the interviewer first met her. Spontaneously, she reports classic vegetative symptoms of depression but not clear-cut hypomania or mania (Q. 62–75). She seems to have experienced severe anxiety in connection with the obsessive thought content. During the interview, overt anxiety is not manifest except in her refusal to talk about her obsessions. The anxiety experienced in the past does not appear to be a clear-cut panic attack.

Diagnosis: The interviewer checks for further symptoms of depression—social withdrawal (A. 51), initial, intermittent, and terminal insomnia (A. 56, 57), and weight loss without body image distortion (A. 59). Q. 62 asks for elation, which she endorses and which lasted for about 3 weeks (A. 63), without imprudent behavior (Q. 65, 66), but increased energy (Q. 67), reduced desire for sleep (A. 68), and push of speech (A. 69–73). These symptoms suggest some elation, but they do not interfere with the patient's life. Only her self-report documents it. No hospitalization or treatment was required. These behavioral changes without symptom value may be within normal limits and experienced as a contrast to her depression. However, they should be remembered because they may predict a different treatment response from clear major depressive disorder.

Q. 76–81: According to the diagnostic hierarchy, the interviewer could challenge his diagnosis of major depressive disorder by finding severe drug or alcohol abuse. Cocaine, amphetamine, and alcohol withdrawal can produce depressive feelings. Therefore, he rules out alcohol and substance abuse.

Q. 82–95: The exploration of obsessive symptoms yields thoughts consistent with depression (harm may come to her daughter). The patient reports repetitive dreams, one abnormal perception, a visual hallucination or pseudohallucination, and some recurring fears about it. The interviewer explores thoughts of infanticide not uncommon in a depressed mother.

The patient admits also to silly intrusive thoughts but is unwilling to elaborate on them. Since these thoughts appear to be linked to her depressive episode and started relatively recently, a preexisting obsessive-compulsive disorder is unlikely. Consistent with this is the finding that she has no compulsions.

Q. 96–103: The patient's symptoms are atypical for panic disorder; she is more concerned about her hallucinations than her anxiety. Vegetative symptoms of a panic attack are missing. Since her fears are associated with a depressive episode, even more typical attacks would not establish the diagnosis of an independently existing panic disorder. Therefore, panic disorder is excluded.

List no. 1 of included disorders is:

- major depressive disorder
- bipolar II disorder
- dysthymic disorder
- cyclothymic disorder
- histrionic personality disorder
- borderline personality disorder
- obsessive-compulsive personality disorder

List no. 2 of excluded disorders is:

- cognitive disorders
- alcohol abuse
- substance abuse
- bipolar I disorder
- obsessive-compulsive disorder
- panic disorder
- adjustment disorder with depressed mood

Phase 3: History and Database

Longitudinal Course

104. I: Were you ever depressed before?
    P: Yeah . . . off and on for a couple days.
105. I: But did you have any long periods where you had to go for treatment or even be hospitalized?
    P: No . . . not before this time.
106. I: When were you first depressed in your life?
    P: About 10 or 11 years ago.
107. I: Have you also experienced some highs during that time?
    P: Yeah, I don't know, probably not as much as I was down. I mean, I was just kind of going along evenly and I was probably down more than I was up . . . or else I was just going even, you know, kind of leveled off.
108. I: Did these bad or good days ever prevent you from doing your work or disturb your family life?
    P: Not really, I may have been more irritable, but that's all.

Premorbid Personality and Social History

109. I: Were you moody . . . as a child or a teenager?

P: I was usually pretty up, you know. I was pretty happy. I had problems with my mom, but as long as I could avoid her, I got along with everybody.

110. I: And earlier on, did you have any problems in your development, such as with walking, talking, or toilet training and so on?

P: Oh no, my mom told me I was real early with all of that.

Family History

111. I: Was there anybody else in your family who was depressed?

P: Well, I have a sister who was in XX. State Hospital, but I don't know what her problems were. She never talked about them.

112. I: Is she older than you?

P: Yeah, she's about 14 years older and she's just had her problems in the past couple of years.

113. I: Is she completely well now?

P: No, she's still seeing a psychiatrist fairly often and taking medication.

114. I: Do you know what kind of medication?

P: No.

115. I: Does she have a family?

P: Yeah, she's got two kids, one is out of high school and the other is a junior this year.

116. I: How many brothers and sisters do you have?

P: Three brothers and three sisters.

117. I: How are they . . . besides your older sister, do any of them have any problems?

P: Well, I have another sister [laughs], she said if she ever went to a doctor, they'd probably lock her up. But she won't go. She has her down days.

118. I: So you have three sisters—that means there are four girls in the family and three boys. Three of you girls have some problems, but the fourth one has no mood swings or problems?

P: I don't know, I'm not around her.

119. I: What about your brothers?

P: They all seem okay; they usually get along fine.

120. I: What about your children? They are young, aren't they? Anything unusual?

P: No. My oldest one just had a few problems in school picking up stuff like her math, but you know, that's just kids. I don't think there is anything to worry about. My other children, too, they are lively, they pick up things and I think they are okay.

121. I: How many children do you have?

P: Three.

122. I: What about your parents—were there any kinds of problems, psychiatric problems, nerve problems?

P: No. They were never treated for anything anyway.

123. I: Any drinking problems?

P: No.

124. I: Your mother had several babies. Did she have problems after the delivery?
        Like did she feel unusually blue or did she have to stay longer in the hospital
        than usual? With any of them?
     P: No. She was in kind of bad health, she had heart problems. With my older
        brother she had a heart attack just after he was born. Outside of that there
        wasn't any problems.

Medical History

125. I: Did you yourself have any medical problems or allergies so far?
     P: Not up till now.

Completion of Database

126. I: You told me a lot about your problems. That helps me to help you. There
        are a couple of things left that I would like to test. Is that alright with you?
     P: Yeah, that's alright.
127. I: You told me that you started to forget things at work. Therefore, I'd like to
        test your memory.
     P: Okay.
128. I: I would like you to repeat four words: gray, watch, daisy, and justice. Can
        you do that?
     P: Gray, watch, daisy, and justice.
129. I: That's fine. Try to remember these words. I will ask you to recall them a lit-
        tle later.
     P: I'll try.
130. I: While we are at it, let me ask you to do some calculations for me.
     P: [with a smile] I was never too good at math, but I'll try.
131. I: I would like you to subtract 7 from 100, and then keep doing it, always sub-
        tracting 7 from the remainder. Let's start. What's 100 take away 7?
     P: 93-86-79-72-63-oh no, it's 65-58-51-54 sorry, 44-37-30-.
132. I: That's fine.
     P: No, I don't think so . . . I have trouble remembering the number that I have
        to subtract from. It confuses me.
133. I: Let's try some other things. How about some multiplication. Like 2 times 48.
     P: Oh no . . . 2 times 48? 86. No, I'm sorry, 96.
134. I: Two times 96.
     P: That's . . . 180 . . . 192.
135. I: Two times 192?
     P: That's 400 . . . 300 . . . and 84.
136. I: Very good. Let me go back to a couple of things that you said earlier. You
        took too many pills . . . Did you ever try to harm yourself before?
     P: No, that was the first time.
137. I: Did you ever think of harming yourself?
     P: [raises eyebrows]
138. I: When you were sad . . . or angry at somebody . . . or frustrated with a situa-
        tion?

P: No, not really. I could have kicked my husband a couple of times when he got me upset, but I usually just shut up or screamed . . . but then later we'd talk about it.

139. I: So this time was really the first time that you tried to harm yourself.

P: I really felt bad then and I still do.

140. I: Can you overcome this low feeling and pretend you are happy and say "I feel really happy"?

P: [looks perplexed] I can't do that. I feel really happy! [awkward shift in facial expression . . . then teary-eyed] Oh, no, I can't talk that way . . . only in the past I felt okay for 2 to 3 years, even after I got depressed.

141. I: I hope we can stop these mood swings for good. Now let's go back to the four words I asked you to remember. Can you remember them?

P: Watch, daisy, and justice. Well, there was another one. Let me see, what was it? It was before watch, I think. Hmm . . . Yes, that's it—gray.

142. I: You are really doing fine.

P: But that's pretty simple stuff.

143. I: Not for everyone. But you did fine. Before we close, are there any questions that you would like to ask me?

P: No . . . they will probably come later . . . after you have left.

144. I: How did you feel during the interview?

P: Oh . . . it was okay. I feel you understand what's going on with me . . .

Rapport: Rapport is good. The patient answers to the point; she elaborates without prodding and does more so as the interview goes on; she feels comfortable enough to reveal some intimate and embarrassing symptoms. Now, she clearly assumes the role of "carrier of an illness" with some distance from her disorder, which makes it easy to interview her about herself and her family. She does not indulge in suffering, or strive to be treated as a "VIP."

To submit to testing requires that the patient trusts the interviewer. Therefore, he prepares her for it and asks for permission (Q. 126). He also prepares her for memory testing (Q. 127) and gets her permission. She agrees without hesitation to be tested, which confirms that the interviewer and the patient have good rapport. A. 144 assures the interviewer that the patient experiences him as an empathic listener and expert.

Technique: The interviewer uses both smooth (Q. 104, 125) and more accentuated transitions (Q. 109–111) to introduce new topics. The patient's goal-directed answers show that she tolerates all transitions well. Q. 104 shifts from a cross-sectional to a longitudinal view, with a smooth transition to keep the patient focused on her depressive symptoms. Q. 107: The interviewer chooses another smooth transition to assess the history of depressive and manic symptoms. More abrupt transitions (Q. 109–111) introduce the assessment of the premorbid personality and family history. They indicate to the patient that the interviewer is changing the topic.

The interviewer summarizes what he has learned and what he is missing, to prepare the patient for testing. He justifies testing by referring to her earlier remarks about her forgetfulness (Q. 126–127).

At the end of this section, the interviewer asks the patient about her feelings during the interview. This shift from data collection to rapport serves two purposes: it concludes the interview, and gives the patient a chance to reflect about it (Q. 144).

Mental status: The patient appears to have more insight into her past mood disturbances as unprovoked mood swings. She also seems to understand the mood disturbances of her family members as disorders and not as environmentally determined reactions, even though she interprets her present mood disturbance as a reaction to outside events. She may not be aware of this inconsistency because she experiences her present mood disorder as ego-syntonic. It will be the therapist's task to create more cognitive distance to her present depressed feelings.

In Q. 140, the interviewer picks up on the patient's statement that she still feels depressed and asks her to emulate happiness. She fails miserably on this important mental status test. Even though the patient shows by the way she reports her history that she has adequate concentration, memory, sentence structure, and flow of speech, indicating at least average intelligence, the interviewer decides to obtain some quantitative measures of functions to document her baseline performance. The patient can repeat four words immediately and recall them after a few minutes. Her series seven backwards shows some mild difficulties with concentration; she makes two mistakes but immediately corrects them herself. Her IQ according to the RAIT (Rapid Approximation Intelligence Test) is in the normal range.

Diagnosis: The history of the present disorder reveals that it is episodic in nature and that the present episode is the first one severe enough to require treatment (A. 105). The proportion of elated feelings to depressed periods— fewer elated than depressed days—concurs with clinical expectations (A. 107).

Q. 109: The interviewer explores the patient's premorbid personality. She seems to have been outgoing and popular with normal early development, which is consistent with an affective disorder and may exclude obsessive-compulsive personality disorder. Q. 111–115: One out of 3 sisters of 11 first-degree relatives has a psychiatric disorder that was remitting and did not affect the marriage. This history is consistent with pure familial mood disorder. The list no. 1 of included disorders is:

- Bipolar disorder II

At the beginning of phase 3 the interviewer had excluded substance abuse, alcoholism, obsessive-compulsive, panic, and somatization disorders. He ponders whether besides borderline, or histrionic personality disorder, cyclothymic disorder may have preceded her more severe depression. The patient's report of at least 2-year intervals between mild but noticeable symptoms of depression exclude cyclothymia however. Her stable marriage and absence of repeated suicide attempts exclude both personality disorders. A. 125 indicates good medical health and *excludes* somatization disorder. List no. 2 of excluded disorders is:

- bipolar I disorder
- alcohol use disorders
- substance use disorders
- obsessive-compulsive disorder
- panic disorder
- obsessive-compulsive personality disorder
- somatization disorder
- adjustment disorder with depressed mood
- cyclothymic disorder
- borderline personality disorder
- histrionic personality disorder

Phase 4: Diagnosis and Feedback

145. I: Let me tell you then what I have learned so far. What you described to me sounds like depressive episodes. They seem to get longer and more severe as time goes on. Since you had a 3-week period with mildly elated mood, you may actually have bipolar II disorder, depressed.

   P: I understand that. But what brings them on? Why do I have them?

146. I: You think it is your work and what happens at home, or your poor sleep. But what makes you sleep more poorly in the first place?

   P: Hmm . . . but there isn't anything . . . maybe my thoughts . . .

147. I: Yes, maybe they change also because you get depressed.

   P: But why do I get depressed?

148. I: I really don't know. All we know is that depression runs in families.

   P: The children learn it from their parents?

149. I: Well, we don't think so. Even when parents with this disorder have their children adopted at birth by another family, these adopted children can develop the same disorder as their biological parents.

P: Hmm, I see.

150. I: Adoptees from healthy parents don't have that risk. Therefore we believe that a disposition for psychiatric disorders is inherited.

P: So, it's all inherited?

151. I: That's probably not the whole story. The environment, such as the upbringing, may contribute to the outbreak and the severity of the disorder.

P: So, what can you do for me if I was born with it?

Rapport: Phase 4 reveals that the patient accepts the interviewer's expertise. She shows interest in his explanation of her disorder, which may lower the risk for suicide. Toward the end of the interview, the interviewer challenges again the patient's insight into her disorder and attempts to use educational therapy for the understanding of her disorder. This improved insight may assure cooperation with treatment.

Technique: The interviewer gives a comprehensive, easy-to-understand explanation of the patient's disorder in the hope that this explanation will aid in her cooperation with treatment. He finishes his explanation with questions that invite her to ask questions of her own so that he can check her understanding of his clarification. This technique works; the patient responds with several questions (A. 145, 147, 148, 150, 151).

Mental status: Mrs. Goodman's partial insight can be influenced by educational efforts, which shows that she is not delusionally fixed.

Diagnosis: Her interest in her treatment may be considered a good prognostic sign, since major depression shows good response to treatment if the patient is compliant.

Phase 5: Prognosis and Treatment Contract

152. I: There is medication that helps you to overcome your depression faster; you may have heard the name of some of these drugs. They are called antidepressants.

P: I don't know . . . sounds familiar. Does that mean I have a chemical imbalance? That's what one of my friends was told who had depressions.

153. I: Some psychiatrists feel that there is an imbalance, since drugs work on depressive disorder.

P: What should I do?

154. I: I'm worried about your overdose . . . I'm also concerned that you still feel
         pretty bad. You also appear worried and puzzled, even though your think-
         ing is pretty clear and your speech sounds good to me. Therefore I would
         really like you to stay in the hospital for a while, relax, and have us take
         care of you. Since I'm in the hospital all the time, I could also see you in the
         morning and evening to get a feeling for your daily mood swings.
    P: Do I really need to stay in the hospital?
155. I: Here we can better watch out for you, we also can give you a higher dosage
         of medication at the beginning. Hopefully, this will make you feel better
         faster. That's really what I would recommend.
    P: If you think so, I'll do it.
156. I: That's the right first step in my opinion. As we get on with your treatment, I
         will tell you how to spot relapse so that you have shorter and less severe
         depressive episodes in the future. The medication has side effects, and we
         will talk about them. We will also discuss some problems that you may
         have.
    P: OK. I'll go along with it.

Rapport: The interviewer explains the treatment plan and prognosis using an educational approach that will help to establish his role as expert.
But he also talks about his concerns for her and what steps should be taken.
Thus, he asks her implicitly to accept his authority by following his advice.
For a patient with some insight into her condition, a good justification for
the treatment plan is to inform her about its advantages. Her response
shows that she is willing to accept the plan.

Technique: In phase 5 the interviewer explains the treatment plan but
makes sure that the patient stays in a questioning mode as an indication of
her interest. He expresses personal concern for her well-being (Q. 154),
thus motivating her to agree to the treatment plan.

Mental status: The patient has insight and is interested enough in her
health to agree to the treatment plan. Her judgment is adequate so that the
prognosis for her cooperation with treatment is good.

Diagnosis: The patient's collaboration with the treatment plan improves
her prognosis.

7. CASE SUMMARY FORMAT

Usually the interviewer gives a written psychiatric evaluation of a patient after the clinical interview. This evaluation has to fulfill specific requirements if

it is presented to the American Board Examination of Psychiatry and Neurology, or when used in a medical record for which reimbursement by Medicare is requested. The chart is also a legal document used in malpractice cases, payment issues, and issues of appropriate care and level of care. Summaries are critically important to organizing the clinical impression obtained in the interview. We therefore give you a step-by-step guide to what you need to include in your psychiatric evaluation.

Adopt a standard format for the summary you will routinely use because it will allow you to organize your data quickly and efficiently, and will prove invaluable.

I. Identifying Data

Summarize the patient's name, sex, age, race, and reason for consultation.

II. Chief Complaint

State in the patient's own words her chief complaint. Alternatively, provide an important, observed sign of the patient's disordered functioning. The interpretative guidelines for HCFA standard 482.61 (b) stipulate the inclusion of the patient's chief complaint recorded in the patient's own words.

III. Informants

List all informants, their reliability, and level of cooperation. Include previous hospital records if available.

IV. Reason for Consultation or for Hospital Admission [HCFA Standard 482.61 (a) (3)]

In case of hospitalization, provide the legal status—voluntary versus involuntary [HCFA standard 482.61 (a) (1)]—and describe why, in your opinion, hospitalization was the least restrictive and safest environment for treatment.

V. History of Present Illness

Start the history when the patient first experienced symptoms, even if this dates back to adolescence or childhood. Give a history of symptoms, signs, and behaviors before you focus on reviewing diagnoses and treatments given by others. Some of these symptoms may have been very mild, and only retrospectively do they appear to signal the prodromal state or the onset of the disorder.

The inclusion of these mild, initial symptoms can be problematic for re-imbursement from insurance companies, even though in the past the pa-tient had no way to recognize these symptoms as part of a potential psychiatric disorder. Insurance companies may take this information as proof to deny payment for treatment of the disorder, claiming it is "preexist-ing." The fight for reimbursement may retard the patient's recovery. Since it is important to include accurate information about the severity of the symp-toms at the time of their first retrospective recognition, you should also point out whether these early manifestations were recognized by the patient as a disorder or not.

Include recent exacerbations of the disorder in this section, especially when the patient is admitted [HCFA standard 482.61 (b) (4)]. Note the onset of illness and circumstances leading to admission, if applicable.

To contrast the patient's psychiatric history, provide a history of the pre-morbid personality that can serve as your baseline of the patient's best level of functioning. You may estimate the GAF score (Global Assessment of Func-tioning) at that time to quantify the decline in general functioning by compar-ing it to the present GAF score. The patient's premorbid personality can also be discussed in more detail in the Social History (compare section VIII).

VI. Past Psychiatric History

This history should cover a psychiatric disorder different from the disorder covered under the present illness. This disorder may not have necessarily ceased at the present time. It may be of less concern than the present ill-ness. However it may significantly interfere with the present disorder. Such an interference occurs if there is a past history of substance abuse that con-tinues into the present, or if a severe personality disorder is present, such as antisocial personality disorder. Since substance abuse is common, its ab-sence should be noted as an important negative history.

The interpretative guidelines of HCFA standard 482.61 (b) stipulate that a past history of any psychiatric problems and treatment be included. This history should give a record of the patient's activities and social, educa-tional, vocational, interpersonal, and family relationships.

VII. Medical History

Give an account of all medical disorders past and present, especially those that can complicate, exacerbate, or mimic a psychiatric disorder [HCFA stan-dard 482.61 (b) (2)]. Some treatments of these medical disorders may also complicate the psychiatric disorder. Review allergies and sexually transmittable diseases at this time. Medical problems that occurred during childhood are of special interest if they involve the central nervous system, such as seizure disorders. In females, exclude pregnancy for safety of psychopharmacological treatment.

VIII. Social History and Premorbid Personality

The social history reflects the impact of the disorder on the patient's life. It should emphasize the psychosocial and environmental problems that may have contributed to the patient's psychiatric disorder, or that the psychiatric disorder has imposed on the patient's life. A thorough social history should also reflect the problems that the patient's personality disorders, if any, have caused.

To highlight the impact of the Axis I psychiatric disorder on the patient's life, you may contrast his premorbid psychosocial functioning with the morbid one. A patient may have a better prognosis if he showed a full range of social activities prior to the onset of his illness rather than being a socially withdrawn, isolated loner. Trace back his functioning to his preschool and early school years, if possible. Early developmental history (developmental milestones) and school history may reflect neurological impairment, disciplinary problems, and learning problems.

IX. Family History

At a minimum, the family history should describe the first-degree relatives, that is, parents, siblings, and children, and their psychiatric history. Since psychiatric disorders seem to have a genetic component, the psychiatric history of older first-degree relatives can serve as a model, which may predict the patient's future. The history of younger first-degree relatives may identify individuals at high risk and may trigger prophylactic interventions.

X. Mental Status Examination

Use a standard format to outline the patient's mental status. Summarize appearance, psychomotor activity, speech, thinking, and thought content. Pay special attention to the cognitive functions of orientation, memory, and intelligence. The assessment of these three functions is demanded by HCFA standard 482.61 (b) (6). Describe the patient's insight and judgment.

XI. Diagnostic Formulation

These diagnostic formulations are used in the Board Examination. They summarize the biological, psychological, and social factors (compare pp. 328–329) contributing to the patient's psychiatric disorders.

XII. Multiaxial Psychiatric Diagnoses

Give information on all five DSM-IV axes.

XIII. Assets and Strengths

According to HCFA standard 482.61 (b) (7), the psychiatric evaluation should give an inventory of the patient's knowledge, interests, skills, aptitudes, experience, education, and employment status, which may be useful in developing a meaningful treatment plan.

XIV. Treatment Plan and Prognosis

Describe the goals of treatment, the psychopharmacological, physical, psychological, and social treatment modalities that are required, their frequency, and their providers. The objectives should be given in descriptive, clearly measurable terms [HCFA standard 482 (c) (1 and 2)]. The treatment plan should include discharge criteria if the patient is treated as an inpatient.

Case Summary

This outline is illustrated in Mrs. Goodman's evaluation.

I. Identifying Data

This is the first psychiatric admission for Mrs. Goodman, a 29-year-old, white female who was brought to the emergency room by her husband because of an overdose.

II. Chief Complaint

"I took all the prescription pills that we had in the house because I was tired and wanted to lay down and go to sleep and not wake up."

III. Informants

The patient, who is reliable and cooperative. Emergency room hospital record.

IV. Reason for Admission or Consultation

Mrs. Goodman was admitted because of a suicide attempt. Her emergency room physician requested a psychiatric consultation to evaluate persisting suicidal tendencies.

V. History of Present Illness

The patient has experienced mood swings of short duration and mild intensity, separated by several years since her late teenage years. Episodes of elated mood, reduced need for sleep, increased energy, and talkativeness alternated with short periods of depression, irritability, and social withdrawal. None of these mood swings impaired the patient either in her normal functions or to such an extent that treatment was necessary.

Approximately 6 weeks ago, the patient was put under increased pressure at work. At this time she experienced family problems, irritability, insomnia with early morning awakenings, anorexia, weight loss of 30 pounds over 6 weeks, obsessive worries, brief auditory hallucinations of somebody calling her name, and social withdrawal. Her feelings of depression became so intense that she overdosed on aspirin in order to get relief from these depressive feelings. The overdose led to the present hospitalization. The affective disorder was not complicated by alcohol or substance abuse.

VI. Past Psychiatric History

The patient has no history of substance abuse or of disciplinary problems.

VII. Medical History

Negative, except for occasional headaches. Patient reports no allergies.

VIII. Social History and Premorbid Personality

The patient reached her developmental milestones without delay. She was an outgoing and popular student with average scholastic accomplishments. She completed high school successfully. She is currently married but experiences discontent in this marriage.

IX. Family History

The patient has 11 first-degree relatives. Only one of three sisters had a psychiatric hospitalization for a disorder unknown to Mrs. Goodman. Her sister recovered but required psychiatric outpatient treatment with medication.

X. Mental Status

Appearance: At the time of the interview the patient is a slightly disheveled, 29-year-old, white, alert female who is initially hostile but cooperates later.

Speech and thinking: She is concentrated throughout the interview, showing good comprehension. Her answers are goal-directed.

Affect: Initially labile and irritable with restricted range of affective expression.

Mood: Depressed but appropriate.

Thought content: Past auditory and visual hallucinatory experiences were of brief duration. Patient had some insight into their morbid nature. Some obsessive worries and fears may still be present, but the patient refuses to elaborate on them. The patient is not homicidal or suicidal at the present time. She denies paroxysmal events.

Orientation: She is oriented to person, place, and date.

Memory: Immediate, recent, and remote memory are intact. Her concentration is slightly impaired on serial seven backwards; she makes two calculation errors. She can multiply 2×192, which shows at least average intelligence. For economic reasons, a confirmation with the Kent Test (Table 5–5) is omitted.

Insight: She has partial insight; it is somewhat impaired concerning the impact of her job on her depression.

Judgment: Seems to be adequate at the present time.

XI. Diagnostic Formulation

Biological factors: The patient has a sister who, out of six siblings (three sisters and three brothers), has a psychiatric history severe enough to have required hospitalization. This sister recovered and has a functioning family life. Mrs. Goodman's parents and her three children have no psychiatric history. The sister's disorder may indicate a genetic disposition to a mood disorder.

  The patient does not mention any prenatal problems. Her mother had a heart attack with her last child. The patient does not report any delayed development. She also denies any medical problems. Therefore, from a biological point of view, a genetic disposition appears to be the only contributing factor to her mood disorder.

Psychological factors: The patient felt that increased work demand had brought on her latest depression. She had experienced a similar increase in work demand in the past when co-workers were on vacation but was then able to cope. This flexibility to adjust to and manage an increased work load disappeared, presumably due to a spontaneously appearing depressive episode. The patient is not able to recognize this spontaneous occurrence, which shows that her insight is limited with regard to a spontaneous mood change. She explains it in the layman's customary cause-and-effect model where the environmental stressor is perceived as an unavoidable psychosocial problem causing a change in mood. The patient perceives herself as unable to cope with the stressor or alter her response.

Transference pattern: Initially the patient projects her discomfort onto the interviewer and treats him like an unwelcome stressor—similar to her perception of her work. She blames herself for being resistant and becomes cooperative at least initially out of guilt feelings. Later she appears to be more genuinely cooperative out of an interest to get help, which shows a rational, adultlike response in terms of transactional analysis. The corresponding defenses appear to be projection and introjection.

Social factors: The patient is married and has three children. She mentions her home life or her husband only a few times. These statements do not reflect any major long-standing problems. Her children do not seem to have any problems. She has been working at the same place for at least 5 years, which shows stability in her social setting.

XII. Multiaxial Psychiatric Diagnoses

Axis I: 1. Major depressive disorder single episode, severe 296.23.
2. Rule out bipolar II disorder 296.89.
    [The following elaborations of the diagnostic impressions on Axis I are not part of the routine psychiatric evaluation, but are examples of discussions that may take place in an oral Board Examination in which the candidate substantiates his or her impressions.]
    Depressed mood is present for at least 6 weeks, also loss of appetite, insomnia, agitation, diminished ability to concentrate, loss of self-esteem, and a suicide gesture (criterion A). There is evidence of temporary friction in her marriage and at work, both of which suggest some impairment in interpersonal functioning (criterion B). There is no evidence that the effects of substance use, or a general medical condition, have directly contributed to

her experience (criterion C), nor is this the result of bereavement (criterion D). All of this suggests that the patient has satisfied the criteria for major depressive episode, which is criterion A for major depressive disorder, single episode. You can rule out schizoaffective disorder, schizophrenia, schizophreniform disorder, delusion disorder, or psychotic disorder NOS. There is no evidence of any manic episodes. However the patient had a possible hypomanic episode.

The longitudinal course of the illness appears to be episodic with mood disorder. Furthermore, there is no evidence of any other disorder that could challenge these diagnoses, such as a cognitive disorder or substance abuse disorder. The obsessive features mentioned by the patient are not sufficient to make the diagnosis of obsessive-compulsive disorder but could be followed up further. The anxiety feelings represent, at best, an isolated panic attack NOS during a depression, rather than an independent disorder.

Axis II: None.

Axis III: 305.90 Status after intoxication with multiple medications.

Axis IV: V62.2 Occupational problem. There is an increased work load at her job due to a temporary reduction of the work force. The work load would be manageable for the patient (as it was in the past) if it were not for her poor reality testing secondary to her depression.

Axis V: GAF = 35. The patient is impaired in her work. She shows poor reality testing with respect to her work, which led to a serious suicide attempt. Her mood is severely depressed. She is unable to relate to her supervisor who was previously supportive of her. While she is presently not acutely suicidal, she is still stress sensitive and could immediately relapse and repeat a suicide attempt if discharged from the hospital prematurely.

XIII. Assets and Strengths

The patient has at least average intelligence. She is not delusional. Therefore she appears to be receptive to an educational approach about the nature of her distorted stress perception and can be convinced that she has a treatable disorder. Furthermore, she has intact support systems in her family and her job. They can be utilized to motivate her for treatment.

XIV. Treatment Plan and Prognosis

1. The patient shall be transferred to inpatient psychiatry because she is still significantly depressed and has poor reality testing and insight in her condition. She may not be able to cooperate with an outpatient treatment plan but force herself to return to work without adequate ability to cope. This could precipitate another suicide attempt.
2. The patient may be started on 20 mg of paroxetine HCL (Paxil) A.M. or any other SSRI and monitored for antidepressant efficacy and adverse effects. A Hamilton Depression Scale or Montgomery-Asberg Scale could help monitor the severity and improvement of the depression. Watch for occurrence of manic symptoms.
3. The social worker should contact the patient's supervisor at work, counteract adverse effects of the patient's suicide attempt, and secure her job. The social worker should also engage the patient and her husband in family sessions to secure his understanding of the patient's condition.
4. The psychologist or psychiatrist should provide cognitive therapy and help the patient understand her misperception about her problems.
5. The pharmacist and psychiatrist shall inform the patient about the beneficial and adverse effects of antidepressants and treatment options and familiarize the patient with the pharmacotherapy of her condition.
6. In group inpatient therapy, the patient should learn from other patients the recognition of her own mood and its impact on her coping skills. She should experience that she is not alone with her condition.

Criteria for discharge in the United States: Today, discharge criteria are determined, in large part, by the patient's insurance plan. Yet, the physician is held accountable for adverse outcome of the discharge plan. Therefore, the physician may share with the patient the discharge options.

In any event, three criteria may be applied in the discharge planning:

1. The patient should acknowledge the value of her life and reasons to live and be free of plans or intent to commit suicide. She should commit herself to challenge her suicidal ideation if such thoughts should return, and inform her health care providers.
2. The patient shall be free of any hallucinatory experiences.
3. Ideally, the patient shall voice that she understands that her depression caused her suicide attempt and that she is committed to continue outpatient treatment.

Prognosis: If the patient can understand her condition and cooperate with the treatment, her short-term prognosis is good.

CHAPTER EIGHT

A DIFFICULT PATIENT

SUMMARY

This interview deals with a patient who initially seemed minimally moti-vated to talk. The patient's short answers do not help the interviewer clarify the psychopathology. He fails to recognize the source of the difficulty and to approach it with fitting techniques. Yet his persistence and empathy do ultimately elicit the source of her suffering and help him to establish rap-port. He garners enough information to make a meaningful differential without being able to convincingly arrive at the principal diagnosis.

▲ ▲ ▲ ▲ ▲

In the United States, man does not feel that he has been torn from the center of creation and suspended between hostile forces. He has built his own world and it is built in his own image: it is his mirror. But now he cannot recog-nize himself in his inhumane objects, nor in his fellows. His creations, like those of an inept sorcerer, no longer obey him. He is alone among his works, lost . . . in a wil-derness of mirrors.

—Octavio Paz, *The Labyrinth of Solitude,* 1985

▼ ▼ ▼ ▼ ▼

The previous chapter showed an interview with a cooperative patient whose symptoms, signs, and behaviors did not obstruct the interview pro-cess. The vast majority of outpatients who seek your help fall into this cate-gory. In a Board of Psychiatry and Neurology Examination, you will most likely encounter a cooperative patient (the organizers of the examination request cooperative patients from the various participating sites). However, throughout your career as a mental health professional you will also en-counter many difficult patients. You find them in the emergency room, on the consultation service, or in your office when a colleague requests a second opinion. We chose the patient represented in this chapter to show you some of the pitfalls with difficult patients.

Difficulties in interviewing patients may stem from at least four sources. First, the patient's symptoms and signs may have a direct impact on the interviewing process and induce the patient to distort the information you seek. Such a patient may somatize or dissociate right in front of you. His high avoidance anxiety may make him shy away from reporting his pathology, or he may befuddle you with dramatic conversion symptoms that appear to be irreversible, at least during the interview.

Second, a psychotic process may dictate the patient's behavior. He presents as stuporous and mute, or attacks you because he has identified you as one of his persecutors.

Third, a cognitive impairment may be developing in the patient. This impairment and his lack of insight conceal his true pathology. Unless you are testing for it, you may miss it. Even if you identify signs of cognitive impairment, you might assume they emerge from a different clinical disorder and not explore them further.

Fourth, the patient may intentionally want to deceive you. He conceals, falsifies, or fabricates information essential to his pathology, or he tries to enlist you to take part in his deceptive strategies.

This book is not designed to familiarize you with how to approach difficult patients. Such advanced challenges are addressed in *The Clinical Interview Using DSM-IV-TR, Volume 2: The Difficult Patient* (Othmer and Othmer 2002).

In the following, we present an unmotivated patient whose pathology interferes with the interview. Basic interviewing strategies do not elucidate fully the nature of her psychopathology. Through the first two-thirds of the interview, the interviewer faces the patient's superficial answers. Only when he opens up to *her* questions and gives her feedback about his observations does his approach become more effective. Now he arouses the patient's interest in the interviewing process and engages her in the diagnostic puzzle.

This interview is with Kelly Jasmin, a 19-year-old, white, slender female. She was referred for a diagnostic evaluation by another psychiatrist.

The patient sits slumped over her crossed legs in the waiting area and does not look up when the interviewer enters. She wears a long-sleeved blouse over skintight pants tucked into boots—all black. Necklaces with big pendants and oversized rings adorn her. Her black hair is spiked, colored red at the tips, and shaved around the ears.

She looks up only after the interviewer addresses her. Her face is pasty white and thick with makeup; her eyebrows are plucked to a thin line.

Phase 1: Warm-Up and Screening of the Problem

1. I: Hi, Miss Jasmin. My name is Dr. O. I'm glad you came over this morning.
   P: Hi.
2. I: [while walking with the patient to the interviewing room] You are still over in the inpatient unit, Miss Jasmin?
   P: No.
3. I: Oh?
   P: [gives a hostile look]
4. I: I thought you were still on the inpatient unit and came over here on a pass.
   P: No.
5. I: So Dr. A. must have discharged you after I talked to him last.
   P: He discharged me last Saturday.
6. I: [entering the interviewing room] Please come in and have a seat.
   P: [sits down without a word]
7. I: Can I get you anything, a coffee maybe?
   P: No. [at this point the interviewer notices that the patient has placed an open cola can on his desk that she must have held in her left hand when he approached her from the right in the waiting room] May I smoke?
8. I: Sure, go right ahead. Here is an ashtray.
   P: Thanks.
9. I: Before we start, what would you like me to call you?
   P: Kelly is fine.
10. I: Has Dr. A. told you what this visit with me is all about?
   P: Yeah [looking at the interviewer with a blank facial expression].
11. I: What did he tell you?
   P: Just what you think about me [blank look].
12. I: Think about . . . [waiting]? Think about what?
   P: [answers quickly without a change in tone] About me cutting myself.
13. I: Yes, he told me he was puzzled.
   P: [shrugs her shoulders and looks down at her knees]
14. I: What do you think about it?
   P: [with a blank facial expression] Nothing.
15. I: Would you like to talk about it?
   P: [shrugs her shoulders] It's OK, I guess.
16. I: When was the last time that you did it?
   P: [looks up at the interviewer] Wednesday, the day before I came to the hospital.
17. I: Why don't you tell me all that happened during the day when you cut yourself?
   P: I got mad at myself [no change in facial expression, posture, gestures, or intonation]. I was angry.
18. I: Angry . . . ?
   P: Yeah.
19. I: Angry about what?
   P: About not getting anywhere.
20. I: Hmm . . . Sounds like [pause] . . . you felt stuck?
   P: Yeah [looks bored].

21. I: Can you tell me more about it?
    P: I don't know. Just with my grades in college.
22. I: Your grades in college . . . which college do you attend?
    P: The XXX community college.
23. I: Hmm . . . What's your major?
    P: I haven't declared one.
24. I: What do you take?
    P: Sculpture [pause] . . . painting [pause] . . . writing . . .
25. I: And what kind of grades do you get?
    P: A's and B's.
26. I: Sounds pretty good to me.
    P: I got a C in weaving [draws down the corners of her mouth].
27. I: How did you feel about that?
    P: Fine, I guess [shrugs her shoulders].
28. I: [displaying surprise in his voice and facial expression] What did you expect
         to get?
    P: At the beginning, a C is fine. There's a lot of technique involved [in weav-
         ing].
29. I: So you are really doing all right?
    P: [silence]
30. I: Then what made you cut yourself?
    P: Just in general.
31. I: I don't understand. Can you explain?
    P: [no change in voice or facial expression] I was just mad.

Rapport: The interviewer quickly notices the patient's inattention and indifference when he enters the waiting room. He decides not to confront her
with her lack of interest by asking her, for instance:

> "How did you feel about Dr. A. asking you to come over here this morning?"

but to wait until he can decide whether the patient's indifference results from
being initially uncomfortable with him, from having a negative transference
to him, or from a clinical or personality disorder. Instead of a confrontation,
he attempts to warm up the patient by reviewing the circumstances of the
referral. Unfortunately, he is not up to date, prompting the patient to correct
him, which she does with a minimum of words. Rapport is not improved
when the interviewer offers her a beverage because he had overlooked the
patient's cola can on his desk. Thus, his offer appears to be routine rather
than a genuine concern for her comfort.

   Not being current on the patient's status and the oversight of the
opened cola would not matter if the patient is eager to talk about her problems. However, this is not the case. It remains the interviewer's task to establish rapport by addressing her suffering (Q. 1–9).

The interviewer probes whether the patient has been adequately informed about the reasons for the referral (Q. 10–12), but this topic does not establish rapport. At this point the interviewer could have asked the patient whether she agreed with Dr. A.'s request to seek a second opinion. This might have caused her to ventilate her feelings about the present interview and to possibly open up. Instead, the interviewer assumes that the patient's cutting is her chief complaint and the center of her suffering. Therefore, he focuses on the emotions that may underlie her self-mutilation. He echoes her emotion (Q. 19) and gives a summarizing interpretation (Q. 20). However, the patient's affect remains restricted and her verbal elaborations scarce.

The interviewer tries to identify frustrating situations that may result in the patient cutting herself, but he draws a blank. No emotional response occurs. Instead, she gives some longer but mainly factual answers. He attempts positive feedback by telling her that he thinks her grades are good (Q. 26). But the praise yields merely the report of a C in weaving. Overall, her answers express reluctance, without overt resistance or refusal to answer.

Technique: The interviewer goes through the formalities of introduction. He reviews the circumstances of the referral and asks the patient how she wants to be addressed (Q. 1–9). He uses four open-ended questions (Q. 11, 12, 14, 17), which are all answered with a short sentence or a single word. When the patient expresses a feeling (A. 17), he echoes this feeling in a client-centered manner (Q. 18, 19) and attempts an interpretation. These techniques do not initiate a spontaneous free flow of information.

Open-ended Q. 21 produces only a vague answer. Follow-up results in answers that do not explain her arm and wrist cutting. Thus, the fact-oriented questions produce diagnostically useless results, yet the interviewer pursues them in the expectation of hitting on a topic that might help to initiate a more spontaneous and productive flow of information. Positive feedback (Q. 26) and two open-ended questions (Q. 27, 28) directed at assessing her feelings about a mediocre grade in school, followed by a summary of her feelings, do not improve upon her one-sentence answers. Probing for the reasons of her cutting (Q. 30, 31) do not reveal a motive. In full circle, the interviewer returns to the topic of cutting without having learned anything significant about her psychopathology.

Mental status: Observation of the patient's attire suggests that she attempts to set herself apart through her fashion statement, and may be searching for her identity. This may indicate that her social judgment is impaired, or that she belongs to a subculture where this look is the accepted uniform.

Her psychomotor movements appear normal except for the lack of a reactive movement—such as looking up—when the interviewer enters the waiting area.

During the brief conversation it becomes apparent that she understands all questions, and answers them appropriately, showing adequate information processing, and no indication of a thought disorder.

Her affect, as expressed in face, gestures, and intonation (Q. 10–20) appears to be restricted. She is indifferent to the interviewer and the topic of the interview, merely going through the motions without being engaged.

She comes for the appointment unescorted and recalls her discharge day, both of which show absence of severe anxiety, gross uncontrolled psychotic excitement, and disorientation to time and place (list no. 3).

The patient is cooperative enough to talk about herself, which allows a progression from conversation to exploration of her current and past problems. Her verbal production shows poverty of response without prolonged latency.

The patient shows ambivalence; she expresses concern about her college grades, but then contradicts herself and reports good grades and satisfaction with a C. This ambivalence reveals an illogical aspect of her judgment.

Diagnosis: The patient's attire, together with her lack of a reactive movement when the interviewer enters the waiting room and her emotionally restricted response during the warm-up period, suggest several psychiatric disorders for list no. 1.

Clinical disorders:

• substance intoxication or withdrawal
• schizophrenia
• bipolar II disorder, depressed
• major depressive disorder
• adjustment disorder with depressed mood

Personality disorders:

• paranoid
• schizoid
• schizotypal
• antisocial
• avoidant
• borderline

Her reluctance to volunteer information may suggest the presence of passive-aggressive personality disorder. Her ambivalence about her grades underscores as diagnostic options schizophrenia, and/or any of the personality disorders of Cluster A in DSM-IV-TR.

It excludes (list no. 2) possibly:

• bipolar I disorder, manic
• adjustment disorder with depressed mood
• dependent personality disorder

The patient's answers do not point to any stressor necessary for the diagnosis of adjustment disorder.

Phase 2: Follow-Up of Diagnostic Impressions

32. I: Any other feelings?
    P: No.
33. I: Did you feel, in any way, down?
    P: No.
34. I: Any other problems?
    P: I don't know.
35. I: How was your sleep during that time?
    P: Okay.
36. I: And your appetite?
    P: Fine.
37. I: Any problems with eating at all?
    P: Sometimes.
38. I: What kind of problems?
    P: Sometimes I eat too much.
39. I: Do you do anything about it?
    P: Like what?
40. I: Did you ever try to starve yourself?
    P: Maybe for a day or so.
41. I: Did you ever do anything else—like trying to vomit?
    P: Yeah, a couple of times but it didn't work.
42. I: What types of things do you eat when you eat too much?
    P: Pretty good food. Lots of fruits and vegetables.
43. I: So you ate all right and slept fine when you cut yourself.
    P: I guess.
44. I: Was anything else going on?
    P: [just looks at the interviewer, then takes out a cigarette and lights it]
45. I: Anything with your friends? Or your boyfriend?
    P: No, we were fine.
46. I: What were you thinking then when you were cutting yourself?

P: I was just mad [no change in tone of voice or facial expression].
47. I: Mad? Mad enough to die?
P: No. Just to cut myself.
48. I: Do you have any idea why you did it?
P: I was angry.
49. I: About . . . ?
P: Myself.
50. I: So you cut yourself when you are angry about yourself?
P: Yeah, and about others too.

Rapport: The interviewer assesses symptoms of clinical disorders that could explain the cutting. Neither reviewing the topics of depressive and eating disorder symptoms nor using open-ended questions enhances rapport and induces more spontaneity.

Technique: The interviewer checks out whether depressive symptoms were associated with the arm cutting. If he keeps the symptom-oriented questions open, the patient makes him specify (Q. and A. 39), or answers them with yes or no as if they were closed-ended (A. 32, 35, 36, 45). His two summary statements (Q. 43, 50) are met with vague consent, which leaves it doubtful whether these summaries establish any facts.

Mental status: The patient reports her arm cutting in a matter-of-fact way. Her affect appears blunted; she displays an inappropriate distance to her maladjusted behavior. She indicates overeating and an attempt to induce vomiting. However, unlike a patient with bulimia, she is not eating junk food but "lots of fruits and vegetables." Overeating those appears to be bizarre and points toward an ambivalence about her eating habits.

Diagnosis: The patient is only reluctantly cooperative and shows no spontaneity. The interviewer decides to verify or exclude some diagnostic options possibly associated with the self-mutilation.

1. Depression. Jasmin denies most depressive symptoms for the time of her last arm cutting, excluding depressive disorder as an explanation.
2. Bulimia nervosa. A. 36–43 exclude that disorder.

The patient's affect appears most consistent with schizophrenia, and/or any of the personality disorders of Cluster A in DSM-IV-TR.

51. I: Tell me what you do when you are angry.
P: I take a razor blade and keep cutting myself.

52. I: And then?
    P: [in a matter-of-fact way] Then I clean the wounds.
53. I: Yes . . . ?
    P: With alcohol.
54. I: Yes . . . ?
    P: I sometimes put some Band-Aids on.
55. I: Hmm . . .
    P: Or I just roll down my sleeves.
56. I: How do you feel then?
    P: I don't know.
57. I: Do you feel any different afterwards?
    P: [without displaying any emotion] A little better, maybe.
58. I: Is this like punishing yourself?
    P: Getting rid of the tension.
59. I: And does it work?
    P: A little.
60. I: Can I see your arms?
    P: [rolls up her left sleeve exposing the forearm. One red scar down along the forearm is visible besides seven or eight pale old scars. The patient points at the red scar] That's where I cut myself last.
61. I: Hmm . . . I see some other scars too.
    P: I have some on the other arm too [she rolls up her right sleeve and exposes a forearm covered with scars running 2 to 3 inches in length].
62. I: You must really go through a lot, that you feel you have to cut yourself so often.
    P: [no answer and no change in posture, gestures, or facial expression]
63. I: How do you feel about that?
    P: [patient shrugs her shoulders]
64. I: How often does it happen?
    P: About every 2 months [her face remains motionless; the inflection of her voice does not change].
65. I: Since when have you been doing it?
    P: For the last 2 years, since I was 17 [throughout, the patient's face remains expressionless and she reports her self-mutilation in a matter-of- fact way].

Rapport: The interviewer switches from assessing the motivation for the cutting to the process of the cutting per se. But the patient's recall does not revive any experiences of anger, pain, hurt, guilt, or satisfaction. Her report remains factual and emotionless.

Technique: The interviewer stays with the topic of arm cutting. By continuation technique he assesses the temporal course of an isolated cutting, the pattern of cuttings over a longer time period, and the associated feelings. He expresses empathy at the end of this assessment (Q. 62), but both techniques fail to induce spontaneous elaborations.

Mental status: The patient's affect is blunted which, in isolation, could be interpreted as *la belle indifférence*. However, a dramatic presentation of life events, ill fate, or other symptoms usually associated with *la belle indifférence* is missing. The patient shows no psychomotor retardation; she talks and moves at normal rate.

Diagnosis: The patient's nonchalant attitude is an expression of true blunting, or a displayed, so-called *la belle indifférence*, which is sometimes described as characteristic of hysteria (somatization disorder in DSM-IV-TR, or histrionic personality disorder). The pattern of frequent arm cutting, whenever the patient feels frustrated and angry, supports the previously considered presence of borderline personality disorder.

66. I: You must really go through a lot of tension.
    P: Just normal.
67. I: Have you ever cut yourself when you have problems with your boyfriend?
    P: Yes. With my last one.
68. I: When was that?
    P: About 9 months ago.
69. I: What happened then?
    P: We broke up.
70. I: How did that make you feel?
    P: Bad.
71. I: Who broke up?
    P: He did.
72. I: And why?
    P: He said, he has to get clear with himself and he doesn't want to have the responsibility of a girlfriend.
73. I: How did you feel then when he said that?
    P: [emotionless] Devastated.
74. I: Were there any other changes?
    P: I slept more.

Rapport: The interviewer expresses empathy for the patient's assumed suffering (Q. 66), but Kelly stays aloof. Up to this point, none of the interviewer's techniques has established emotional rapport: open-ended questions, reflection on and echoing of the patient's feelings (Q. 18–20), positive feedback (Q. 26), or expression of empathy (Q. 62, 66).

Technique: The interviewer makes a smooth transition; he focuses on the patient's relationship with her boyfriend to evaluate its intensity. She appears to have intense feelings for at least one of her boyfriends; however, the assessment of this emotionally laden topic does not result in a spontaneous verbal eruption.

Mental status: Neither the expression of empathy nor the review of a stressful life event expand the patient's restricted affect. She shows no increase in latency of response, which could indicate psychomotor retardation and depressed mood rather than blunted affect.

Diagnosis: Following up on the impression that the patient may have a borderline personality disorder, the interviewer focuses on her intense and unstable relationship with her last boyfriend. However, an emotional ambivalence in the present relationship (which is thought to be a characteristic of borderline personality disorder) is not apparent.

The previously discarded option of an adjustment disorder resurfaces for the time period of the breakup with her last boyfriend (A. 73, 74). However, it cannot explain the repeated self-mutilation, which is more consistent with a clinical disorder or a personality disorder.

75. I: Were you down so much that you started to hear things that were not really
there?
P: [hesitates]
76. I: Like voices?
P: [stares into her lap, blinks as if waking up] A couple of times, maybe.
77. I: Can you describe them?
P: Somebody called my name a few times.
78. I: Any other voices?
P: Maybe. I'm not sure. I think I'm in a daze when it happens.
79. I: Hmm . . .
P: Just my thoughts.
80. I: Do you hear them now?
P: They are just inside my head.
81. I: Do they sound like a voice?
P: Just like my own.

Rapport: The patient appears to dissociate when she talks about her voices (A. 76, 78). This disturbance may prevent her from being emotionally more engaged, or more detailed about her problems.

Technique: The interviewer checks for psychotic symptoms associated with the breakup of her relationship. He does not follow up on her signs of dissociation.

Mental status: The patient admits to having phonemes, which are voices inside her head. They seem to occur only occasionally without being intrusive, and when she is in a daze, an indication of dissociation.

Diagnosis: The interviewer probes whether a major depression was associated with the breakup. The breakup could either have been caused by a
depressive episode, or could have been a precipitating event for a depression. The interviewer focuses on hallucinatory experiences because, if present, they would clearly exclude an adjustment disorder. Indeed, he gets a
report of some hallucinatory experiences. It is, however, not clear whether
these experiences were associated with the breakup and therefore indicate
a brief psychotic episode, or whether they were related to a major depression, or are even present on a more permanent basis as in schizophrenia or
borderline personality disorder or dissociative disorders. DSM-IV-TR criteria
for borderline disorder list: transient, stress-related paranoid ideation or severe dissociative symptoms that include hallucinations.

82. I: When this happened, did you take any street drugs?
    P: Not lately.
83. I: And before that? What did you take?
    P: Everything.
84. I: Like what?
    P: Oh, speed, pot, downers, hashish, crystals, bennies, heroin, cocaine, mush-
         rooms . . .
85. I: Yeah . . .
    P: Lots of alcohol too.
86. I: For how long?
    P: For a few months or so.
87. I: When was the last time that you took it?
    P: Not since I broke up with my boyfriend. He was very much into that.
88. I: Did you like any of these drugs more than others?
    P: I liked them all.
89. I: Do you do any with your present boyfriend?
    P: No.

Rapport: The interviewer stays with a symptom-collecting approach,
which enables him to include and exclude disorders without the benefit of
the patient's spontaneity and a genuine affective expression of her suffering. He enjoys a rapport comparable to that of a computer program that
checks off symptoms and diagnostic criteria.

Technique: The admission of psychotic symptoms leads the interviewer
to assess possible causes for the hallucinations. Therefore, he asks for essential symptoms of substance and alcohol abuse, but does not follow up
on dissociative disorders.

Mental status: The fact that the patient took different types of street drugs indiscriminately in the past but not at present—because her former boyfriend was a drug abuser—underscores her field dependence and her vulnerability to being influenced by others, which points to suggestibility.

Diagnosis: The patient admits to a period of indiscriminate polysubstance abuse. Her former boyfriend seems to have exposed her to street drugs, which the patient did not continue to abuse after she broke off with him. Her drug abuse is therefore a *folie à deux* and reveals more her dependency on and suggestibility by others than an autochthonic abuse disorder. Her arm cutting is not limited to the periods of substance abuse; therefore, the abuse is not responsible for the cutting.

90. I: How are you getting along with your present boyfriend?
    P: Fine.
91. I: Can you describe this relationship?
    P: We are getting too close.
92. I: Do you love him?
    P: Yeah.
93. I: Do you have any other feelings for him besides love?
    P: [takes a puff from her cigarette and then swallows]
94. I: Do you fight?
    P: We argue a lot.
95. I: Have you ever hurt each other?
    P: Not physically.
96. I: Are you jealous of him?
    P: Only if he is jealous of me.
97. I: You said you were too close?
    P: Yeah, we were together all the time. We did not see anybody else.
98. I: And?
    P: We are going to change this now. We are going to meet other people.
99. I: Do you usually have more than one boyfriend?
    P: Yes, I do. Three or four.
100. I: Do you sleep with them too?
    P: No. Just with my main boyfriend. I don't believe in sleeping with anybody else.
101. I: Has your boyfriend also girlfriends other than you?
    P: Usually not.
102. I: And if he does?
    P: It hurts a little . . . but not any more.
103. I: Not any more?
    P: No, I do the same thing.
104. I: Is there a reason why you like more than one boyfriend?
    P: I'm getting too close if I have only one. I can't handle it.
105. I: Have you ever cut yourself because of your boyfriend?

P: Yes, 2 months ago.
106. I: Would you like to talk about it?
P: No, not really.

Rapport: The interviewer talks about her relationship with her boyfriend. This potentially personal and intimate topic does not engage her emotionally. Notice that the patient does not treat the interviewer as an empathic listener in whom she confides, nor does she treat him as an expert who can help her fix what's wrong. She relates to him as if he is a hostile, interrogating authority with whom she has to comply.

Technique: The interviewer makes a smooth transition from past to current drug abuse, which she denies. He invites her to describe her relationship with her current boyfriend but ends up with a one-sentence answer. Frustrated, he continues to get a feeling for this relationship by using closed-ended questions. Interviewing a patient about a close relationship often results in emotionally laden verbal outpour, but not so here.

Mental status: It appears that the patient can become very dependent on a boyfriend, and develops an intense relationship. She is unable to handle the intensity of these feelings and escapes into alternate relationships without becoming promiscuous.

Diagnosis: The patient has an acceptable college record. Her substance abuse is limited to the duration of her relationship with the last boyfriend only, and she denies promiscuity. All three facts exclude antisocial personality. The interviewer explores whether the patient is predominantly involved in intense but ambivalent heterosexual relationships, which would point to borderline personality. The patient admits indeed that she gets very close to her partners and may get so angry that she cuts herself. This report is however obtained in a piecemeal fashion; it lacks spontaneity to be taken as a testimony for an intense ambivalent relationship. Therefore, it remains questionable whether the patient's behavior indeed fulfills criteria for borderline personality disorder.

107. I: I notice that most of the time you just answer my questions, but you don't
          want to talk about it on your own.
P: That's right.
108. I: How does it make you feel talking to me?
P: Just nervous and tense.

109. I: Yes, I noticed that. Is there any reason why you feel so tense when you talk about these things?
    P: I don't know, I just don't like it, I guess.
110. I: Anything that concerns you?
    P: Yes.
111. I: What is it?
    P: I'm not getting anywhere. I wiggle all the time. I cut myself. And I get those downs.
112. I: So that is what you are concerned about?
    P: My mother is.
113. I: How are you getting along with her?
    P: Fine.

Rapport: The interviewer confronts the patient directly with her unwillingness to talk about her problems and tries to assess the reason of her resistance, but the patient does not provide an explanation. From an analytical point of view, her admission of nervousness and tension suggests that defense mechanisms are at work. From a descriptive point of view, it may indicate that a clinical or personality disorder interferes with rapport (see below).

The interviewer attempts to shed the role of an interrogating authority by confronting the patient with her resistance, hoping she may accept him more as an empathic listener, but he fails to bring about this transition.

Technique: The interviewer confronts the patient with her resistance to elaborate freely (see Rapport).

Mental status: The patient describes herself as nervous and tense, which may contribute to her guardedness. She first reports that she is concerned about wiggling, cutting, and having downs, but quickly assigns these concerns to her mother, which shows that she is ambivalent about her problems, has only partial insight into them, and projects them onto her mother.

Diagnosis: The patient's downs introduce a new diagnostic element. Depressive disorder was already excluded previously as a sufficient reason for the cutting. But the patient's report of downs raises the possibility of depressions occurring independent from the cutting.

114. I: Do you also think there is anything wrong with you?
    P: Maybe the lows. I don't like the lows.
115. I: Has anything helped you with the lows?
    P: Maybe the Zoloft a little.

116. I: When you are low, in what way are you changed?
     P: I sleep more. Don't want to do anything.
117. I: Anything else?
     P: That's it.
118. I: Do you still care what you look like when you are down?
     P: Usually not.
119. I: Anything different with your friends when you are low?
     P: I don't think so.
120. I: Do you stay away from them?
     P: No, not really.
121. I: Do you still enjoy sex?
     P: Yes.
122. I: Even when you are down?
     P: [emphatically] I enjoy it a lot [looks as if she relives a sexual experience, shivers as if freezing].
123. I: Do you care for other people when you are depressed?
     P: Yes, I do.
124. I: Who are you close to?
     P: My mother, my sister, my stepfather, and my real father [stares into space and presses her elbows into her sides].
125. I: Anybody else?
     P: [shrugs her shoulders]
126. I: You did not mention your boyfriend.
     P: [swallows]
127. I: I notice you swallowed.
     P: [blushes] I just didn't get around to him.
128. I: Hmm. How do you feel about him now?
     P: I'm a little mad. But it's really okay.
129. I: How are you getting along with your stepfather?
     P: I stay away from him.
130. I: Hmm.
     P: I stay away from him. He is an alcoholic and he shouts a lot.
131. I: Has he ever abused you?
     P: [firmly] No, just screamed a lot.
132. I: How about your real father?
     P: [stares through the interviewer . . . startled] He's in Austin.
133. I: When did he last live with you?
     P: [painful squinting, then flat, empty expression] When I was real little.
134. I: You say you have some lows. Does anybody else in your family have lows?
     P: My mother does.
135. I: Anybody else?
     P: [shrugs her shoulders]

Rapport: The interviewer attempts to get the patient's view of her disorder (Q. 114). This question produces a two-sentence answer, an admission that she suffers from lows. However, the follow-up does not induce the patient to elaborate spontaneously, nor to become emotionally involved. Instead, she returns to short, one-sentence answers.

Up to this point, the patient's lack of emotional involvement suggests four interpretations:

1. The interviewer has not tapped the patient's suffering—probably because he mistook her initial report of the cuttings as her true chief complaint, and therefore, he has no access to material that is of emotional importance to her.
2. It is possible that the subject of cutting is emotionally highly charged and anxiety provoking for the patient. Therefore, she uses the defense mechanisms of denial or isolation to defend herself against feelings that would otherwise overwhelm her.
3. The patient has a disorder characterized by a blunted affect (see below, Diagnosis).
4. The patient dissociates and has only incomplete access to her suffering.

Technique: The interviewer, frustrated with the patient's short answers, attempts again (Q. 116) an open-ended question followed up with, "Anything else?" (Q. 117). But the patient replies "That's it." To get more data the interviewer resorts to symptom-oriented, circumscribed even though open-ended questions. They produce short, appropriate answers limited to a minimum of information, making the interview boring and dry; every detail is pried out of the patient. He misses following up on her signs of dissociation.

Mental status: The patient shows an emotional response when she emphasizes that she enjoys sex even when depressed. At the same time, she appears to dissociate (A. 122). She also does when she is asked about abuse by her father (A. 124, 132–133). She also shows an affective change when the interviewer confronts her with not mentioning her boyfriend as a person she cares about.

Diagnosis: The patient admits to low mood, low energy, hypersomnia, some neglect in dressing and hygiene, but no decrease of sex drive or social withdrawal. The interviewer does not assess enough symptoms to establish the diagnosis of major depression over dysthymia. He obtains some evidence for a positive family history of a mood disorder in the patient's mother.

136. I: I asked you a lot of questions. Is there any question that I can answer for you?

   P: [leans forward, flirtatiously] Yes. Can Dr. A. or you ever diagnose me? [with emphasis and determination in her voice] I want to know what my diagnosis is. [with a challenging expression] Do you know?

137. I: Very good . . . So you would really like to know what we think about you.

   P: [her facial expression appears animated, and with her left hand she taps on the desk] Oh yes, very much. Can you tell me what you think about me?

138. I: Well, I don't know enough about you yet, but if you help me . . . You said already that you have some lows and that you don't like to have them. I have no idea how long they last.

   P: [quickly] Oh, up to several months. Are those real depressions?

139. I: I don't have any idea how bad they really get.

   P: Pretty bad. I feel silly, I can't do anything. I can't put my mind to anything . . . I tried to kill myself twice and I ended up in the ICU twice—I overdosed.

140. I: We would call that a depression. You seem to suffer from real depressions. But I don't know whether you have real highs also.

   P: Yes, I do. They last a short time. I'm full of energy, my thoughts are real fast, I can't keep up with them and I talk too fast. I don't sleep a bunch but I don't feel real good. Are these real highs?

141. I: Real negative highs! That's what a patient of mine calls them—negative highs. You seem to have them.

   P: That's exactly it—that's a good word.

142. I: So—experts call your condition a bipolar condition where you have both highs and lows, but I don't really know when you have those highs.

   P: Both before and after my lows.

143. I: Besides your bipolar or manic-depressive problem, there may be something else going on . . . But I don't know enough about it. You did not tell me enough about it . . . [pause]. Your cutting and your getting so angry and your relationship to your boyfriends, they seem to be intense. But it doesn't seem that it is all love. Do you have some other feelings?

   P: Yes, my boyfriend—I hate it. I hate it that I get so close to him.

144. I: Hmm.

   P: I have no control over my feelings. They just come and make me do things. They make me do things that I don't want to do.

145. I: I don't know how long that has been going on.

   P: All my life.

146. I: For your diagnosis, we would probably say that you also have a personality problem, especially with your cutting.

   P: [shaking her head] But I'm not worried about my cutting. That's not my worry. I just have to stop it.

147. I: Can you?

   P: I just have to. Dr. A. told me he will put me into a State Hospital if I don't stop.

Rapport: The interviewer asks whether the patient has any questions for him. And she does. Her first question verbalizes her worry whether the interviewer can diagnose her. This question shows that she struggles with a valid evaluation of her behavior. She experiences herself as "normal" except for the depressive episodes—but her mother criticizes her and points to her pathological features. This discrepancy between her experience of herself and her mother's criticism is her true point of suffering. As soon as the interviewer identifies this point, rapport changes dramatically; the patient spontaneously elaborates on her answers and begins to ask questions—rapport is finally established.

What has happened? Here is an observation that Jamie Smith, ski teacher and member of the Jane Gang at Winterpark, Colorado, reported on working with children and teenagers. While riding up the Challenger ski lift at 5°F, we compared notes on the teaching of nonlinear processes. He said:

> "I can't teach children and teenagers skiing until they are ready. I just ski with them, get them through the bumps, and hope that they will imitate me. Finally, they start to ask questions. How do you go so fast? How can you turn so easy? How do you do it? Then I know they are ready, I have their attention, they are open to listen, and I can teach them."

Jamie Smith refers to the same strategy that is important for interviewing patients: you have to find their point of suffering. With the statement:

> "Do you have any questions for me?"

the interviewer had tapped the patient's true point of suffering—"What is wrong with me? Am I normal, or not?"

Retrospectively, it becomes clear that the interviewer had taken the self-mutilation as the chief complaint when it first emerged but he failed to confirm this with the patient. He mistook pathology impressive to him, but not to her, for her chief complaint and ended up in laborious data collection not fueled by the patient's emotional engagement.

To keep the patient aware that a diagnostic evaluation is only possible if she engages herself in the process, the interviewer introduces several of his questions with the phrase "I don't know enough about you" (Q. 139, 140, 141, 143, 144, 146). This humble reminder of his need for her cooperation stabilizes rapport.

A transition has occurred in the roles of the patient and the interviewer. The interviewer is no longer treated as the interrogating authority to whom the patient was referred by her psychiatrist who in turn was backed by her mother, but as an expert who can give her some understanding about herself. Through his role as expert, he can also gain footage as empathic listener.

Technique: Often, interviewers use the technique of having the patient ask questions at the end of an interview. Here, it is used in the middle to mobilize the patient's interest in the interviewing process and to break the monotonous "short question-short answer" format. And the technique works—the patient herself starts to ask questions (A. 136–138, 140). Her true chief complaint emerges—not the cutting but her question about her normality: "Am I crazy or not?"

The interviewer keeps her in this questioning mode by making statements about her that he introduces with the phrase "I don't know," which appears to animate her. It works because the interviewer has found the patient's interest in the interview, *her* point of suffering. She is now interviewed from *her* point of view. The interviewer fails to elicit sexual abuse, possibly by her father, to examine her hypnotizability, and to entertain the possibility that her hallucinations are at least partly a dissociative rather than a classic psychotic phenomenon.

Mental status: This segment shows that the patient is capable of detailed and goal-directed verbal elaboration without thought blocking, circumstantiality, or flight of ideas. Suddenly, she shows appropriate changes in posture, gestures, facial expression, and intonation. One single question has brought about that change, which shows how much she is field-dependent.

This section shows that the patient has difficulties with insight. She recognizes her mood swings, but she considers only her lows as a disorder. It appears that the patient experiences a switch in personality, but the interviewer fails to explore this option.

Diagnosis: The patient describes spontaneously (A. 139) a host of depressive symptoms of sufficient duration (A. 138) to support the diagnosis of major depression. Furthermore, she gives enough evidence (A. 140, 142) for mania, which may precede or follow a depressive episode.

A. 143–146 suggest the possibility of borderline personality disorder supported by the ambivalent relationship to her boyfriend and by her cutting. An alternate explanation for the cutting is that this act represents an impulse control disorder NOS. This diagnosis is suggested by the patient's statement that she feels many uncontrollable impulses; cutting seems to be the dominating one. The interviewer has learned so far that the patient usually is angry prior to the cutting, that she feels some relief afterward, and that the impulse is ego-syntonic. However, he fails to assess whether this impulse is irresistible. Also, he has not elucidated other impulses that the patient has difficulty controlling. Alternatively her arm cutting could represent an act of dissociation.

148. I: So cutting does not worry you. What worries you then?
    P: [with low, soft voice, as if mystified] That I have delusions and hallucinations.
149. I: What kind of hallucinations do you worry about?
    P: My voices.
150. I: I don't know enough about your voices to give you your diagnosis. You said before it was just your thoughts—so I don't know.
    P: [shaking her head, bending forward, whispering but with animated facial expression] No, no. It is like a voice that comes from the back of my head and it tells me what to do and what not to do. Is that crazy?
151. I: Hmm . . . Does it also tell you to cut yourself?
    P: [eyes move rapidly sideways, back and forth] It does. But that's the least that worries me. That's just one of many things. It tells me all the other things to do or not to do.
152. I: Can you turn it off?
    P: [frowns] No. It's there all the time. All I can do is try to ignore it but I cannot turn it off.
153. I: Usually people can turn off a thought. So your voice is more than a thought? Is it your own voice?
    P: It is, because it comes from the inside of my head. But it does not sound like my voice.
154. I: What does it sound like?
    P: It sounds like a neutral voice. Not male, not female. It has no sex and it has no age. So it isn't really my own voice, is it?
155. I: Hmm . . . Is it there at any time of the day?
    P: Yes, mostly.
156. I: Is there more than one voice?
    P: At times there are. Then it is as if you argue back and forth with yourself. But there are many parts and they all talk back and forth. Isn't that crazy?
157. I: I don't know whether you can control them.
    P: No, they just happen to me. Should I be able to control them?
158. I: Well, are there any times when these voices occur more frequently?
    P: Yes, they are all there when I have my highs.
159. I: And when you are in a low?
    P: Then I hear my name called once or twice. That's all.
160. I: I don't know whether you have any other hallucinations besides the voices. Do you also see things?
    P: Yes.
161. I: Like what?
    P: [lights a new cigarette and puffs on it] Funny faces.

162. I: How does my face look to you?
     P: It moves. It makes grimaces. Things pop out. Your mouth pops out. Some-
          times I think I can see the atoms of everything and how they move. Every-
          thing is changing. I see movements. I can feel my thoughts. They are like
          electric shocks flashing through my head. Is this normal?
163. I: I don't know how bad it gets. For instance, have you ever seen blood com-
          ing out of people's faces?
     P: [after a long pause] No, I don't think so, just parts of the face popping out.
164. I: So you have visual distortions. What happened to these distortions when
          you took street drugs?
     P: With most drugs they became more intense. Especially with acid. With acid
          things become real bright and real loud—real brilliant colors.
165. I: You also said you had delusions? What do you mean by delusions?
     P: All the time I think I will be famous one time in my life. Very famous. I
          thought this as long as I can think back. I was always convinced that at one
          time I will be famous—that I'm special. I'm convinced that I'm a genius. Do
          you believe that I'm a genius? Or is this a delusion?
166. I: Why do you think this is a delusion?
     P: My mother says so and Dr. A. thinks so. Do you think so too, or do you
          think I'm a genius?
167. I: I don't know enough about you. What do you think?
     P: I just don't know. I had these voices all my life; I had these visions all my
          life. I don't know any different.

Rapport: This remains good during this section; the patient continues to
elaborate freely. She reveals her hallucinatory experiences and talks about
her grandiose delusions, while the interviewer displays expertise in asking
the right questions, which may or may not be noticed by the patient. She appears to become more trusting in the interviewer's expertise, as evidenced by
her many questions. Her formulations and lack of guardedness suggest that
now she experiences him also as an empathic listener.

Technique: Since the patient's interest has been tapped, as evidenced by
her frequent questions (A. 150, 154, 156, 157, 162, 165, 166), open-ended
questions that did not work before now produce spontaneous elaborations,
and the interviewer can stay with the problems that she introduces. First, he
follows up on her auditory (Q. 149–159) and then on her visual hallucinations (Q. 160–164). Thereafter, he returns to her delusions (Q. 165–167).

Mental status: At present, the patient has auditory hallucinations and visual illusions if not hallucinations. The hallucinations are congruent neither
with a depressive nor a manic mood, even though they increase during a
high. However, during a high period the patient seems to have more halluci-

natory experiences than during relative normality, or during a depression. She has permanent grandiose delusions mood-congruent with mania. Presently, the patient is not manic. Therefore, it appears that her hallucinations and delusions are somewhat permanent and not limited to periods of affective disturbances. Furthermore, this section shows her partial insight into her hallucinations and delusions, which she has difficulty in accepting as part of an illness. Her grandiose delusions affect her judgment and impair her social adjustment and future planning. Her permanent mood-incongruent hallucinations may represent a dissociative process (Kluft and Fine 1993).

Diagnosis: Manic and depressive mood disturbances together with mood-incongruent hallucinations fit best the diagnostic criteria of schizoaffective disorder, bipolar type. However, there exists a controversy whether this diagnosis predicts a more chronic schizophrenic-like disorder, or a more episodic, affective-like disorder. Since the bizarre thoughts and hallucinatory experiences reach back to her childhood, a personality disorder may have preceded a schizoaffective disorder.

One of the readers of our first edition wrote us in response to the interview with Kelly Jasmin that he considered the diagnosis of dissociative identity disorder because of the patient's "self-mutilation, inner voices, feeling split into different parts, evasiveness, mood swings, mad feelings, eating disorder symptoms not meeting the criteria of either bulimia or anorexia, substance abuse, child abuse . . . prolific writing or other artistic productions under therapy, in intense often chaotic relationships with significant others." We agree with his assessment and add dissociative identity disorder to the diagnostic list. In *The Clinical Interview Using DSM-IV-TR, Volume 2: The Difficult Patient* (Othmer and Othmer 2002), we describe techniques useful for the interview of patients with dissociative disorders.

So far, the interview reveals some evidence for a borderline and/or schizotypal personality disorder. The patient's intense and intimate relationships exclude schizoid personality disorder. She also reports neither severe jealousy nor suspiciousness, which excludes paranoid personality disorder.

The patient's initial reluctance to communicate freely with the interviewer had also suggested avoidant personality disorder. But since she opened up after the interviewer tapped her source of suffering, and since he found no evidence that she is afraid of being criticized, the diagnosis of avoidant personality disorder is unlikely.

The only other coexisting disorder may be impulse control disorder NOS, which would account for her arm cutting.

168. I: Artists sometimes seem to have different experiences. Vincent van Gogh, for instance, painted things as if he could see them grow. Maybe he really saw them growing. He seemed to be fascinated by light and bright colors.
    P: I see things move, move all the time. Am I a genius?
169. I: I guess when you can express how you see things so that others can see it too and can feel how you feel, you may have some part of a genius.
    P: I can express it sometimes. I have to learn more about it. I take creative writing next term. I am all excited about it.
170. I: Van Gogh hurt himself too, he cut off his ear. But I think there is one thing that bothers you about your experiences. You cannot control them. They make you do things that you don't want to do. So, therefore, we would call some of your experiences hallucinations. Has your medicine helped with them?
    P: A little.
171. I: Which one? The Zoloft or the Loxitane?
    P: I don't know.
172. I: You can express your visions and your feelings sometimes?
    P: Yes, sometimes.
173. I: How?
    P: With my sculptures, with my poems, and maybe with paintings.
174. I: When you feel your tension coming on, when you want to cut yourself, can you put this tension on a canvas rather than on your forearms?
    P: I can try.
175. I: I'm interested in how well you can express yourself. Can you bring me your poems and your pictures and whatever you think is the best you have done, where you think you have expressed yourself?
    P: I will bring them.
176. I: There have been artists like van Gogh who had depressions and had to go to an asylum, and there were also psychiatric patients who often lived in mental institutions who could express their visions. Have you ever seen those paintings?
    P: No.
177. I: I will bring some along and show them to you, if you like.
    P: I would love that very much [smiles].
178. I: I would like to know more about you to answer your question about diagnosis. Would you like to meet again?
    P: Yes. I would like that. I would like to talk about my experiences and get your opinion about it.
179. I: That's great, Kelly. I would like to meet with you again.

Rapport: This remains good, since the patient is interested in the artwork that the interviewer introduces toward the end of the interview. He brings up the topic of art in an attempt to show expertise in her problems by linking her experiences to her need for artistic expression. Since she feels her hallucinations and delusions are part of her existence as an artist, this topic is concordant with her level of insight. The interviewer is capable of understanding the patient's view of herself. He can adopt a vantage point that allows him to interview her from *her* viewpoint, rather than from that of an outsider who makes it apparent that whatever she reports is abnormal from his point of view. Since the patient has some interest in expressing herself artistically, the interviewer attempts to channel her impulse to cut herself into a more sublimated acting out in her artwork.

At the end of the interview the patient indicates that she would like to meet again. The interviewer has turned a reluctant patient—who had only followed the pressure of her referring psychiatrist to see him—into an engaged, cooperative patient.

From a role point of view, the interviewer attempts to establish himself as an authority knowledgeable in art and in the artistic expression of unusual experiences, which the patient seems to accept. At the end of the session, rapport in its different aspects is established, even though the diagnostic interview is not completed with all its phases.

In an interview, you can postpone the completion of the phases and the diagnostic process at any time, but you cannot postpone the establishment of rapport, simply because the patient may not return. Therefore, if you meet a resistant patient, attempt to establish rapport within the first session even if you have to compromise the completeness of your diagnostic assessment.

Technique: The interviewer establishes a link between the patient's hallucinatory experiences, her need to express herself artistically, and the painter Vincent van Gogh who presumably also had a mood disorder and/or substance abuse disorder with psychosis (Arnold 1992). This link fits into the patient's present level of insight, where she cannot acknowledge her voices as being the expression of an illness, and where she has no distance to her grandiose ideas (see Rapport above).

Mental status: This section highlights further the patient's impaired reality testing, her inability to judge what is a disorder and what is not, and to evaluate her creative potential. Her clothing and elaborate jewelry appear to be an attempt to establish her identity as an artist. Her ambivalence about her school record expressed at the beginning reflects her doubts about that identity. She probably compensates for her lack of success in her artistic work with an "artistic life-style."

Diagnosis: The patient seems to be cooperative and motivated to learn more about her condition. These factors affect her prognosis positively. No new diagnostic information emerges in this last section; therefore, the diagnostic considerations given previously may suffice.

Epilogue

Since the interviewer could only obtain the patient's emotional engagement in the last third of the session, this interview is incomplete as far as the phases are concerned. The diagnostic impressions are not substantiated by sufficient examples and details. The longitudinal view with social, medical, and family history is almost entirely missing. Data are not complete; tests of handedness, attention, and concentration are desirable. Feedback has only been touched on. The treatment contract is reduced to an agreement on a return appointment.

The interview with Kelly Jasmin shows the main point of this book: interviewing is a nonlinear process—many events occur simultaneously. The phases are of heuristic value; they indicate what type of topics have to be covered in a complete interview. When you master these topics, feel free to jump back and forth from screening to family history to feedback and to verification of impressions as the patient's responses urge you to do.

Do not get hung up on the idea that you have to complete your interview during the first visit. What is essential in the first interview is to establish rapport and determine the patient's immediate need for treatment, especially in regard to safety for herself and others. The difficulty in this interview arises from the fact that the patient dissociates and that the interviewer does not identify this behavior and use it for the diagnostic process. Such an advanced technique is presented in *The Clinical Interview Using DSM-IV, Volume 2: The Difficult Patient* (Othmer and Othmer 2002).

CHAPTER NINE

DISORDER-SPECIFIC INTERVIEWING: CLINICAL DISORDERS

SUMMARY

Chapter 9 shows how to modify interviewing strategies for symptoms, signs, and behaviors that interfere with rapport and the information-gathering process for some clinical disorders. These modifications may help you to overcome some typical problems emerging with these diagnoses.

▲ ▲ ▲ ▲ ▲

The first step toward a knowledge of the symptoms (of mental disease) is their locality—to which organ do the indications of disease belong? What organ must necessarily and invariably be diseased where there is madness? Physiological and pathological facts show us that this organ can only be the brain.

—Wilhelm Griesinger, [1845] 1882

▼ ▼ ▼ ▼ ▼

The "standard" interview is appropriate for patients who have enough insight into their symptoms to describe them (Chapters 7 and 8). They are able to see their symptoms as due to the disorder and, as a result, do not usually interfere with the interview process. This more straightforward interview is therefore feasible with patients who, for instance, suffer from milder forms of mood, anxiety, somatoform, substance-related, or sleep disorders.

Modify your interview for clinical disorders if the patient's pathology interferes with either rapport or the diagnostic assessment process—for example, when you encounter the following:

1. perplexity and memory problems, as seen in the cognitive disorders,
2. deception as seen in alcohol dependence or abuse,
3. hyperactivity as seen in bipolar disorder,
4. suspiciousness as seen in delusional disorder,
5. avoidance as seen in phobia,
6. disbelief and embarrassment as seen in panic disorder,
7. persecutory ideas as sometimes seen in mental retardation,
8. laziness as sometimes seen in narcolepsy.

These eight pathological features are specific for a group of disorders; for instance, hyperactivity, besides occurring in bipolar disorder, can occur in alcohol intoxication, amphetamine use, or attention-deficit/hyperactivity disorder. They are core pathology, each typical for some clinical disorders. Similar characteristic features exist for personality disorders. We will propose how to interview for both sets of features in the next two chapters.

We will point out, for the disorders discussed, what to look for and what special strategies may work in establishing rapport, assessing mental status, keeping the interview going, and with it the diagnostic process. The format we use to highlight our method is a running commentary, which we insert at key points to emphasize the four components of the interview.

1. PERPLEXITY AND SUSPICIOUSNESS IN DEMENTIA

To diagnose advanced dementia is easy, even for the novice. The patient is disoriented; he is unable to memorize three words, to count, spell, or name all months of the year backward and displays aphasia, apraxia, or agnosia and disturbances of executive functions (see Chapter 4: Mental Status and Chapter 5: Testing).

In contrast, beginning dementias (due to mild diffuse cortical lesions, especially of the nondominant hemisphere) are considerably more difficult to spot. A key sign for these lesions may be perplexity. The patient is bewildered by everyday situations because he cannot understand them. For him, everyday events roll by like isolated still frames of a movie. He perceives the pictures but cannot connect them, and therefore cannot comprehend the intent of the actions. He recalls elements of situations without integrating them logically. For instance, he may not understand what happened when he and his family left the house in the morning. He did not grasp where and why things were placed in a certain way. He is perplexed by the unfamiliar look of the house when he returns in the evening. He often explains the "newness" in a persecutory manner:

"Things are strange. I can't figure out what's going on. I have to be on the lookout to protect myself."

Therefore, if you detect signs of perplexity or suspiciousness in an older patient, either in his history or during the interview, add dementia to your differential diagnoses.

In interviewing such a patient, the strategy is to recognize his perplexity and accept his misinterpretations without challenge. Try not to scare him or arouse his suspiciousness. Let him describe in detail his observations and show your interest in them. Carefully explore how he interprets events. Express empathy for his struggles. If you can win his trust, he may become less guarded toward you. Don't examine him as if you doubt his reports and explanations. Avoid distancing yourself from his account. For instance, a question such as:

"What did this mean to you?"

implies that it means something else to him than to you.

"How did that make you feel?"

implies that you might feel differently. Alienation may result and the patient may stop cooperating. Ask instead:

"What were they up to?"
"What did you do?"

Also, use short sentences, because the patient may not remember long ones. Use simple, concrete words. Use his vocabulary, and connect questions by smooth transitions, so that he can follow your train of thought without becoming irritable or frustrated. If he shows signs of becoming tired, stop the interview and continue later.

> Mrs. M., a 60-year-old, African-American widow, is presented by a female social worker who is concerned that the patient might be exploited by her relatives. According to the patient, her relatives go through her belongings in her absence. They leave the house in disarray, and sometimes take her checks and money. The daughter reports that her mother was hard to deal with during the last 2 years and that she accused family members of robbing her.
>
> When the patient enters the room, she grabs the arm of the social worker who accompanies her.

1. I: Hi, Mrs. M., your social worker, Dr. B., has told me about your problems [the patient looks at the social worker and smiles]. I would like to learn more about them. How long have you been coming here?
   P: Oh, I started about 9 months ago [information is correct]. I could not get along with my daughter any more.
2. I.   How often have you been coming?
   P: About every other week [information is correct].
3. I: Did you miss appointments sometimes?
   P: No, I don't think so. I keep good track.
4. I: So, you have a good memory. You always know what date it is?
   P: Sure.
5. I: Let me see, what date is it today?
   P: [gives the correct date]
6. I: Who brings you here to the clinic?
   P: Sometimes I come alone. But mostly my daughter or my son-in-law brings me.
7. I: They bring you?
   P: Yes.
8. I: Who tells them about your appointment?
   P: I do. I call them up and tell them.
9. I: Do they have the time to do it?
   P: No, not really. My daughter takes off from work.

Rapport: The presence of the social worker relaxes the patient because she considers her an ally.

Technique: Simple questions that require recent memory about apparently peripheral circumstances of the clinic visits are designed to gauge the patient's ability to interact with the interviewer. In case of a memory disturbance, he can branch out to the mental status examination and focus on the remote history. If memory is intact, he can assess more recent problems.

Mental status: The interviewer starts small talk that seems to explore only the peripheral circumstances of the clinic visits and the patient answers openly without suspiciousness. What the interviewer actually does is use conversation as a tool for the examination of the patient's recent memory and orientation (the clinic visits can be verified from the record). Both appear to be intact. The interviewer does not pick up on the clue in A. 1 (difficulties with her daughter) because he expects this topic to resurface later.

Diagnosis: The patient's grossly intact memory excludes the diagnosis of dementia at a more advanced stage (list no. 2).

10. I: So your daughter brings you here. She seems to be concerned about you.
    P: I'm not sure. She seems to keep track of me.
11. I: How's that?
    P: She wants to know where I'm going.
12. I: Has she always done that?
    P: I don't know. It just dawned on me. I just found out about it.
13. I: Can you tell me what happened?
    P: One time when I went out, things did not look the same when I came back to the house. One of the tiles in the ceiling seemed to be removed. Somebody had tampered with my closet. They didn't even close it. And I could not find my money. They must have taken it.
14. I: What did you do about it?
    P: I tried to hide it, so they cannot find it. But then it is gone anyway.
15. I: Why does your daughter do it?
    P: I don't know.
16. I: Do you have any other examples?
    P: Yes. Things never look the same when I come back home. I can tell somebody is tampering with my things.
17. I: Do you know who?
    P: Only my daughter has a key.
18. I: What did you do about it?
    P: I asked her to give it back. I asked her not to tamper with my things. She looked at me kind of strange. And she lied to me. She lies and says she is not doing it.

Rapport: The patient is neither guarded, nor delivers angry and revengeful tirades; instead, she levels with the interviewer and shares her concerns, which is contrary to a patient with persecutory ideas due to a delusional disorder.

Technique: With a smooth transition, the interviewer reintroduces the subject of the patient's daughter but challenges the patient by stating that her daughter seems to be concerned about her, contrasting what the patient had said in A. 1. He uses this technique to stir up an emotionally charged response necessary to explore her feelings about her daughter (Q. 11, 13, 16) with factual What? How? Why is it done? questions (Q. 13–15).

Mental status: Mrs. M. seems to be perplexed; she seems to misperceive and suspiciously misinterpret events. If her daughter actually stole money from the patient, she probably would not take off from work to bring her mother to a psychiatric clinic.

Diagnosis: The persecutory feelings are of recent onset. They do not show a depressive or manic flavor or an organized paranoid system, such as the belief that she is singled out and discriminated against. Instead, the persecutory ideas reveal bewilderment and mild derealization (A. 13, 16, 18), suggesting impaired information processing.

List no. 1 of included disorders is:

- dementia of the Alzheimer type with early onset, with delusions
- vascular dementia, with delusions
- substance-induced persisting dementia
- psychotic disorder due to a general medical condition, with delusions
- parent-child relational problem.

List no. 2 of excluded disorders is:

- mood disorder due to a general medical condition
- schizophrenia, paranoid type
- delusional disorder.

19. I: Are there any other things going on?
    P: Strange things.
20. I: Can you tell me about that?
    P: Yes.
21. I: Okay?
    P: It is with my grandson. He likes to come to my house. After his visit I took him to the door and a yellow car was stopping. It stopped right at the corner.
22. I: What did this have to do with your grandson?
    P: Well, he went over there and they talked to him.
23. I: What else happened?
    P: They talked to him and he got in their car.

24. I: Did you know the people?
    P: No, I haven't seen them before in my life.
25. I: What happened then?
    P: I was scared. I thought they had kidnapped him.
26. I: Did you do anything about it?
    P: I called my daughter. I told her about it and she just laughed. I felt like they are tricking me.
27. I: Hmm.
    P: Later I called again and they denied it. They said he was already home. They said a friend's daddy had brought him home.
28. I: Was he home?
    P: They somehow got him. They must have.

Rapport: The patient supplies the interviewer with desired details without censoring.

Technique: The interviewer explores perception and ability to interpret everyday events. The patient tells her story in short segments. She has to be prodded to elaborate. Three types of questions help: time-related questions, for example: "What happened then?" (Q. 23, 25, 27); questions that tie elements of the story together, for example: "How is A related to B?" (Q. 22, 28, 32); and questions that ask for more details, for example: "How did it look?" "What do you know about it?" (Q. 24)

These questions reveal whether the patient can interpret an event accurately as a chain of cause and effect. The most powerful of these questions addresses the patient's interpretation:

"Why did that happen?"
"What does this mean?"
"What did you do about that?" (Q. 26)

Mental status: The patient could not grasp her grandson's new social relationship. This reveals a deficit of her recent memory not apparent from the initial assessment of her orientation and memory. The patient can reproduce the sequence of events, but misunderstands their social significance.

Diagnosis: The patient's impaired learning points toward a cognitive impairment. A depressive disorder in an elderly patient could explain such a deficit, if attention and concentration were disturbed and if psychomotor retardation and social withdrawal were present. In their absence, a cognitive process is the more likely culprit.

29. I: Why?
    P: They let me talk to him [the grandson]. But his voice sounded strange.
30. I: Sounded strange?
    P: Yes.
31. I: Did those things happen again?
    P: Another time the same car came by and stopped. They picked him up again.
32. I: Was the car waiting?
    P: No, it was just driving by.
33. I: How did they know when your grandson leaves your house?
    P: Oh, they must have known. He must have called them. I heard them whispering on the telephone.
34. I: Did you ask him?
    P: No, I did not want to. I just wanted to see what happened. And there the car came again and picked him up.
35. I: What do you know about the people in the car?
    P: Nothing, but they already had another kid in the car and they let my grandson in too.
36. I: Could he be a friend of your grandson?
    P: No, I don't know him. My daughter says he is, but I don't know. I think something is going on.
37. I: Do you have any idea what that could be?
    P: No, not really. It's just strange.
38. I: Do you feel they are after you?
    P: I don't know. I think they might be. But I'll be on the watchout. And I have my windows nailed down and bolts installed on the doors.
39. I: Would there be any reason why they would be after you?
    P: No, I have not done anything.
40. I: What are they after?
    P: Maybe my money.
41. I: Who would they be?
    P: Oh, I think maybe my daughter and maybe the people in the car.

Rapport: The patient trusts the interviewer. She reveals her fears, concerns, and feelings of insecurity.

Technique: The interviewer focuses on the patient's interpretations of events (except Q. 31, 35), which reveal the patient's lack of comprehension, but also her delusional thinking.

Mental status: The patient continues to interpret events in a persecutory manner, delusional not organized. For instance, she cannot explain why the parents cooperate in the kidnapping of her grandchild. The patient perseverates on the theme that these people and her family are after her money.

Diagnosis: Adequate verbal production, together with a deficit in recent memory and understanding of social situations, and the presence of non-organized persecutory delusions support the diagnosis of dementia with early onset with delusions.

In the remainder of the interview the interviewer excluded the presence of depressive symptoms, alcohol abuse, and use of any medication known to interfere with mental functions such as anticholinergics. Further mental status examination revealed also that the patient had difficulties interpreting proverbs, counting backward by two, and copying a cube (Fig. 9–1).

These results plus further workup—including an electroencephalogram, brain scan, Wechsler Intelligence Test, Shipley-Hartford Test, and Halstead-Reitan Neuropsychological Test Battery, which together confirmed a cognitive impairment—supported the initial impression of

Axis I:
1. **Dementia of the Alzheimer's type, without behavioral disturbances, with early onset, DSM-IV-TR 294.10.**
2. **Psychotic disorder due to Alzheimer's disease, with delusions, DSM-IV-TR 293.81.**

Axis III: Alzheimer's disease 331.0.

Since dementia due to Alzheimer's disease is a diagnosis of exclusion, we must rule out the other types of dementia. Furthermore, the patient's suspiciousness leads to behavioral disturbances (e.g., accusing relatives) that seem to be due to the delusion and not to the dementing process. Therefore, we coded this case vignette "without behavioral disturbance." The concomitant recording of the medical condition causing the dementia is coded on Axis III.

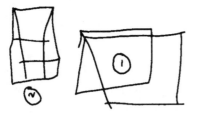 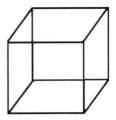

Figure 9–1.   Constructional apraxia: draw a cube.

2. DECEPTION AND DENIAL IN ALCOHOL ABUSE AND DEPENDENCE

There are a number of presentations of alcohol abuse and dependence that seem to appear over and over again:

1. The homeless, street alcoholic who openly admits his drinking. Often he checks into a hospital for detoxification in exchange for food and housing but refuses to give up his drinking. He often brings contraband to the ward and drinks secretly.
2. The younger patient with alcohol abuse/dependence and antisocial personality disorder who reports truancy, bad school and work habits, violent behavior, lying, stealing, multiple traffic tickets, or a police record. His sociopathic symptoms may overshadow the drinking.
3. The middle-class patient with alcohol abuse/dependence and mood disorder who reveals depressive symptoms but downplays drinking.
4. The middle-aged professional or executive with alcohol abuse/dependence who continues to fulfill his or her social functions, maintains the veneer of a happy home life with spouse and children, and talks about the stress he or she endures but denies excessive drinking.

While the first two types are easy to interview because they admit their drinking, the latter two have an active interest in concealing their alcohol dependence.

To overcome these obstacles, you first have to detect the patient's drinking in spite of the denial. You should therefore look for:

1. a past history or family history of drinking, alcohol abuse, or alcohol dependence;
2. a history of frequent short-term illnesses and absenteeism;
3. signs of intoxication or withdrawal during the interview; and
4. liver function tests, GGT (gamma-glutamyltransferase) above 30 units, CDT (carbohydrate deficient transferrin) above 20 units, and elevated MCV (mean corpuscular volume).

If you suspect alcohol abuse/dependence, but your patient denies it, pursue it. Insist on this topic tactfully, and frequently. Bring it up again and again until the patient admits little by little the full story.

Be careful not to make the patient lose face by being caught lying or by being accused of misleading you. Understand the motivation for lying: individuals who abuse alcohol usually have the perception that they are not truly alcohol-dependent; that they could indeed stop drinking if they seriously wanted to; that their spouse, employer, and physician unfairly exaggerate and overemphasize their drinking habit in a dogmatic, nonunderstanding way. They may claim that they drink for relaxation, which they are entitled to in order to compensate for the pressures of family life and job.

Second, when you have established a drinking pattern, discuss the advantages and disadvantages of drinking. Induce the patient to admit to its good and ill effects so that you can fully explore the impact of the alcoholism on his or her life. Work toward this goal by asking whether any family member, colleague, or friend considers him or her an alcoholic. The patient may grudgingly admit to such criticism. Then ask whether the critic's point of view is well taken. The patient may get angry, defensive, and quote examples of "those bum alcoholics" who are "the true alcoholics" who should be criticized. It may take more than one interview to reach a stage of admission and insight.

Even when a patient admits that he is an alcoholic and assures you that he will stop, expect secret denial. Translate this "cooperation" into its real meaning:

> You expect me to admit that I have a drinking problem. I am willing to admit it, not because I think you are right, but because you don't know any better. When I tell you that I want to stop drinking, I mean: "Get off my back." I say, "I will stop drinking" to pacify you but I will hide my drinking better so that people don't get the wrong impression.

If you have collected enough evidence for the patient's alcoholism, there is no use in pressing the patient to give lip service to the well-known dual therapeutic premise to admit his alcoholism and promise abstinence. He has to be convinced first that drinking is indeed wrecking his life.

The alcoholic patient is most sensitive to the loss of a support person. If such a loss is imminent, use it to make the patient see the damage drinking inflicts on him. Approximately 25% of suicides are committed by alcohol abusers; they often follow the loss of a support person (Goodwin and Guze 1989). If suicide is a gauge for the importance of support, use the support person as leverage in your interview.

> Here is an interview with Mr. Harold B., a 58-year-old professor of economics. Mr. B. had a history of severe alcohol dependence, his wife had threatened divorce, and the dean had notified him that he might lose his tenured position if he did not curb his drinking. After such warnings—according to the wife—the patient had indeed stopped drinking during the last year. After

the wife had returned home from a 2-week vacation that she had taken without her husband, she found him in an "awful" state. He was referred for electroshock treatment because of severe symptoms of depression.

The patient was sitting barefoot on his bed. He was unkempt, unshaven, and the rancid smell of body odor hung in the room.

1. I: Hi, Mr. B. Dr. A. has asked me to talk to you [Dr. A. is in charge of the patient's treatment].
   P: Hi [patient avoids eye contact and looks down at his hands. He is sweating. His face is somewhat puffy and blotchy with mild peripheral edema. His hands are tremulous].
2. I: Did Dr. A. tell you that I was going to see you?
   P: I guess . . . he may have.
3. I: Do you remember what he told you?
   P: Told me what?
4. I: About why I should see you?
   P: I don't know. Maybe something for treatment of depression [there is no prolonged latency of response].
5. I: When did he talk to you about it?
   P: Didn't he tell you? You should know. Aren't you the doctor? Why ask me all these stupid questions?
6. I: Well, it is important for me to find out how well you can remember things.
   P: There is nothing wrong with my memory. I'm just sick. Can't you see that? Do I have to tell you what's wrong with me? You should know [starts trembling].
7. I.   You must feel awful. The way you look tells me that you feel bad; but it's also the way you talk.
   P: What do you mean?
8. I: It seems to bother you to talk with me.
   P: No, that's okay.
9. I: You seem to be irritable.
   P: That's not because of you. Everything just bugs me. Sitting here. Nobody does anything. Nobody cares in this whole damn hospital.
10. I: You must really feel bad.
    P: That's no joke. I don't need any wisecracks [blushes].
11. I: Let me get you something that will calm your nerves.
    P: What do you want to give me?
12. I: Some Librium and a shot of vitamins [physician calls the nurse and gives the order for Librium 50 mg po and thiamine 100 mg. He takes the patient's pulse. It is 108]. When you have the medication, it will be easier for you to talk to me. You want me to come back in a little while?
    P: No, it's okay. It doesn't make any difference. Let's get it over with.

Rapport: The apparently peripheral questions (if and when the treating physician has discussed the consultation visit, Q. 1–4) irritate the patient (A. 5–6). So, the interviewer switches to statements that express empathy for his suffering (Q. 7–12) to find cooperation. The patient becomes less irritable and more agreeable.

Technique: The opening questions assess recent memory. The patient is evasive and resists this line of questioning, which prompts the interviewer to assure rapport (see above).

Mental status: The patient's appearance and poor hygiene suggest either major depression, severe, or—with the background of alcohol dependence— a withdrawal state. Increased pulse rate, sweating, puffiness, and fluency of speech support alcohol withdrawal. The patient's irritated refusal to answer questions that assess his recent memory strengthen this impression. Therefore, the interviewer orders chlordiazepoxide (Librium) to abate withdrawal, and thiamine (vitamin B_1) to prevent Wernicke's syndrome, a vitamin B_1 deficiency.

Diagnosis: The mental status in combination with the history strongly suggests alcohol withdrawal. During this state an underlying depression is difficult to assess.

13. I: When did you come in?
    P: Must have been the day before yesterday.
14. I: Do you know what time?
    P: Must have been in the evening [records show that he came in 1 day ago in the morning].
15. I: Why did you come in?
    P: My wife and her sister brought me. They must have thought I was sick. I felt sick to my stomach. I was just sitting around. I had not gone to work for a while. They came back from a trip. So they brought me here.
16. I: How well did you sleep last night?
    P: I was exhausted, but I could not sleep. I tossed and turned. I had to get up several times during the night to drink. I drank a lot of water.
17. I: Just last night?
    P: Maybe the nights before too.
18. I: When did you get up in the morning?
    P: Oh, these nurses made me get out of bed and have breakfast. But I was not hungry. I just drank coffee.
19. I: How much coffee did you have?
    P: You mean today?
20. I: Yes.
    P: Eight or ten cups. I don't know [the nurse brings the Librium 50 mg, water, and the syringe. The patient takes the Librium without any comment and washes it down with the water. He then starts to pull his pants down for the shot].

21. I:	What are you doing?
    P:	Didn't you want to give me a shot?
22. I:	Yes. You look shaky to me. But don't you want to know why I'm giving it to you?
    P:	You do what you want to do in this hospital. What's the sense in asking?
23. I:	Well, let me tell you then. I read in your chart that you had a drinking problem. I think you are drinking again and that it's rough for you to get off that stuff. That's why I'm giving you Librium.
    P:	What makes you think that? I'm not drinking anymore. I quit.

Rapport and technique:	The interviewer uses the improved rapport to assess some symptoms of alcohol withdrawal in a straightforward checklist manner to prepare the patient for more direct questions about his drinking, which he starts in Q. 23.

Mental status:	The patient has some mild disturbances of recent memory and restlessness with insomnia. He is not interested in his present treatment and denies drinking.

24. I:	You mean, you have not had a drink recently?
    P:	I quit last May, the 18th of May, precisely.
25. I:	You mean, you had your very last drink then?
    P:	Yes, that's when I went to the hospital.
26. I:	What happened when you came out?
    P:	I was fine all summer. But I did not feel so hot when the semester started.
27. I:	What happened?
    P:	Well, I just slowly went downhill. My wife thinks I'm depressed again.
28. I:	Well, what do you think?
    P:	She may be right, I guess.
29. I:	So, when you felt depressed, did you take up drinking again?
    P:	I could not sleep.
30. I:	Does alcohol help you sleep?
    P:	Yes, it did in the past. At least in the beginning.
31. I:	Did it help this time?
    P:	I try not to drink anymore.
32. I:	You mean you slowed down?
    P:	My wife told me she would leave me if I started up again.
33. I:	So you are scared that she will leave you?
    P:	I may also lose my job. They may fire me.
34. I:	Well, what do you do when you need a drink during the day or when you can't sleep?
    P:	I try not to do anything.
35. I:	Okay, and if that does not work?
    P:	I sometimes go to my study and sleep there.
36. I:	In your study?

P: Yes.
37. I: So you sneak out to your study? Is that where you have your stuff?
P: What do you mean?
38. I: Well, you told me that you will lose your job, if you are found drinking again and that your wife will leave you. So you have no choice. You have to hide it.
P: Well, I sleep in the study, so that my wife does not smell it. I have switched to vodka. They say it smells less. But I take it only when I can't sleep, when I need it for my nerves.

Rapport: The interviewer expresses interest in Mr. B.'s mental state during the last year and shows empathy in his concern that the patient may lose his wife and job if he is found out drinking again. This concern helps to maintain rapport.

Technique: The interviewer vacillates between collecting the recent history of increased alcohol consumption and expression of interest in the patient's worries (see Rapport). This approach keeps the patient talking and slowly admitting his return to the bottle.

Mental status: The patient's denial melts away.

Diagnosis: The interviewer fills in details of the recent history of alcohol abuse and dependence.

39. I: Hmm.
P: You really don't believe me, do you?
40. I: Well, I am trying to understand you. I know once you start drinking, you need more and more to make it work. And you told me that you started again when the semester began in August. Now it's January. You are right back into it and now it got too much.
P: You are worse than my wife. You can ask her. She has not said anything about drinking anymore. She has not even talked to the dean. Nobody has said anything about me drinking.
41. I: So what is your main problem?
P: My main problem is depression. I feel awful.
42. I: I know you do. But I'm afraid we'll do you a disservice by not caring about your drinking problem.
P: I really don't have that problem anymore.
43. I: Well, you told me you are hiding your drinks now. What do you do when you are at work and your nerves bother you and you feel shaky and can't concentrate?
P: I told you I have slowed down.

44. I: I know, but when you had a drink in the evening and you feel rotten in the morning, what do you do?

    P: I just have coffee.

45. I: Okay, but if that does not work? Do you have anything in your office for an emergency?

    P: I'm not crazy. I don't want to lose my job. What do you think would happen if they found it?

46. I: So what do you do?

    P: [silent]

47. I: I can help you better if you level with me. In the meantime, let me give you the shot [he gives the vitamin shot]. If you don't want to level with me, why don't you talk with Dr. A. about it.

    P: I don't need anything about my drinking in my chart.

48. I: I won't write anything in your chart. I will just talk to Dr. A. and recommend that we detoxify you. In a few days I would like to look at you again and see how much is left of your depression.

    P: You really don't believe me.

49. I: I know that you are under a lot of pressure, that you are scared you will lose your wife and your job and I don't want you to lose anything. I want to help you as much as I can.

    P: You all say that. But nobody really understands how I feel. Nobody understands the pressure I am under.

50. I: I know you are under a lot of pressure . . .

    P: If my wife sees me having a drink, she exaggerates and thinks I am an alcoholic. And that's the only reason why I hide it. She has not said anything anymore.

51. I: I know. I read the admission note and talked to Dr. A. Your wife did not mention your drinking when you came into the hospital this time.

    P: So don't you believe her?

52. I: I have not talked to her directly.

    P: Why don't you give her a call? She will tell you that I have not touched the stuff.

53. I: Oh, I believe that.

    P: Why is that?

54. I: I think there are some good reasons for her to tell me that.

    P: Why should she? Do you think I hide it that well?

55. I: Maybe. But maybe that's not all.

    P: What do you mean?

56. I: I don't think she wants you to lose your job either. What is she going to do when you are out of work?

    P: Why would she bring me here?

57. I: Well, I think she notices your condition. She wants some help for you without naming the problem "drinking." If you don't trust me, there is no reason for me to talk to you . . . Although there is . . .

    P: What should that be?

58. I: That I take better care of your interests than you do. You don't gain anything by hiding your problem from your doctor, if you really want help.

    P: So what else do you want to know?

Rapport: The interviewer is nonjudgmental and expresses repeatedly that he wants to help.

Technique: The interviewer neither confronts nor interprets Mr. B.'s attempts to use his wife as an alibi for his claimed abstinence to assure his slowing down in drinking. He also bypasses the patient's attempts to downplay his drinking and pursues in detail the patient's recent drinking history, thus wearing down his denial.

59. I: I want to know what you do at work when you need something for your nerves.
    P: You are back on that again.
60. I: If you tell me that, we can drop it for good.
    P: I told you I have slowed down.
61. I: Yes, you slowed down, you try to control it better, and you try to hide it better. So where do you hide your stuff during the daytime?
    P: Oh, just a few days before I came in here, I had one bottle left. After I bought it, I did not want to bring it into the house. So I left it sitting in the car.
62. I: You mean, it just sits in the car so that anybody can see it?
    P: Of course not. I put it where the spare tire is and I wrapped a rag around it.
63. I: So you hide your stuff in your study and in your car.
    P: Not really. My wife often goes into the study. There is not that much room to hide anything.
64. I: Where did you hide it in the past, when you were drinking more?
    P: Then? I had a whole collection in the basement.
65. I: You mean it is all gone now?
    P: Oh no, it is still there. But I have not touched it.
66. I: I understand how you feel and the pressure you are under. I will talk to Dr. A. I think we will give you a few days' rest and good food. Then we will see how your depression is doing. I will give Dr. A. my recommendation.

Rapport: The tactic of extracting the alcohol history little by little prevents the breakdown of rapport. Even though the interviewer is not accepted as an ally during this first interview, he has laid the groundwork for future therapeutic alliance. The task is to achieve the patient's full insight into his drinking problem. With many alcohol and drug addicts this is a long-term rather than a short-term goal that requires prolonged therapy often punctuated by relapses.

The interviewer's active pursuit of the alcohol history places him in an authoritative role, which he will give up when the patient has full insight and accepts the goal of abstinence.

Technique: The interviewer's task is to deal with the defense mechanism of denial. In this interview the denial of any drinking was replaced by the admission of drinking a little bit, occasionally, when under duress. Obviously, the patient's withdrawal state contradicts this assertion. However, it is a long process to break down this defense.

Mental status and diagnosis: Concerning the present admission, the differential diagnosis includes alcohol abuse and major depressive disorder. In spite of this patient's denial of drinking, the interviewer assumes that the patient drank heavily ("I had not gone to work for a while") during the wife's absence, but had stopped drinking on her return to avoid marital conflict. This led to his "desolate state." The essential features of beginning alcohol withdrawal are visible: nausea ("I felt sick to my stomach"), trembling, autonomic hyperactivity (sweating, tachycardia), malaise, depressed mood, irritability, anxiety, and fitful and disturbed sleep. He showed dehydration and a dry mouth ("I drank a lot of water"). He admits to hiding alcohol at home and in his car to use at work.

The intoxicated alcoholic has often an acute amnestic syndrome, which may have been responsible for Mr. B.'s inability to recall the time of his admission.

Diagnosis

DSM-IV-TR diagnoses: Alcohol dependence 303.90 and Alcohol withdrawal 291.81.   This interview intended only to show one way to deal with denial by an alcoholic. It did not assess other alcohol- or non-alcohol-related disorders. Such a differential usually poses no difficulty and the format of the standard interview can be applied.

3. IRRITABLE HYPERACTIVITY IN BIPOLAR DISORDER

Lack of insight, control, and goal orientation, together with elevated drive, all result in irritable hyperactivity and interfere with the interview of the patient with bipolar disorder, manic episode. This patient's lack of insight prevents you from using rational arguments and confrontation with his altered mood in order to influence him. Handle him like an unpredictable explosive ready to go off at any time.

The lack of insight makes him distractible. A random noise in the corri-

dor may attract his attention. He may be stimulated to excessive mono-
logues by the doctor's overall appearance or her shapely legs, only to
comment in the next moment on the orderly's beard. From compliments he
may switch to profanities. No topic stays in focus. His thinking is unpredictable and erratic.

The elevated drive and disinhibited control make the patient with mania talk, shout, persuade, swear, holler, or sing. Blinded by energy, he feels
angry, happy, or excited, but above all justified in insisting on whatever he
pursues at the moment. Whoever opposes him is his foe. He has some
vague feeling that things don't go his way. This ticks him off. The manic
cannot realize that his enormous drive is bewildering, frightening, or amus-
ing to the bystander. He has no insight into how he affects others.

How Do You Interview Such a Patient?

The best approach is to make his elevated drive work for you. Discern his
point of view, identify with his goals, and appear to adopt them. If you help
him in the pursuit of his goals, his mood will remain elated. If you oppose
him, you may arouse his anger and hostility and prevent compliance. If he
wants to leave the hospital, you can tell him you want him out even faster
but permanently. If he wants to talk to you at this moment, you really
wanted to talk to him an hour ago. In short, you agree with him and support him rather than become the obstacle to his goals, contradict him, pull
rank on him, and cross him.

How Do You Collect the
Facts to Make a Diagnosis?

The patient with bipolar disorder, manic episode has little insight into his
feelings but is aware of his actions. He knows that he is sleeping less and
can get into fights and arguments, and realizes that others have brought him
to a psychiatrist. Even after remission this patient typically talks about his
past manic attacks in terms of behavioral (and not mood) changes. He seldom realizes or remembers that he feels or felt abnormally high or elated:

> "I wrote more letters; I spent more money than I had; I wrote bad checks; I
> enrolled in three health clubs at the same time; I bought $6,000 of pottery for
> my house; I walked out on my girlfriend; I picked up a nurse, a secretary,
> and a go-go dancer; other people told me to shut up—so I must have talked
> more; I really don't know how I felt, reasoned, or thought. I didn't feel sick or
> out of control."

Let the patient with mania describe his behaviors, but don't expect him to admit that there is anything wrong with him. He feels better than ever. Use his distractibility to redirect him when you reach an impasse. Don't argue and don't try to persuade him, but distract him.

In the following example, the patient insists on being discharged (heightened drive). The interviewer agrees with him but lets the patient repeatedly know that he can only be discharged if certain conditions are met. He may tell him that he wants to do more for him than just discharge him: he does not want him to be returned to the hospital. He reminds the patient that he had been readmitted before when released prematurely. If the patient recalls an angry outburst against the police, or the friends who he thought betrayed him, or the doctor who played a dirty game, the interviewer will agree with him and insist that this should never happen again. He tells him:

> "I want to help you to cope better with others and not be their punching bag. You see, you shouted and screamed and pushed them, and even struck out at one of them. That's how you ended up in the hospital. I want to help you so that you don't have to scream, shout, and push! Then those people won't bother you anymore."

A description such as "You screamed, kicked, and shouted" works—as mentioned above—better than introspection such as "You feel restless, angry, and excited, we have to calm you down," because the patient may not experience himself as restless, angry, and excited. But he remembers that he shouted and kicked.

Mr. Brendan R., a 38-year-old, white, married patient was transferred to the psychiatric ward from another hospital where he had punched a doctor. His hands and feet were handcuffed to a stretcher. In the accompanying report he was diagnosed as a schizophrenic. "Bizarre actions" and "paranoid delusions" were mentioned, but precise descriptions of the patient's behavior were missing.

Establish Rapport

1. I: What happened to you?
   P: [silent, angry looks, breathing hard]
2. I: What happened? Why are you tied down?

P: Screw it. Let me out of here. I'm not talking to you. Just let me out. God will not tolerate it. I want to help mankind, set them all free—we are free creatures—we are equal to God. God will free the creatures—we are equal to God. God will see to it. Seeing is believing. I see! I see! Let me out. Now, now, now. Now is now, and now is ever. Now is not never [straining on his cuffs].

3. I: I don't want to keep you here. I want you out, too, after you stop shouting, screaming, and kicking.

P: Get me out! Get these cuffs off, get them off, off, off! Bitch! [shouting].

4. I: I want them off, too. But I don't want to put them back on again. So when you stop shouting, we can take them off.

P: Then take them off! Take them off now!

5. I: I will take them off if I don't have to put them back on again.

P: I want out!

6. I: I want you out too. Understand? You can come out when you talk calmly. I want to know what brought those cuffs on.

P: I don't want to talk to you, woman, I want out.

7. I: Okay, I'll get you out. But tell me, why are you in them in the first place?

P: I hit him. I hit that doctor, because he told me I could not get out. He can't do it, he can't do it, he can't do it.

8. I: You will get out. But you are too loud. You shout, you don't talk.

P: [lowers voice] I can talk. Take the cuffs off [wriggling on the restraints].

9. I: I want to take them off, but I don't want to put them back on. I want to make sure that you don't strike out.

P: Then do it.

10. I: Okay, but I first have to help you talk calmer.

P: Calm me down? I'm tied down. That makes me shout.

11. I: I will give you a shot so that we can take off the cuffs, so that you don't shout and scream, so that you can talk to me.

P: I don't need no shot, nobody needs a shot. I'm nailed to the cross. God's son was nailed to the cross, Jesus was our savior.

12. I: I want you off the cross. Let me help you. Here is the shot so you can get off the cross.

P: Okay, hurry up. I want out. [interviewer gives the patient a shot of 50 mg chlorpromazine im without the patient objecting]

Rapport: The interviewer establishes rapport with Mr. R. by agreeing with him to have the restraints removed. Since the patient has no insight into his excitability as a symptom of a disorder, the interviewer does not express any empathy with the patient's excited state. In this respect the approach taken with the irritable patient deviates from the second step described in Chapter 2: Rapport. Statements like "It must be awful to be strapped down" may sound sarcastic to the patient and ignite his hostility rather than kindle rapport.

Technique: The interviewer agrees with the patient's goal but attaches the condition that he has to stop shouting first. She does not present this condition as a restraint but as an assurance that the patient does not have to be put back in handcuffs. She avoids talking about the patient's mental state in which he has no insight but addresses only his behavior, which the patient can recognize even though he perceives it—unlike the interviewer—as justified.

Mental status: The patient is alert and shows hostile excitement with flight of ideas and thematic perseveration on the goal to be uncuffed.

Diagnosis: All disorders associated with an excited state have to be considered, such as:

- dementia due to a general medical condition
- intoxication with PCP, cocaine, amphetamines
- delirium, substance-induced or due to a general medical condition
- bipolar I disorder, most recent episode manic
- schizophrenia, paranoid type
- schizophreniform disorder
- schizoaffective disorder, bipolar type

Rule Out Dementia and Delirium

13. I: When did you come in?
    P: Too long ago. Two sunrises ago.
14. I: On Sunday?
    P: [laughs] It was a Tuesday, cutie, not the sunny Sunday. Two days ago was a Tuesday, because today is Thursday.
15. I: Of what month?
    P: Of what month, of what month? I'm not dumb. Leave me alone.
16. I: I will go, but give me the month first. You gave me the day.
    P: I give you nothing. I give you everything. Give, give, give. God gives and forgives.
17. I: The month?
    P: The month, month, month! What is the month? Not July, not September. But the month in between, is what I remember [accurate].
18. I: When did you start to get so restless?
    P: I could not sleep. God wanted me to preach. I want to preach [stares at the physician]. You are tied down too. Do you have tied down tubes?
19. I: When did you start to preach?
    P: One and a half weeks ago. I was helping everybody. I was helping mankind, but they caught me. The soldiers of Pontius Pilate caught me.

20. I: Have you preached before?
    P: Two years ago. I was in a hospital. They said they kept me because I was a schizophrenic or something like that. I spent all my money on an invention, I made mock collars and cuffs. Get these cuffs off. [interviewer gives order to remove the cuffs]

Rapport: The interviewer seems to engage in small talk and gets cooperation.

Technique: The interviewer explores and tests recent memory, a technique described as part of the mental status examination.

Mental status: Mr. R. is oriented with intact recent memory. He shows a tendency to rhyme, to pun, and to perseverate on words like "month." His thought content shows religious preoccupation. The investment in an invention where he lost all his money shows bad judgment.

Diagnosis: Mr. R.'s answers exclude the presence of dementia or delirium and suggest a recurrent psychiatric disorder, most likely bipolar disorder, less likely periodic substance intoxication.

Rule Out Substance Abuse

21. I: Let's walk around. Let me show you the place. Let's go.
    P: Doc, you are cute. Let's go all the way.
22. I: Yes. We'll go all around. I want to know more about you. Tell me, when you preach, do you take any drugs?
    P: I never take drugs. I didn't even take what the doctors gave me. I want to be clean. I don't want to be doped. Dopidopidoo [starts dancing and singing]. Dopidopidoo.
23. I: Do you drink?
    P: I don't need drinks. I can feel good without them. I feel so good, so good, so good [giggles and laughs].
24. I: What did you do before you came in?
    P: Worked as a tailor. Made good money. But I can do better.
25. I: What do you want to do when you get out of here?
    P: I want to help mankind with my inventions. Nobody has to buy a shirt anymore. They just wear a collar and cuffs.

Rapport: The interviewer offers to walk around with the patient to give him a chance to relieve his restlessness, which the patient appreciates.

Technique: The interviewer checks symptoms in a straightforward manner. A more open-ended approach would be less productive because Mr. R. is distractible and shows flight of ideas.

Mental status: The patient continues to show flight of ideas with word games. After the removal of the handcuffs, the irritable mood is replaced by elation, demonstrating situation-dependent lability of mood. The thought content shows grandiose ideas. Future plans reveal poor judgment.

Diagnosis: All of the above exclude the diagnosis of substance intoxica- tion or substance-induced mood disorder and support bipolar disorder, manic episode.

Confirm Bipolar Disorder

26. I: You have such big plans now. Have you ever felt discouraged, have you ever felt down?
    P: Have I felt down, down, down? Down in the dumps? Oh yeah. I first worked on my invention and then I got so down, stayed in bed all the time, did not want to move, I felt so bad [starts crying].
27. I: It's all right. You are not feeling bad now.

Diagnosis: A. 26 confirms bipolar I disorder. At this point more history can be obtained following the format of the standard interview.

Diagnosis

DSM-IV-TR diagnosis: Bipolar I disorder, current episode manic, se- vere without psychotic features 296.43.

4. SUSPICIOUSNESS IN DELUSIONAL DISORDER

The patient with persecutory delusions experiences life events and every- day happenings as directed against him. He suspects he is persecuted be- cause of his "special knowledge," "insights," or "gifts."

   There are two difficulties in interviewing the patient with persecutory delusions: First, he may become suspicious of you because any of your re- marks, gestures, or facial expressions can trigger his feelings of being perse- cuted by you. The patient may be convinced that you communicate and collaborate with his enemies, that you are a member of a secret brother- hood that is out to hurt him. If he decides that you are part of "them," he will become scared or hostile, and stop cooperating. The paranoid patient may not complain openly about your plotting against him; he may hide his suspicions in order not to tip you off that he has found out about you.

Second, he fears that you will think him crazy. He may therefore be guarded and withhold information. The giveaway is his interaction with you. He will track you closely with his eyes, give short, vague, and evasive answers with underlying hostility, or reply with counterquestions.

How Do You Interview Such a Patient?

The basic strategy in interviewing this patient is to handle his persecutory ideas not as something strange, but share the suffering that these ideas cause him and sympathize with his mental anguish. Treat his delusional interpretations as if they were true. Approach them not from the outsider's but from the patient's point of view.

The novice finds that a difficult task. He is more comfortable with an "outsider" approach, which works best with patients who had delusions in the past but are not acutely ill now. Questions like:

"Do you have a tendency to be suspicious?"
"Do you feel easily harassed?"
"Are you pretty paranoid?"

will leave you empty-handed with a patient who is presently delusional. Also, neutralizing statements such as:

"Since when have your neighbors, in your opinion, harassed you?"
"Where else do you believe injustice has been done to you?"

may arouse his anger and lead to objections:

"What do you mean with 'in my opinion.' Don't you think it's true? I don't just believe it; it really has happened!"

Such a response is plausible, since the patient is used to skepticism, ridicule, and rejection by family and friends when he ponders his suspicions. However, if you reassure the patient that you understand his side, he may trust you. When he experiences your empathy, he will become more cooperative and show a need to share his problems with you. Questions that take his suspicious feelings seriously may assure cooperation:

"How have you been treated by others?"
"Have you ever been harassed, unjustly treated, or discriminated against?"
"Is it your experience that people don't seem to like you?"
"Have you ever been subjected to humiliation?"
"Who else did injustice to you?"

This strategy fails if the patient feels "tricked" or "buttered up" and if it makes him feel that you are taking his side in a phony way just to pump him for information and fool him.

Some interviewers resist taking the patient's side. They feel that they reinforce the patient's delusions by pretending to share his poor reality testing and that they violate their professional integrity. If you have such scruples, remember that delusions are fixed, false beliefs that cannot be corrected by logical arguments which only evoke the patient's antagonism and destroy rapport.

Persecutory delusions, like other delusions, mellow with neuroleptic treatment or with time. Their intensity can be measured by the five stages of insight (see Chapter 4, section 3: Exploration, Perception). Adjust your interview style to the patient's stage of insight. At Stage V the patient acts on his delusion. Handle the delusion as if it is true. Tell the patient that treatment (medication) is given in order to blunt the effect of those "harassments."

When he does not act on his delusion but merely talks about it (Stage IV), or refuses to talk about it any more (Stage III), or claims it was only true in the past but has stopped now (Stage II), show the same distance to the delusion. Finally, when the patient dismisses his past delusion as factual and recognizes it as part of an illness (Stage I), express the same view and discuss its morbid nature with him.

Examples: A patient may ask you:

"Do you really believe that my neighbors are after me or do you think it is all in my mind?"

You have several options to choose for your response. If you believe that the patient basically has no doubts in his delusion and is simply testing you, respond like:

"The main thing is that you are convinced that the neighbors are after you. And this conviction of yours is very real for me. I take it seriously. I will help you to deal with it and get you some relief."

If you feel that the patient is starting to question his own delusion and is on the verge of shaking it off, you may proceed by:

"What makes you ask me that question? Are there any doubts in your mind? I'd like you to tell me more about your doubts. Do you feel differently about your past experience now?"

Then help the patient to accept reality and to recognize his past delusion as pathological. However, keep track of the vanishing delusion, because it often returns later during a follow-up period. Tell him:

> "It is not always easy to tell whether one has really been wronged or if one tends to exaggerate because one feels hurt so badly. Therefore, I'd like you to discuss these thoughts right away with me when they appear, so that we both can sort out what to think about them."

The following interview was conducted with Mrs. Frances S., a 52-year-old, white, female outpatient. She was presented by the social worker who wanted to rule out any psychiatric disorder. According to the social worker, the patient had become increasingly discouraged because of difficulties finding a job as an executive secretary. Similar to the social worker, the resident was not certain whether a psychiatric disorder was present or not. The patient's complaints had been vague. She had said that "the deck of cards was stacked against her," and had refused to elaborate.

1. I: Mrs. S., I have heard from Dr. A. [social worker] and Dr. B. [resident] that you had some problems finding a job. I understand that you are very discouraged about that.
   P: Yes, it does not seem to work out anymore.
2. I: How do you support yourself?
   P: I have some savings. They may last for another 2 or 3 months and then I'm finished.
3. I: What will you do then?
   P: I'll just be finished. I can't do anything.
4. I: That sounds real bad.
   P: Well, it is.
5. I: When you say you are finished, what does that mean?
   P: I don't know. It's just over with.
6. I: Do you plan to do anything about that?
   P: I have thought about it.
7. I: Like what?
   P: Like jumping. Just smash myself.
8. I: Are you at this point now?
   P: Not now. But in 2 months I will be if things don't change.
9. I: That sounds very depressing to me.
   P: Well, it is. I keep on fighting. But I have a feeling that it is coming to an end.
10. I: That must be on your mind day and night.
    P: Well, it is.

Rapport: The interviewer takes three opportunities (A. 1, 4, 10) to express empathy and win the patient's trust.

Technique: Mrs. S.'s chief complaint (she cannot find a job) suggests an occupational problem that can be approached by exploring why the problem developed and what the expected outcome might be. The interviewer chooses to explore the patient's expectations and future plans to get a feeling for her judgment.

Mental status: The patient's expectation about the future is negativistic and her judgment appears impaired, since suicide does not appear to be a rational solution.

Diagnosis: Disorders with suicidal ruminations or behaviors have to be considered (list no. 1, see Chapter 6), such as:

- major depressive episode
- bipolar II disorder, depressed
- alcohol abuse
- other substance use disorders
- somatization disorder
- dependent personality disorder
- borderline personality disorder.

11. I: Does it affect your sleep?
    P: My sleep is alright. I forget it all when I'm asleep.
12. I: And your appetite?
    P: I'm cutting back because I don't have the money. But I like to eat.
13. I: Well, I'm sure Dr. A. [social worker] can help you to explore how to get some assistance from Social Security, or the Welfare Office.
    P: Really?
14. I: What you really need is a job.
    P: That's right.

Diagnosis: Mood disorder is one of the most common psychiatric disorders in middle-aged females. Therefore, the interviewer explores vegetative symptoms of depression but comes up empty-handed.

15. I: Tell me what happened at your last job interview.
    P: I came in for the appointment and the secretary was real nice. But I had the feeling it won't work out.
16. I: This must be terrible to know already that it won't work out and you still go through the motions.
    P: Yes, it is.
17. I: How do they ruin it for you?
    P: They don't give me the job.

18. I: Do you have any idea why they did not give it to you?
    P: No. Not really. I don't know.
19. I: Well, what's your feeling? Is there anything going on?
    P: I don't know. It happens too often.
20. I: You mean it happens over and over again?
    P: Yes.
21. I: I admire you that you still keep trying.
    P: Well, yes. I hope some employer may not know and will hire me.
22. I: You say may not know?
    P: Hmm.
23. I: Can you tell me about that?
    P: Well, I don't know. But I think it has to do with the computers.
24. I: What about the computers?
    P: Well, they are everywhere. If you go on a bus trip, they put your name on a computer. When you book an airline ticket, they put your name on a computer. They store all the information about you on a computer.
25. I: Hmm.
    P: They have [with emphasis] everything on a computer.
26. I: And why don't they hire you?
    P: Because I know about their computers . . . that's their way to get back at me.
27. I: That puts you in an awful bind. You know about it, but you still need a job from them.
    P: Yes.

Rapport: Again, the interviewer expresses empathy with the patient's situation in order to maintain rapport (Q. 16, 21, 27). When he hits on some persecutory thoughts, he puts himself in the patient's shoes and explores details from her vantage point (Q. 17, 19, 24, 27).

Technique and mental status: The interviewer probes for details of the patient's job interview and invites her to speculate about the reasons of her rejection (see Chapter 3, section 1: Complaints). Presumably, since he expressed compassion for her situation, the patient reveals her persecutory delusional explanation for her rejection. Otherwise, she may have been more guarded, since patients with persecutory delusions are exposed to disbelief and ridicule and learn to hide their delusional beliefs.

Diagnosis: The persecutory delusions add to the list of included disorders (list no. 1, see Chapter 6):

• dementia of the Alzheimer's type, early onset, with delusions
• psychotic disorder due to a general medical condition
• schizophrenia, paranoid type
• delusional disorder.

The interviewer has excluded another option, namely the presence of a depression with persecutory delusions, by showing the absence of vegetative symptoms of depression (see Q. 11, 12).

28. I: You always have to fill out an application and they put that on the computer. They know everything about you. Tell me, when did you notice it first?
    P: Oh, that was still when I was in Junction City. I made an appointment with an employer and I went in to see them, but I did not get the job. They already knew about me.
29. I: Was that the very first time?
    P: Yes.
30. I: So everything was fine before you went to Junction City. Where did you live before that time?
    P: We were in Arizona and lived in Phoenix. I was still married then.
31. I: Did anything happen in Phoenix?
    P: No, everything was fine.
32. I: And you had a good job in Phoenix?
    P: No, I really didn't.
33. I: But did you find one eventually?
    P: No, not really. Maybe it was in Phoenix when all this began. This was 18 years ago.
34. I: Tell me about it.
    P: When I went to Phoenix I made an appointment for an interview and when I got there the boss was not even there.
35. I: So he was out of the office?
    P: Yes, and all of a sudden I knew there was something fishy going on and it never stopped thereafter.
36. I: You lived with your husband before it started?
    P: Yes.
37. I: How was your marriage?
    P: Not very good. He was under the influence of his mother.
38. I: Did she live in Phoenix?
    P: No, that was in Illinois. Before we went to Phoenix we lived with his folks in Illinois.
39. I: What happened?
    P: His mother was always against me. She did not say anything, but I felt it. And I told her that I knew. So it did not work out and my husband and I went to Phoenix.
40. I: And that's where it started with the job problems?
    P: Yes. Whenever I applied for a job, they ran my name through a computer and they knew who I was and that I know everything about their computers. So, they got back at me by not hiring me.

Rapport: Since the interviewer continues to interview Mrs. S. from her point of view, without expecting her to have any insight into the falsehood of her beliefs, he maintains good rapport.

Technique: The interviewer uses continuation and smooth transition techniques to explore the beginning of her delusional thinking, and he is able to trace back her delusions until at least 18 or more years ago.

Mental status: The persecutory delusion appears to be well organized and long-standing. During the course of the conversation the patient shows no evidence of formal thought disorder. Everything she says is logical if her delusion were true.

Diagnosis: This segment reveals suspiciousness about the mother-in-law. The long-standing nature of the delusion further supports the notion that a mood disorder is probably not responsible for its occurrence. The persisting delusion also excludes any of the above-mentioned personality disorders as reason for the patient's problems, since personality disorders by themselves do not produce delusions or hallucinations.

41. I: You have gone through a terrible ordeal. It must be awful to know that they won't give you a chance. Does your mood ever get affected by this?
   P: I get angry, but I try to show them that they can't wear me down.
42. I: Do you ever hear them talking about you?
   P: No, but I know they are there.
43. I: Have there been times when they haven't bothered you?
   P: No, it's there all the time. I try to ignore it, but I don't seem to get the job that I should.
44. I: You did not tell all this to Dr. B.?
   P: Well, I thought she would think I'm paranoid.
45. I: Is that what people think?
   P: Yes, they think I'm crazy.
46. I: What do you think?
   P: I don't think—I know it's true and they are wrong. They just cannot understand it. You are the first one who seems to believe me. You don't talk to me as if I'm crazy.

Rapport and technique: The interviewer uses a smooth transition from Q. 40 to Q. 41. Again, he expresses empathy for the patient's ordeal (Q. 41) to maintain rapport and to prevent his becoming part of her delusional system.

Mental status: The interviewer excludes auditory hallucinations (Q. 42) and documents further a lack of insight on the patient's part.

Diagnosis: The absence of hallucinations and a formal thought disorder allows the interviewer to exclude schizophrenia, paranoid type.

47. I: Thank you. I'm glad that you feel that I understand what you went through.
    P: You can say that!
48. I: When you were under so much stress, did you find that any kind of medica-
         tion or even a drink would help you or relax you?
    P: Why do you ask this? Do you think I am a drunk?
49. I: No, I don't think you are a drunk. But when people feel under stress like
         you do, they sometimes try to do something about it—they may have a glass
         of wine and feel relaxed.
    P: I don't like alcohol.
50. I: Have you ever taken any other kinds of drugs?
    P: Like what?
51. I: Any kind and for what problems?
    P: Maybe an aspirin for headaches or so.
52. I: Were there ever times when you had to take something to stay awake?
    P: No, I may drink a cup of tea. I don't even like coffee.
53. I: Have you ever had a problem with your weight and taken something for it?
    P: You mean amphetamines or so?
54. I: For instance.
    P: I don't like drugs, okay? And I don't like your questions either. I don't like to
         be accused!
55. I: You are right, you went through enough without me making it worse for
         you. But I don't mean to accuse you. If it sounded like that, I have to apolo-
         gize.
    P: I don't understand why you think I abuse liquor or take uppers. I don't
         know what you are driving at.
56. I: Maybe you can tell me why these questions bother you.
    P: You think I'm paranoid from drinking or taking uppers.
57. I: You are right, when you take uppers regularly they can make you sensitive
         to rejection and can make you suspicious.
    P: Do you think I'm suspicious and paranoid?
58. I: You said employers are against you even before they meet you; just know
         you through the computers. Sometimes uppers can make you feel that way.
    P: I'm not taking any uppers. What I feel is real.
59. I: I believe you. I believe it feels very real what you went through. I believe
         you that you do not take any drugs. I believe also that you went through a
         lot, and I want to help you!
    P: Then stop accusing me!

Rapport: Rapport deteriorates when the interviewer explores alcohol and
substance use. Smooth transitions do not prevent the patient suspecting that
the interviewer interprets her problems as a result of substance or alcohol
abuse. It makes her aware that he does not believe in her delusional explanations. This stirs her anger and distrust. The interviewer's confidence in his
rapport with her is shown to be wrong. When you neglect the patient's
stage of insight and express indirectly or directly any doubt in her percep-

tion, the suspiciousness of the patient with delusional disorder can emerge at any time. If you fail like the interviewer did, save the situation, assure the patient, as shown above, that you believe her, that you are on her side, and that you want to help her.

Let's rescue the interviewer—from 20/20 hindsight. A more intuitive - interviewer may have used the patient's delusional system to explore alcohol and substance abuse. Let's replay Q. 48 and following questions:

48. I: All these employers seem to check with the computer. Is there anything put into that computer record to harm you?
    P: Must be. Otherwise—why wouldn't they give me a job?
49. I: Do you have any idea what that could be?
    P: No. But maybe something about me knowing about computers . . . that I can't be fooled . . . that I may be dangerous to them.
50. I: Could there be anything else? Something to bad mouth you? Something like dealing with drugs or cocaine, or taking it, or maybe secretly drinking alcohol?
    P: They couldn't do that. That would be a lie. I hardly even take aspirin and I can't stand any liquor.
51. I: Is there a possibility that they could have gotten any kind of a hint where they saw you drinking a glass of wine or where you bought diet pills?
    P: Nonsense. No way. Nobody would believe that about me. I don't touch anything.

Here you get into an ethical dilemma. Accepting a delusion as a patient's reality is one thing. Using it for diagnostic purposes is another. If it benefits the patient without any chance of harming her, one might use her delusional thinking to obtain clinically useful information; otherwise, you may want to discuss the problem with a medical ethicist.

Mental status: The original section Q. 47–59 showed how easily the patient's suspicion can be aroused and how quickly she can turn against you. A patient who may appear disinterested in nearly any subject and show blunted affect through most parts of the interview often shows strong affect if her delusion is challenged: the delusion is affect-laden.

Differential Diagnosis (DSM-IV-TR)

1. Schizophrenia, paranoid type 295.30 versus delusional disorder 297.1.
The patient's age of onset (about 34) is compatible with both schizophrenia, paranoid type and delusional disorder. The onset of schizophrenic disorder is usually in adolescence or early adulthood, before age 25 in males and af-

ter age 25 in females. In schizophrenia, paranoid type however, the onset tends to be later in life (middle or late adult life) just as in delusional disorder. Clear and orderly thinking is better preserved in delusional disorder than in paranoid schizophrenia. The patient's delusions lack the bizarre flavor common in other schizophrenic subtypes; they are isolated and systematized rather than fragmented, multiple, and intrusive in all types of behavior as found in other schizophrenic subtypes. There is also no evidence of prominent hallucinations, incoherence, loosening of associations, or negative symptoms. Therefore the diagnosis of schizophrenia, paranoid type is rejected in favor of delusional disorder.

2. Major depressive disorder, severe, with psychotic features 296.34 versus delusional disorder 297.1. Persecutory delusions are common in both disorders. The persecutory delusions of depressed patients usually contain an element of guilt. Previous failures or sins are named as the reason for the persecution. The above patient names her knowledge of computers as reason for her persecution, which has more a grandiose than a depressive flavor. The depressions rarely persist for more than 2 years. The decisive difference between the two disorders however is the presence of affective symptoms in major depressive disorder but not in delusional disorder. The patient denies affective symptoms; therefore the diagnosis of major depressive disorder with delusions is not supported.

3. Paranoid personality disorder 301.0 versus delusional disorder 297.1. Easily provoked suspiciousness is common for both delusional disorder and paranoid personality disorder. Both disorders exist in the absence of a mood disorder. Persistent psychotic symptoms, however, such as delusions are not part of the paranoid personality disorder. Therefore this diagnosis is rejected.

4. Psychotic disorder due to a general medical condition, with delusions 293.81 versus delusional disorder 297.1. To make the diagnosis of a psychotic disorder due to a general medical condition requires the demonstration of such a specific condition judged to be responsible for the development of the delusions. Further probing into the patient's history, searching for ictal phenomena, demonstrating focal neurological signs or symptoms, laboratory tests, and a brain scan did not produce any evidence for a medical condition to account for her delusions. Therefore, by exclusion, the working diagnosis was delusional disorder.

Final Diagnosis (DSM-IV-TR)

Delusional disorder, persecutory type 297.1.

Epilogue: The patient began taking a neuroleptic. After 6 weeks of treatment she was still convinced that computers were running her life, but she could hide this delusion well from other people. She talked about it only to her psychiatrist and social worker. She found a job as an executive secretary and functioned adequately, while being continued on neuroleptic medication.

5. AVOIDANCE IN PHOBIA

Difficulties in interviewing patients with agoraphobia and social phobia arise from both the patient's embarrassment that the fear is silly and an avoidance of discussing this fear.

You can overcome this avoidance behavior with two tactics: 1) chiseling away at it by asking short, specific questions, often closed-ended, especially when you find that open-ended questions encourage evasiveness, or 2) attempting to make the patient comfortable with supportive and accepting statements trying to reduce both her anxiety and avoidance.

Here is an example where short, closed-ended questions were used.

Ms. Brenda P., a 23-year-old, white woman, was referred by a psychiatrist who had left the outpatient group practice. Her record was vague; paranoid feelings were mentioned, but the diagnosis was deferred. She had been treated with 50 mg thioridazine (Mellaril) tid without a change in her complaints.

1. I: You have seen Dr. V. for quite some time. He had given you Mellaril but it did not seem to help you?
   P: Yeah. Maybe I was a little calmer, but I don't think it made much difference.
2. I: Please tell me, why did you come to a psychiatrist in the first place?
   P: I don't know. It is because of other people [patient looks downward].
3. I: Other people?
   P: Yeah [long silence].
4. I: What is it about other people?
   P: I don't know. Maybe it's my stepfather [again avoids eye contact].
5. I: Your stepfather?
   P: Yes, I can't speak up when he's there.
6. I: Why can't you speak up?
   P: I'm all bottled up. I can't get a word out [looks away].

7. I: You can't talk to him?
   P: I think he'll hurt me.
8. I: Has he ever done anything bad to you?
   P: No, he was always nice to me. I have no reason . . . He probably thinks I'm weird.
9. I: How long have you had this stepfather?
   P: Just the last 2 or 3 years.
10. I: Did you have trouble with other people before that?
    P: Yes.
11. I: What do you think they'll do?
    P: They'll do me in.
12. I: Do you in?
    P: Yes.
13. I: In what way?
    P: Just hurt me.
14. I: How does that make you feel?
    P: I don't know. I really don't want to talk about it. I just try to stay away from it [looks down again].
15. I: Are they really out to get you?
    P: I don't know. I think I'm silly. But I can't help it [looks to the side].
16. I: Have they ever tried to plot against you?
    P: Oh no, they don't plot against me. I'm not paranoid. I just have that . . .
17. I: That . . . ?
    P: Fear. It's silly, but I really don't want to think about it.

Rapport: On the surface, rapport appears to be adequate. Ms. P. is neither hostile nor fearful but vague, which may indicate that she is concealing something.

Technique: The interviewer uses short, pointed questions, which she answers in an equally short but vague way. Then, he echoes the patient's statements in Q. 3, 5, 6, 7, 12 to pursue her to open up, but to no avail. He probes with symptom-oriented, closed-ended questions (Q. 15, 16) whether persecutory feelings are responsible for her vagueness. Her answers reveal that unexplained fear but not persecutory feelings lead to her avoidance behavior. Looking at the interview, it is obvious that the interviewer missed an earlier opportunity after A. 8 to assess an unfounded, silly fear that points to a phobic disorder. Instead of Q. 9 he could have asked:

> "Your stepfather is nice, yet you are afraid of him and think that this is weird?"

Her answer could have very well excluded a persecutory delusional fear in favor of a phobic fear.

After A. 14, the interviewer could have confronted the patient with her tendency to be short and vague, or provoked her with the interpretation that she is concealing something. Such an intervention could have sped up the interview, leading directly to the discussion of phobic avoidance. But it would also have carried the risk of activating the patient's defenses.

Mental status: Ms. P. is alert, giving goal-directed but short and vague answers without latency of response. There is no evidence of a formal thought disorder. The reasons for her vagueness are neither persecutory feelings nor the inability to express herself but tendencies to avoid her silly, phobic anxiety. Her statements show that she has full insight into the morbid nature of this anxiety.

Diagnosis: Ms. P. reports a "silly," "unfounded" fear (Q. 8, 15) that she avoids discussing. Her full insight is typical of the anxiety disorders.
List no. 1 of included disorders is:

- social phobia (social anxiety disorder)
- panic disorder with agoraphobia
- agoraphobia without history of panic disorder
- panic disorder without agoraphobia
- avoidant personality disorder.

List no. 2 of excluded disorders is:

- schizophrenia, paranoid type
- delusional disorder
- paranoid personality disorder

The task now is to uncover the phobic stimulus, if any.

18. I: I want to understand what makes you suffer.
    P: [looks away] I'm okay, when I'm by myself.
19. I: You mean, it's only there when you are with other people?
    P: Yes.
20. I: Are there any people in particular you are afraid of?
    P: [glances at interviewer] I don't think so. It's just all the time [looks down].
21. I: What about me?
    P: [blushes] I'm afraid you'll laugh at me, and think that I am making a fool of myself.
22. I: With me?

P: [looks interviewer in the eyes] Yes.
23. I: Is that what you are afraid of?
P: [maintains eye contact] Yes.
24. I: And with everybody else?
P: I'm just scared. I don't dare say anything [still looks at interviewer].
25. I: Does it make any difference who is there?
P: No.

Rapport: The interviewer expresses his empathy for her suffering (Q. 18), but she rebuffs it and points out that she is not suffering when alone (A. 18). After the interviewer has explored to what extent he himself is a phobic stimulus for her, rapport improves. She answers more specifically and maintains eye contact.

Technique: The interviewer screens with closed-ended questions for the objects of her phobia (Q. 19, 21). She reveals her fear: to be ridiculed by other people.

Mental status: The patient had previously concealed overt expression of anxiety and had avoided eye contact. After being confronted with the discomfort toward the interviewer (Q. 21–23), she expresses her social anxiety.

26. I: Or how many there are?
P: It gets worse when more people are there. I feel lost and dizzy. My heart pounds. I get all sweaty.
27. I: How do you manage at work?
P: Oh, I try to sit all by myself.
28. I: How about going to the cafeteria?
P: I don't go. I bring food from home and eat at my desk.
29. I: You mean you can't go out to eat?
P: No. I haven't been out for the last few years.
30. I: Do you ever go to the movies?
P: No. I seldom go. When I go, I go late. I slip in when it's dark.

Technique: The interviewer presents a laundry list of phobic stimuli that Brenda acknowledges as relevant for her.

Diagnosis: A. 26 shows that she may experience panic attacks. Since she also avoids crowded places, she may qualify for the diagnosis of panic disorder with agoraphobia.

31. I: When did all this start?

P: Oh, it started back when I was in school. I couldn't finish high school. After the summer vacation I was scared to go to school. I couldn't stand it. So I never did go through my senior year.
32. I: Why didn't you tell anybody?
P: I was scared to. I think it's so silly, people will laugh at me and think I'm crazy.

Diagnosis: A. 31 reveals that the patient had suffered from separation anxiety disorder of unusually late onset, but a mild form may have been present before that time. The interviewer does not follow up on clarifying this point.

33. I: Did this ever affect your mood? Did you ever get depressed?
P: I'm low most of the time.
34. I: Does this affect your sleep?
P: Mostly my sleep is OK.
35. I: Does it affect your appetite?
P: No, my appetite is fine.

Diagnosis: The interviewer excludes the presence of a mood disorder.

36. I: When you get scared, do you ever get really panicky so that you can't catch your breath?
P: One time I did that. I was all upset. I couldn't breathe, I got all sweaty.
37. I: Did you feel your heart?
P: It was pounding in my throat and my chest hurt. I thought I was going to die. It hit me all of a sudden on a Sunday morning, out of the blue.
38. I: How often did you have this?
P: I've only had it once. But I feel scared an awful lot.

The interviewer now proceeds to a standard interview.

Rapport: Remains adequate.

Diagnosis: The interviewer attempts to assess presence and frequency of panic attacks. There is only evidence of one clear-cut panic attack (A. 38), even though statements in A. 26 suggest that at least milder forms occur more often.

Diagnosis

DSM-IV-TR diagnosis: 1. Social phobia (social anxiety disorder) 300.23.   Ms. P. expresses fear of other people and tries to avoid them (criterion A of social phobia). She also recognizes that this fear is excessive and unreasonable but still cannot overcome it (criterion C of social phobia). The presented interview section does not allow the interviewer to rule out avoidant personality disorder (301.82). If the patient avoids public social exposure and performance because she feels disapproval and embarrassment, has no or only one close friend besides first-degree relatives, and exaggerates the difficulties of some ordinary activity, she would qualify for this personality disorder in addition. This aspect is not explored further.

2. Agoraphobia without history of panic disorder (300.22).   The patient avoids restaurants and movie theaters (criterion A), and is isolated and constricted in her life (criterion B). There is no evidence obtained that she avoids public places out of fear of having a panic attack. The patient does report one spontaneous panic attack. DSM-IV-TR requires recurrent, unexpected panic attacks with fear of having another one, persisting for at least one month, to qualify for panic disorder with agoraphobia. The interviewer fails to assess whether she had that persisting fear after her first attack. Therefore, he cannot establish the diagnosis of panic disorder with agoraphobia.

There is no evidence for major depression, paranoid personality disorder, or schizophrenia. Obsessive-compulsive disorder was not assessed in this part of the interview.

Follow-up: With the diagnosis of social phobia and agoraphobia without history of panic disorder, the patient was prescribed paroxetine (Paxil), an SSRI. After 6 weeks, she felt much better. She was less scared to talk to individual people but still avoided crowds. She was able to identify her feelings clearly as unreasonable fears rather than as persecutory ideas. The interviewer developed a plan for deconditioning her agoraphobia. She agreed to visit crowded shopping centers, movie theaters, and crowded restaurants on a regular basis, with stays of more than 1 hour at a time.

6. DISBELIEF AND EMBARRASSMENT IN PANIC DISORDER

Clinically, panic disorder shares some symptoms with generalized anxiety disorder: motor tension, autonomic hyperactivity, apprehensive expectation, and hypervigilance. According to DSM-IV-TR, comorbidity of generalized anxiety with panic disorder ranges from 15% to 30%. If these anxiety symptoms affect daily functioning, patients accept diagnosis and treatment (even though they may claim that they are not really psychiatric patients).

In contrast, patients who suffer from panic attacks without generalized anxiety between attacks often believe they have suffered a heart attack and are convinced of the physical origin of their disorder. They have full insight into the morbid nature of the attacks, but they have difficulty in accepting them as a psychiatric disorder. This conviction may become the obstacle to rapport and therefore to diagnostic assessment.

Adjust your interview to the patient's beliefs:

1. Tell him that the attacks are metabolic in nature with a genetic component. Assure him that the attacks are not just in his head or an expression of a weak character.
2. Combine educational statements with symptom exploration. To win the battle for his confidence, show him that you are an expert on the disorder.
3. Intersperse supportive statements to relax him.
4. Tell him that his condition can be treated by medication.

"I'm glad you came to see me. It is good that we finally know what's going on. I think we can help you with your problem."

Mr. Christian X. is a 23-year-old, 245-lb., muscular, 6'4" male who stated that he would only agree to see the director of the outpatient clinic.

1. I: Hi, my name is Dr. O. I understand you requested to see me.
   P: Yes.
2. I: My secretary told me that you didn't want to see anybody but the chief of the clinic.
   P: Right.
3. I: Was there any particular reason why you wanted to see only me?
   P: Yes.
4. I: [looks at the patient quietly and attentively]
   P: Well, I thought you must know best.
5. I: Hmm.
   P: I wanted to be certain that I get the best opinion.
6. I: Hmm.
   P: I figured you must know best, because otherwise you would not be the head of the clinic.
7. I: It must be of concern to you to get the best opinion.
   P: That's right.

Rapport: Whenever a patient makes special requests, explore them; they give important clues. Mr. X.'s request reveals both apprehension about misdiagnosis and difficulty in accepting his disorder as psychiatric.

Technique: The clue "I want to see the head of the clinic" is followed up by clarification and interpretation (Q. 7).

Mental status: Answers to Q. 4–7 reveal apprehension and possibly some distrust.

Diagnosis: Apprehension and distrust are compatible with:

- all anxiety disorders
- mood disorders
- adjustment disorder with anxiety about a physical illness
- obsessive-compulsive personality disorder
- dependent personality disorder.

8. I: Tell me what made you come here in the first place.
   P: I did not want to come. My doctor sent me.
9. I: It does not sound like you really agree with your doctor.
   P: No, I don't.
10. I: May I ask who your doctor was?
    P: Dr. H.
11. I: The cardiologist?
    P: Yes.
12. I: Did he explain to you why he wanted you to see me?
    P: Not really . . . I guess he may have.
13. I: You don't really remember?
    P: No. It's not that. But I was so upset. I could not really listen when he talked to me.
14. I: Okay, maybe we can start at the beginning.
    P: I was so upset and angry. I felt like a nut. I could not listen. I don't remember a word. But he said something like that you are more familiar with my condition than him. And if I want to get rid of it, I'd better see you. So, why not? And I have to get over it, because I want to make the team and can't just crack up.
15. I: What is it that upset you so much? You say you felt like a nut?
    P: Yeah, I thought Dr. H. thinks I'm nuts, that I imagine things and that it's all in my head. But I'm not a guy like that. I can knock the daylight out of those offensive linemen. I don't need to imagine things.
16. I: What Dr. H. told you must have really hurt your pride.
    P: That's darn right. I felt like I got too many hits on the head and then cracking up—all these jokes they make about being a wimp . . .

Rapport: Mr. X. has a problem with insight. It is unclear whether he denies being sick, but it is clear that he rejects having a psychiatric disorder and therefore he has no reason to see a psychiatrist. He has the common misconception that "psychiatric patients are nuts; they imagine things." Later, this misconception should be corrected to gain trust, cooperation, and compliance; however, presently the interviewer knows too little about the patient's condition to make such an educational effort. Since the patient is motivated enough to wait for a diagnosis, he gives sufficient information without having to be urged to accept his condition as psychiatric.

Mental status: The patient is tense, talks a lot, and shows some mild flight of ideas in Q. 15 and 16.

Technique and diagnosis: The interviewer attempts twice to take a history (Q. 8 and 14). He fails because the patient shows resistance to seeing a psychiatrist—he is too upset. The interviewer allows him therefore to ventilate his feelings about having to see a psychiatrist rather than pushing him to give historical information. He uses clarification and interpretation techniques (Q. 15, 16), which release the patient's tension.

17. I: Let me suggest again that we start at the beginning. What made you see Dr. H.?
    P: Okay, let's start there. It happened at spring training. It was our first meeting and all of a sudden I felt that chest pain. I felt choked and sweaty. I trembled and my heart pounded like crazy. I thought that's it, I am having a heart attack. I felt I had to die. It was just awful.
18. I: Do you mean it came in the middle of a workout?
    P: No, that's the embarrassing thing, and it's so frightening. We hadn't even started yet. And I just zonked out.
19. I: What happened then?
    P: They gave me oxygen at the camp and then they rushed me to the hospital. There they started to draw blood and ran an electrocardiogram (EKG). And then the EKG did not show anything, but they said it's safer to put me in a cardiac intensive care unit because sometimes those changes show up later. They told me later that my blood was normal and that I did not have a heart attack.

Rapport: The patient has sufficient rapport to give a history of events.

Mental status: The patient is colorful and dramatic in his description, with adequate recall of details indicating intact recent memory.

Diagnosis: The patient describes a panic attack. Panic attacks can occur during:

- alcohol withdrawal
- amphetamine and caffeine intoxication
- major depressive disorder
- schizophrenia
- somatization disorder
- panic disorder

Besides alcoholism and depression, general medical conditions for a panic attack need to be considered:

Cardiological
- paroxysmal atrial tachycardia
- angina pectoris
- mitral valve prolapse

Endocrinological
- hyperthyroidism
- pheochromocytoma
- hyperparathyroid disease
- hypoglycemia

Other medical conditions
- vestibular dysfunction
- seizure disorders

Associated medical conditions
- asthma
- chronic obstructive pulmonary disease
- irritable bowel syndrome

20. I: And then Dr. H. told you to see a psychiatrist?
    P: No, not really. He just said he would like to get a psychiatric consultation.
21. I: Okay?
    P: I told him if he did that, I would sign out right then.
22. I: So that really hurt your pride?
    P: Just because they didn't find anything doesn't mean that I'm nuts and that it's all in my head and that I'm imagining things!
23. I: I agree with you. But did Dr. H. really say that you imagined it?
    P: No, but he thought so. Why else would he want me to see a psychiatrist?
24. I: So you think going to a psychiatrist means that one imagines things?
    P: Isn't that right?
25. I: Well, not really. So you refused to let a psychiatric consultant evaluate you and you didn't want to see a psychiatrist on the outside later on?
    P: Absolutely not!

Rapport: With Q. 20 the interviewer continues history taking, but introduces again the topic of psychiatric disorder. Q. 22 gives an interpretation, and Q. 23 and 25 assure Mr. X. that psychiatric disorders are not imagined. Such statements emphasize that he has a "respectable" disorder. It allows the interviewer to split off the sick part of the patient and build an alliance. It prepares the patient to accept a psychiatric diagnosis and to comply with treatment, if he will accept the interviewer as the expert and authority.

26. I: What made you change your mind? You are seeing me now.
    P: Well . . . I had another spell. It came out of the blue just 5 days ago. I was just sitting there watching TV and it came.
27. I: So you decided then to call up here and see me?
    P: Well, my mother kind of pushed me to do it. But I thought if the XX (professional football team) found out that I'm loony, that would be the end of my career.
28. I: I'm glad that you came.
    P: [stares at his hands]
29. I: [waiting] Is there anything making you feel uncomfortable?
    P: Well, I guess I should tell you that I really did not call here right away. I was just thinking about it.
30. I: But you are here now.
    P: The darnest thing is . . . It was Monday night, no really Tuesday morning. I woke up early . . .
31. I: Yes?
    P: And I had another spell. I thought then I can't live like this. The hell with what they think in XX, if they want to scrap me, okay. But I can't take it. I can't go around having those spells and feeling like dying. I just can't. It was that morning that I called your clinic.
32. I: Why didn't you go to another cardiologist?
    P: Well, Dr. H. is the best man in town, they say. And it has happened to me before. That was when I still was in college. Way back then they could not find anything either. So I thought I would just give it a try.
33. I: I am glad that you are here. So when you had these three attacks, you were really scared?
    P: Yes, I really thought I would die.
34. I: And how is that now?
    P: Well, I still think it might have been a heart attack. Maybe they just did not see it.

Rapport: A. 27 and 31 show Mr. X.'s embarrassment and how only the frequency of attacks made him finally come to see a psychiatrist without giving up his internal resistance to this step (Q. 34). The patient is given support (Q. 28, 33) to encourage him to cooperate further.

Diagnosis: A. 32 reveals that Mr. X. may have had a longer-standing history of panic attacks than originally reported.

35. I: Tell me more about the attack in training camp.
    P: I just got drafted as a rookie. I was a ninth-round draft choice for the XX. I tried hard to make the team as a defensive end. And that's when it happened, when all of a sudden my heart started to pound, I felt choked, I could not breathe, fought for air, had horrible chest pain. Everything looked blurry, I was sweating and trembling all over. They all must have thought I had a real heart attack and now it's nothing. What will they say when they find out that I see a shrink? [hides his face in his hands]
36. I: Is that why you came a few hundred miles to Kansas City?
    P: No, my parents live here. When I got out of the hospital, the coaches wanted me to take a break.
37. I: How long ago did this happen?
    P: About 2 weeks ago.

Diagnosis: A. 35 describes the main symptoms of a panic attack. The last three attacks occurred in the last 2 weeks (A. 37).

38. I: Before you had that attack, was there anything happening?
    P: Like what?
39. I: Do you have any other problems?
    P: I don't know what you mean.
40. I: Well, let me ask you a few things. Did your appetite change?
    P: No, I could always eat like a horse. Only when I'm tired and exhausted, I only want to drink then.
41. I: Drink?
    P: No, I don't mean liquor. Just water or soft drinks. I don't care much for alcohol.
42. I: And how was your sleep?
    P: Pretty good. Never had any problems. But the night before the tryout I may have tossed and turned. I just worried if I can make it.
43. I: Did you feel in any way down or depressed?
    P: No, I was really excited, because XX is a really good football team and if I could make it, that would just mean a lot to me.
44. I: Did you take any kind of drugs?
    P: No. There were some guys who took speed—you know what they say about football players. But I try to stay away from it. I tried some pot in college, but I even quit that.
45. I: And you don't drink liquor either?
    P: No, not really . . . I may have a couple of beers with the guys, but no hard stuff.

Technique: Open-ended questions (Q. 38, 39) do not yield a precipitating event. They do not work too well for this patient. Closed-ended questions produce believable answers and not merely yes/no responses.

Diagnosis: This section works on list no. 2 of excluded disorders as causes for panic attacks:

- major depressive disorder
- alcohol abuse
- substance use.

46. I: Did anybody in your family have problems that made them see a psychiatrist?
   P: No.
47. I: Was there anybody in your family who may have had a heart attack?
   P: Well, I don't know. I think my Dad mentioned something like that.
48. I: Do you know more about that?
   P: Well, see, when my Dad was younger, he had a drinking problem. I think he mentioned something about thinking he had a heart attack, but they didn't find anything.
49. I: I see.
   P: Does that have anything to do with me? I tell you I don't have a drinking problem.
50. I: But you have those spells.
   P: Well, I thought my Dad thought that those spells came from drinking too much.
51. I: What about your mother, did she have any drinking problems or spells?
   P: No.
52. I: Did she ever see a psychiatrist or psychologist?
   P: I don't think so, not that I know of.
53. I: Do you have any brothers or sisters?
   P: One older brother and two younger sisters, but they are all right. I am the only one.
54. I: I understand. I want you to know that those spells often occur in more than one member of a family.
   P: You mean they are genetic?
55. I: We don't know for certain. But it is possible that you may have been born with such a condition. Strenuous exercise can bring it on. It has something to do with the buildup of lactic acid in the blood. And that happens often when you exercise very hard. There are several drugs that can help you. What you had is called a panic attack. They feel real because they are real.
   P: You say drugs can help it? You mean I have to take heart medication all my life?
56. I: Well, it's not exactly heart medication that you need. But a drug that is a muscle relaxant and an antianxiety drug, or another one that is a so-called antidepressant may help you. And there is indeed also one medication that one could call a heart medication. It is called propanolol or Inderal. This may also be helpful for your condition. Would you say that you are an anxious person?

P: Well . . . when I was younger . . . my mother always said I was hyper or
      headstrong. Yes, I remember now, she used to say: "You are always so ap-
      prehensive." Apprehensive, I think that is a pretty good word.
57. I: I think we can help you with both these things, your spells and your appre-
      hensiveness. Now, let's go over some of the things that you may have expe-
      rienced when you were a child and teenager.

Rapport: Q. 56 educates Mr. X. about the nature of the disorder to make
the condition more acceptable to him and to encourage him to comply with
treatment. Somatic treatments are emphasized in Q. 57. The patient is now
willing to describe himself as "generally anxious." Full rapport is established.
Mr. X. accepts the interviewer as the appropriate expert and authority to treat
his condition. The remainder of the interview follows the standard format.

Technique: The interviewer informs the patient about panic disorder and
combines his teaching with questions that confirm this diagnosis if answered positively. This strategy reduces apprehension and permits the patient to describe "embarrassing symptoms."

Diagnosis: The family history reveals possible alcohol abuse and panic
attacks in the father. The description of general anxiety is compatible with
the diagnosis of panic disorder. A workup to exclude some of the above-
mentioned medical conditions may complete the diagnostic process.
      Mr. X. reports the essential features of panic attacks: discrete episodes
of dyspnea ("I feel choked"), palpitations ("my heart pounded like crazy")
and discomfort ("I felt that chest pain"), choking sensations, sweating, and
trembling. He describes 7 out of 13 symptoms for panic disorder; required
are only 4 out of 13 during at least one attack. Not mentioned were the
other symptoms: dizziness, feelings of unreality, paresthesia, hot and cold
flashes, nausea, fear of dying, and fear of going crazy. DSM-IV-TR calls for
recurrent, unexpected panic attacks with concern about future attacks and
for one or more attacks followed by a period of at least a month of persistent fear of having another attack. Our football player meets these criteria.
He has an adolescent onset and possibly a positive family history.
      He does not meet diagnostic criteria for other mental disorders such as de-
pression or somatization disorder, and there is no association with agoraphobia. The only associated feature the patient admits to is apprehensiveness.

Diagnosis (DSM-IV-TR)

Panic disorder without agoraphobia 300.01.

7. PERSECUTORY FEELINGS IN MENTAL RETARDATION

To interview a patient with mental retardation is not difficult: the patient talks in simple sentences and uses concrete words. Once you suspect it, a few tests (see Chapter 5: Testing) help to confirm your impression. However, a mentally retarded or dull normal patient is more difficult to diagnose if she is keenly aware of her deficiency, and tries both to overcome and to hide it. She is extremely sensitive when she feels anybody alluding to her deficiency. She develops self-protective suspiciousness and hypersensitivity.

Such a patient is under chronic stress. Everyday situations test her limits. She seems to be in a perpetual "adjustment" situation of the "dull among the smart." To appear smarter than she is, she may pursue schooling fanatically, gather a broad vocabulary, and copy behaviors, tastes, and themes of conversation of people she considers smart. She hides her inability to think abstractly behind learned phrases. And she can fool the unsuspecting—Swiss psychiatrists have coined the term *Verhältnisblödsinn* for such patients (Bleuler 1972). This word indicates that the patient's goals are out of proportion to her capabilities (intelligence).

Usually, such a patient comes to the attention of a psychiatrist when she develops symptoms such as dysphoria, anxiety, or suspiciousness. At times it is difficult to discern whether she has an independent generalized anxiety disorder, mood disorder, delusional disorder, or symptoms in reaction to being chronically overtaxed.

What are the characteristics of this type of patient? She is frequently the offspring of middle- or upper-middle-class parents. She often has retarded intellectual development resulting from a birth injury or other unknown factors. These disturbances may not have affected all intellectual functions equally; they rarely impair ambition and the hunger for success.

In our outpatient clinic, psychiatric residents, social workers, and psychologists have misdiagnosed this condition. They have often entertained a diagnosis of a mood disorder but were surprised that antidepressants worked less than satisfactorily. May is one of these patients. She was invited for a diagnostic conference in which five residents participated. Her treating resident psychiatrist described her as depressed and resistant to treatment with antidepressants, such as SSRIs, bupropion, tricyclics, and MAOIs.

Ms. May M., a 30-year-old, boyish-looking, small, single, white woman, with sharp facial features, enters the conference room. Her straight brown hair is unevenly cropped; she is casually dressed in blue jeans and a beige jacket, giving the impression of a graduate student. She glares at the interviewer, who stands up from the conference table where he and five residents are sitting and walks toward her. The patient reaches out to shake hands.

1. I: My name is Dr. O. I'm the director of the outpatient clinic. Your name is May M.? Please sit down. Have you been told what this meeting is about?
   P: [sits rigidly on the chair with shoulders back, head poised arrogantly, piercing the interviewer with her eyes] Yeah, I know—you're gonna ask me a bunch of questions—and give me some advice!
2. I: [moves his chair closer so that he can touch Ms. M.'s arm if assurance is needed] Well, this is a weekly conference with the residents. Each time we invite one of our clinic patients so that we can see her progress. Today you are that patient. Does it bother you to speak in front of a group?
   P: [answers quickly, looking only at the interviewer and not at the group] Dr. O., I've been lookin' forward to this for 2 weeks.
3. I: Have you met any of these doctors before?
   P: [looks around the room, examines everybody carefully, and points with her finger] These two. I used to see another doctor, but I guess she isn't here anymore.

Rapport: At the beginning of the interview the patient's body language signals a conflict: she shakes hands and seeks eye contact, but expresses a reserved, even hostile attitude in her posture. Since Ms. M. avoids eye contact with the group, the interviewer invites her to look at the group members, thus including them in the interview process.

Technique: The interviewer includes the group to reduce Ms. M.'s tension somewhat, and to make her talk spontaneously.

Mental status: The concreteness and shortness of Ms. M.'s first answer may point to a difficulty with abstract thinking. The rapid and short second answer without eye contact to the group suggests anxiety as the most likely affect. Ms. M. recalls the interviewer's name, indicating that she has good short-term memory, or that she had rehearsed his name prior to the interview to avoid failure. Ms. M. recognizes her past resident physicians—obviously her recent memory is intact. She stays relaxed while facing a group of people, which demonstrates that she has no extreme social avoidance.

Diagnosis: Ms. M. interacts with the group, without avoidance behavior as seen in a phobic patient or guardedness as seen in patients with persecutory delusions, or joking interaction with individual group members as seen in patients with mania.

List no. 1 of included disorders is:

- generalized anxiety disorder.

List no. 2 of excluded disorders is:

- bipolar disorder, current episode manic
- schizophrenia, paranoid type
- delusional disorder
- social phobia (social anxiety disorder)
- paranoid personality disorder
- avoidant personality disorder.

Shift to Diagnosing

4. I: How long have you been coming to the clinic?
   P: For about a year.
5. I: What was your problem when you first came here?
   P: [stiffens her back and seems to shoot out of her chair] What d'ya mean, problem? You think I got a problem?
6. I: [touches her arm and looks in her face for a second until the patient relaxes] Maybe I should have said "reason" you first came to the clinic.
   P: [appears dumbfounded, rolls her eyes sarcastically] You're the doctor, you're s'posed to know what's wrong with me [pause].
7. I: Can you tell me how I can help you?
   P: [indignantly] I didn't need help—my math teacher—she says I need help.
8. I: Your math teacher?
   P: [more jovially] Yeah, we was playin' some tennis one day and she came up to me and she says: "May, you don't talk about things anymore"; I said to her: "I don't?" And she says, "You need to see somebody." And so here I am.
9. I: Did you agree with that? Did you also notice a change while in college?
   P: Well, yeah, because I started getting bad grades.
10. I: Was that a change from high school?
    P: Change? Of course it was a change! I made all A's and B's in high school.
11. I: Were you an honor student in high school?
    P: No.
12. I: What kind of grades did you have in high school English?
    P: English? I hated that rotten subject—I got a C out of the course—and I worked so hard for it.
13. I: What about math?
    P: [with increasing hostility] What year?
14. I: Senior year.
    P: Well, I put in a lot of time but the teacher hated my guts and that's why I only got a C [looks down at her knees with an angry expression on her face].

15. I: What about social studies?
    P: [with a hostile peek at the interviewer] That's the worst course, most of the
         stories don't make any sense. I read lots of books for it. I hated that course
         worse than any of them. I got a D out of that course [bites her lower lip and
         breathes heavily].

Shift to Rapport

16. I: I notice that you feel bothered by my questions.
    P: Darn right! Why do you have to pick on my weak spots? Can't you be nice
         for a change?
17. I: You are right. I should really ask you what courses you liked in high school?
    P: [sighing with relief] I loved basketball and choir.

Rapport: Ms. M. feels attacked by words such as her "problem" (Q. 5).
The interviewer therefore substitutes "reason" for "problem" and touches
her arm to calm her down but to no avail. She changes her attitude immediately when she can tell her story—showing that her irritation is not rooted
in persecutory delusions (Q. 8). She resumes a hostile attitude when she
feels cornered by questions about her grades (Q. 11–15). The interviewer
shifts therefore from diagnostic history taking back to rapport and makes
her aware of her emerging hostility (Q. 16). Only when he asks her about
her strengths does she blossom.

Technique: Closed-ended, directive questions and deliberate probing
into Ms. M.'s intellectual weaknesses provoke her anger and tension. Therefore, the interviewer shifts to open-ended questions, allowing Ms. M. to
choose the topic (Q. 17).

Mental status: Ms. M. interprets "problem" and "help" concretely as accusations. The rapid switch in her attitude from hostility to trust, when given
the opportunity to tell her story, reveals that her hostile suspiciousness was
not delusional but situational and self-protective in nature. These misinterpretations of words highlight her inability to abstract. Her concrete thinking
surfaces again, when she does not summarize but repeats the complete dialogue with her math teacher—as a child would do—without going beyond
the most literal meaning of the words (A. 8). Ms. M. also accepts and follows
without questioning her math teacher's advice. All indicate low intelligence.

Diagnosis: Her misinterpretation of words followed by hostility and her
poor abstraction point to concrete thinking with persecutory ideas. Since
these signs surface in a young person, they may indicate borderline mental

retardation. Since her persecutory ideas or ideas of insecurity may reach back to her high school days, they point to a personality disorder. The social withdrawal (as noticed by her math teacher) indicates either superimposed adjustment reaction with depressed mood, or a major depressive disorder.

List no. 1 of included disorders is:

- dementia not otherwise specified (NOS)
- mental retardation
- generalized anxiety disorder
- personality disorder NOS
- adjustment disorder with depressed mood
- major depressive disorder.

List no. 2 of excluded disorders is the same as that given above.

Shift Back to Diagnosis

18. I: How did you get along with the other students in high school?
    P: I was the most popular one.
19. I: What about teasing each other?
    P: [proudly and emphatically] Yeah, I did all the teasing.
20. I: Can you tell me a little bit about your friends?
    P: Well [pause]. I don't have many. Maybe one or two.
21. I: How did this happen?
    P: Because I hate people—they're rotten and they stab you in the back. I get all the bad breaks in life.
22. I: Could you tell me about some of your bad breaks?
    P: [pleased] Do you have all day? [laughs]. Well, here's one of them. In college I was friends with the English prof and we were playin' tennis and he said I should take his class, so I did. At first, I was makin' A's and then B's, and somehow he gave me a D out of the course. I don't get it—he gave me a D on this last paper I wrote and then I gave it to a friend for her class—I knew it was cheatin' and all, but I felt sorry for her—well, she got an A out of the course and the teacher said it was the best paper he ever read! So, is that a bad break or what?

Shift to Rapport

23. I: Sounds like it. You must have felt really awful. She gets an A and a mention of the best paper, when you get a D for the same thing. I can understand your anger and disappointment.

P: Yeah . . . Let me tell you another one! Once I had a girlfriend and I told her that I kinda liked this guy and before I knew it I found out she was sleepin' with him!

24. I: You told her your secret and she took advantage of it. That must have torn you up.

P: You better believe it. I'm never gonna talk to that bitch again. I am through with her for life, Dr. O.

Shift to Mental Status

25. I: Do you feel there is a reason behind why you get all these bad breaks?

P: Like what?

26. I: Is there anybody who has it in for you?

P: What do you mean?

27. I: Like somebody who doesn't like you and plots against you.

P: It looks like it, but I guess it's just bad luck.

Shift to Diagnosis

28. I: Any other bad breaks that you would like to tell me about?

P: Yeah, I was workin' for the police in the animal care department and what happened was that the officer there hated my guts, and then he told me to go over to a house and pick up these dogs. So I went over there and picked 'em up. He called me in later and said: "May, what have you done? You went into a man's backyard and picked up his dogs!" But that is exactly what he told me to do and I told him so, but he just said, "Get the hell out of here—you're fired!"

29. I: Is there anything else you would like to tell me?

P: I could sit here for 20 years and tell you about my bad breaks, because I have them all the time. My car just blew up and I don't have any money. My parents hate me and my sisters are always putting me down. I felt so low, nothing turned me on anymore.

30. I: Ms. M., you got hit with so many bad breaks—did that ever affect your appetite at all?

P: Yeah, some months back there were weeks where I didn't want to eat a thing.

31. I: Did you lose any weight?

P: Must have, 'cause my jeans were baggy.

32. I: How was your sleep?

P: I didn't. You wouldn't either, if you had so much on your mind.

33. I: So you must have really felt bad. Did you have any friends to talk to?

P: No, shit, I didn't want to talk to anybody.

34. I: Did you have a boyfriend then?

P: I had no interest in guys or sex, are you kidding? I had no fun with nothin'.

35. I: How is your sleep and appetite now?

P: Oh, it's really much better since I take those pills for depression. Now I eat too much and oversleep. But I still don't care for other people.

Shift to Mental Status Examination

36. I: [pause] Ms. M., can I ask you some questions that will help us to assess the way you think?
    P: [indignantly] Dr. O., I am not here for my thinking. I'm here to get your help. Why are you trying to cut me down like everybody else?

Shift to Rapport

37. I: Ms. M., I don't want to cut you down. I think you can stand on your own. I just would like to ask you these questions to help you better.
    P: I don't want to do that right now.
38. I: Okay, Ms. M., that's fine. I would like you to know that I think you have a lot going for you. You speak up, you are quite motivated, and I think we can help you. Thank you for coming in.

Rapport: By referring to "all the bad breaks in life," the interviewer encourages Ms. M. to complain and to reveal her suffering. When he shows empathy, she is no longer hostile, and continues to open up and elaborate on further frustrations. However, when the interviewer wants to test her intellectual functions, Ms. M. resumes a hostile and defensive attitude. Instead of taking this examination as part of the interview, she misinterprets it as criticism. To finish on a positive note, the interviewer summarizes the patient's assets. She is grateful for the personal feedback and leaves the office head up and with a big smile (Q. 36–38).

Technique: The interviewer forgoes scrutinizing Ms. M.'s claim of being popular. He avoids breaking through her denial (which could endanger rapport). Instead, he focuses on her "bad breaks," and probes the borders between suspicious, delusional, and illogical thinking. The switch to open-ended questions allows Ms. M. greater freedom to express herself.

Mental status: The patient reports "bad breaks," a perception that is not due to persecutory delusional thinking or overvalued ideas (Q. 25–27), but to her inability to understand events around her as results of cause and effect.

Ms. M.'s monosyllabic, simplistic, and concrete word choice again underscores her limited intellectual capacity. Taking things literally impairs her judgment, for example, she does not realize she could pick up only stray dogs and not dogs in someone's backyard. Her concrete thinking fosters misinterpretations and suspiciousness. They lead to anger and frustration.

Differential Diagnosis (DSM-IV-TR)

1. Major depressive disorder, in partial remission 296.25: Ms. M. fulfills diagnostic criteria for major depression. A restricted affect and lack of emotional tone are still noticeable. The diagnosis of depression excludes—according to DSM-IV-TR—an alternate or additional diagnosis of adjustment reaction with depressed mood (Q. 30–35).

2. Borderline intellectual functioning V62.89 (coded on Axis II; see American Psychiatric Association 2000, p. 740): Continually poor performance in high school and college, concrete thinking, and poor word choice support this diagnosis.

3. Paranoid personality disorder 301.0: Ms. M. made persecutory interpretations, and is defensive and hostile when she feels threatened. Denying any need for help, because she wants to appear competent and self-sufficient, limits her insight. Her paranoid tendencies may originate in her borderline intelligence. The diagnosis of a delusional disorder cannot be made because delusions were not detected.

4. Academic problem V62.3: College exerted continual pressure to perform that she could not master.

5. Generalized anxiety disorder: Not adequately assessed because the above diagnoses explain the patient's initial apprehension and anxiety.

Comment: This is an incomplete diagnostic interview. It did not address diagnoses such as: substance-related disorders, bipolar disorder, anorexia nervosa, phobias, panic disorder, and schizophrenia, paranoid type. Furthermore, the course of present disorders, and family, social, and medical history were not assessed. Feedback to the patient was not given by the interviewer, but was later provided by the resident.

Later, Ms. M.'s birth record was obtained. It supported the impression of a medical condition responsible for her borderline intellectual functioning. She was born prematurely (7 months), and needed prolonged care in an infant intensive care unit—a possible reason for her below-average intelligence. A Wechsler Intelligence Test taken later confirmed the clinical impression. Of further diagnostic relevance would be:

1. premorbid history from outside sources
2. neuropsychological testing

3. assessment of so-called "soft neurological signs," which may be indicators for brain insult at birth

This interview shows that without the index of suspicion of mild mental retardation, the lack of improvement could not be understood. Ms. M.'s mental status and the nature of her psychosocial and academic problems revealed her impairment in thinking, problem solving, and judgment.

8. LAZINESS IN NARCOLEPSY

Some psychiatric disorders are relatively rare. Some sleep disorders—such as narcolepsy—belong to this group. The prevalence of narcolepsy in the general population is estimated as .02–.16 (DSM-IV-TR) but may be much less recognized. Patients also lack insight and understanding. As a result the presentation of the patient's problem is sometimes misleading, circumstantial, and confusing to the interviewer, especially if she is not familiar with the many different forms sleep disorders assume.

A sleep disorder such as narcolepsy drives home the point that the interviewer needs to know both the criteria of psychiatric disorders as well as their various clinical manifestations (DSM-IV-TR). Their real-life presentation is best learned through clinical experience. We present the case of Mr. Cassius W.

> Mr. Cassius W., a 25-year-old African American, comes with his wife (W), father (F), mother (M), and 5-year-old son (S) to the emergency room.

1. I: Hello! I'm Dr. B. [looking at the whole family and her intake sheet]. Who is Mr. Cassius W. [looking at the older male]?
   W: It's him [pointing at the younger adult male in blue overalls]. That's Cassius.
2. I: Hi! Mr. W., would you like to follow me?
   P: [remains sitting] Call me Cass.
3. I: Would you like for any member of your family to come to the examination room with you?
   W: We'd better all come. He may not tell you what's really going on [all follow the interviewer to the examination room and sit down].
4. I: Well, Mr. W . . .
   P: [slightly annoyed] I'm Cass, OK?
5. I: Cass, what's up? What got you all in here tonight?
   P: [shrugs his shoulders] I don't know. I got kinda upset, I guess.
   W: [excited] Kinda upset? For heaven's sake! He took his gun! That man wanted to shoot himself!

S: [gets up and jumps into the middle of the room] Daddy has a big gun. Bang! Bang! Bang!

M: Come back, Rodney. You sit down here with me! Sorry, Doc.

S: He has a big gun! A real big one!

M: [getting up and grabbing the child by the hand, pulling him over toward her] Hush, Rod!

6. I: Well, Cass, sounds like you did some upsetting things?

P: I don't feel like shooting myself no more. Lakeisha told me that she loved me when she saw me grab the gun. She told me she will stay with me for now.

7. I: She wanted to leave you?

P: [ignoring the question] And then my Dad came over and said that he loved me and he never told me that in my whole life [starts crying].

F: That's right. I was hard on Cass. [to Cass] Sorry, son. [to the doctor] I was givin' him some awful time. I didn't know what to do with him. He was so lazy. Kinda wanted to whip 'em into shape, sort of stir him up.

8. I: [to the patient] So you got some beating from your dad and now Lakeisha wanted to leave you? What was going on?

P: You see, Doc, I lost my new job—I got fired. And I had just quit my other job. [pointing at his mother] My folks had just given me money for a truck, so that I could have a good job doing deliveries for XX company.

W: [interjecting] I got real upset with him. He can't hold any job. I do all the working. Besides my regular job, I work as an agency nurse. I can't work any more. We can't pay back the truck without him working.

P: I'm sorry [puts his head in both hands, sobbing, suddenly slumping forward].

W: There! You see? He's doing it again! Pretends as if he is falling, when he hears what he doesn't like.

9. I: So what's going on?

P: [sitting up] I'm sorry. I'm feeling weak and I shouldn't, shouldn't.

10. I: Weak?

P: I felt weak just now. I'm getting weak once in a while, but it's getting better. I just need to drink more coffee.

11. I: Tell me more about your weak spell. Are you getting dizzy?

P: No, not really [pointing at his family]. Maybe they're right that I'm just lazy.

12. I: Just lazy? What do you mean? Can you tell me?

P: Yeah. I got fired today. My boss saw me dozing off. I was in my truck. He said, "I can't work with a lazy bum like you who lets his customers wait so that you can take your nap." And then he called me a name. He's a real racist. And I got mad. I know I shouldn't. That was the end of me.

13. I: I'm sorry to hear that. What got you so tired?

P: Must have been my lunch. I ate that nine-piece chicken dinner today.

14. I: Well, have you gotten sleepy like this before?

P: Yes, I have. I got fired before. This time, when I told my wife, she got bent all out of shape. She said she was going to leave. And when she said that, I just wanted to do away with myself.

W: It wasn't just that. He was shouting. He does it all the time. It cost him his army career.

15. I: [to Cass] Your army career? What happened?

P: I got mad with my lieutenant. He kicked me and then he called me a lazy bum. So I grabbed that son of a . . . well, I shouldn't say that. But he had called me names before and he's black himself.

16. I: So, what was happening?

P: I was dozing off on my watch and we were out there in the desert and the Iraqis could have come over and gotten us all.

17. I: So you fell asleep on duty?

P: Yeah. I do that kind of thing but it was only the second time he caught me.

M: I tell him not to eat so much. He slept a lot when he was still in high school from all that food. Already then he was 230 pounds and he's not that tall.

18. I: So you have that sleepiness.

P: [sitting up straight] I'm going to lose some weight, go to the gym, and drink more coffee. I'll get it licked.

Rapport: In the emergency room the interviewer sometimes has to handle a family because they feel that their troubled family member cannot do it on his own. In that situation, the interviewer has to decide whether to have a session with the patient only or with the entire family. If the patient appears distressed, the family may provide stability and support during the interview, make the patient more manageable, and contribute to the information gathering. The downside is that the family may distract from the task at hand, cause the patient embarrassment, prevent the interviewer from pursuing certain lines of questioning, present their own problems to the interviewer, or certainly their own interpretation of the patient's problems. If the negative factors begin to dominate, the interviewer can always excuse the family.

Technique: In our case, the family volunteers information about the patient's long-lasting history of laziness and sleepiness. They also offer their own interpretations of his problems (A. 7, 17). The family's insights help more than hinder and the interviewer is able to isolate the chief complaint: sleepiness and some weak spells.

Mental status: The patient appears to have adequate recent memory, because he gives a history that agrees with the family members' observations. He seems to have labile affect because he admits that he became angry and that this had grave consequences. The patient has a spell of weakness during the interview.

The Clinical Interview Using DSM-IV-TR

Diagnosis:

1. Seizure disorder. The weak spell could be an atypical atonic seizure.
2. Syncope. The patient could experience episodes of low blood pressure.
3. Antisocial personality disorder. The patient may be unmotivated and malinger, as his wife seems to think.
4. Major depressive disorder with hypersomnia, which may cause the patient to be more sleepy but also irritable.
5. Episodic dyscontrol disorder because of the anger outburst.
6. Substance use. The patient may take downers and feel sleepy. He may abuse cocaine or stimulant drugs and may appear exhausted.
7. Narcolepsy because the patient has sleep attacks and spells of weakness, which may be cataplectic attacks.

Establish a Psychiatric Diagnosis

19. I: Tell me more about that sleepiness.
    P: Well, they pulled chapter 15 on me but I still got an honorable discharge.
20. I: Did you see a doctor or a psychiatrist before they discharged you?
    P: Yeah, I did. He told me that he doesn't want to help any malingerer, or something like that, and that it is too dangerous to keep irresponsible people around. And he wrote something about an antisocial trait in me.
21. I: Tell me about these sleep attacks. Is there anything that brings them on?
    P: No, just my laziness. I can't watch television. I even got real sleepy when I had to drive the jeep in that hot desert.
    W: He does not want to drive either! It makes him sleepy! So I was against it when he wanted to drive that delivery truck.
    P: I made good money! If I had my nap, I'm okay for at least 3 hours.
22. I: How long have you had that?
    P: I guess Mom's right. I had it in high school. I fell asleep in class.
23. I: Did it get worse since then?
    P: I don't know. Every day, off and on, I suddenly feel sleepy.
24. I: Does anything happen when you go to sleep?
    P: [startles, licks his lips, looks anxious] Like what?
25. I: Do you see or hear things?
    P: [startled] What do you mean? I'm not crazy! First I'm lazy and then I'm crazy, hey, Doc?
26. I: Don't worry, Cass, I don't think you're crazy. But some people who have those sleep attacks have like a dream before they doze off.
    P: I don't know, Doc. Are you tricking me, or something like that?
27. I: Why are you so worried, Cass?
    P: Because that's what the doctor psychiatrist did in the desert. First, he told me I should tell him everything that's on my mind, and I told him that I saw these camels with wings in the desert. Then he told me I should cut it out. He's not giving me a medical discharge for schizophrenia, if that's what I'm after. He said, we just get rid of you with a general discharge.

28. I: What do you mean?
    P: They gave me the honorable discharge but they put chapter 15 in my pa-
        pers. And when I wanted to join the police force, they wouldn't take me be-
        cause of that.
29. I: Do you have those visions now before you go to sleep?
    P: Sometimes.
30. I: Also with your naps during the day?
    P: Yeah, once in a while.
31. I: And when you wake up, has it happened then too?
    P: I have some bad nightmares and they are still going on when I'm awake.
32. I: Do you see things at any other time?
    P: When I'm not going to sleep or waking up?
33. I: Yes.
    P: Never. I'm always falling asleep or just waking up from a dream.
34. I: How does your body feel when you have those nightmares?
    P: Well, just the other night I read about the Doberman who killed that
        2-year-old. Then I dreamt he was chasing me. I woke up and couldn't move.
        I was scared.
35. I: Has it happened other times?
    P: What do you mean? Sometimes I feel weak when I wake up.
36. I: You slumped over before, when you were sitting here.
    P: Sometimes when I laugh hard or get mad, I feel kind of weak.

Substance Abuse

37. I: Are you taking anything?
    P: My dad is a Southern Baptist. He's even doing some preaching. I never got
        into drugs.
38. I: What about liquor?
    P: Even if I have just one beer, I get real tired.
39. I: Have you done any uppers or downers?
    P: I don't need any downers. I sleep without them. In Desert Storm, I tried co-
        caine once. It gave me a head rush and I got scared. I couldn't even smoke
        marijuana. Even that makes me sleepy.
    M: He drinks an awful lot of coffee. But he can sleep on it.
40. I: What about uppers?
    P: After the coke I got scared. I never tried them.
41. I: Have you done any sniffing? Like glue or gasoline? Anything like that?
    P: Nope.

Family History

42. I: Does anybody else in your family have sleep attacks or weak spells?
    F: [interjecting] Nobody in my family! I was in the army too. I wouldn't dare fall
        asleep. Sleeping on the job? Ha, they would get rid of me in a second at the
        post office.
43. I: [to the patient's father] And those visions? Do you have anything like that?

    F: Oh, I dream. But I have no weak spells.
    M: He just has that tic that he tries to drive me crazy with. He kind of drops his
        jaw down and tries to look real dumb.
    F: Oh, shut up. I don't do that on purpose. It's just a nervous tic.
44. I: [to the patient's father] So your jaw drops down?
    F: Isn't that strange? If I get in a real heated argument, my jaw kinda drops
        down. I sound as if I'm drunk.
45. I: Well, your son has the same thing. Just worse. You both have a real illness
        called narcolepsy. [to the father] Cass got it worse than you. [to Cass] The
        good news is it can be treated. I hope you won't lose a job over your sleep
        attacks any more.

Rapport: Rapport is not an issue other than that the patient does not understand his symptoms and wants to conceal them from others out of embarrassment. The interviewer's expertise and familiarity with the disorder
help Mr. W. to overcome his embarrassment and entrust her with his problems.

Technique: The technique is straightforward and dictated by the search
for the classic tetrade of narcolepsy: sleep attacks, hypnogogic and hypnopompic hallucinations, sleep paralysis, and cataplectic attacks. These signs
characterize a normal Rapid Eye Movement (REM) dream during which every individual experiences paralysis and has visual images. Once you as interviewer understand the physiology of sleep and dreaming and the fact
that the dream mechanism can be turned on fully or partially in a forceful
manner during wakefulness, you can interview for this disorder.

Mental status: Mr. W.'s mental status shows labile affect and he seems to
have labile mood. He has a cataplectic attack during the interview. He describes the symptoms well but does not understand their nature.

Differential Diagnosis (DSM-IV-TR)

1. Narcolepsy 347:   The interviewer established the presence of this syndrome. The patient's father had symptoms of cataplexy, a finding that confirms the diagnosis in his son, since 5%–15% of first-degree biological
relatives of individuals with cataplexy have narcolepsy and 25%–50% have
primary hypersomnia.
    To confirm the diagnosis, the interviewer ordered a multiple sleep la-
tency test, which should show sleep onset after 5 minutes (pathological
sleepiness) and rapid eye movements (REMs) at sleep onset in at least two

out of five scheduled naps. Additionally, human leukocyte antigen (HLA) typing should show the presence of HLA-DQB1*0602 in almost all individuals with narcolepsy and cataplexy compared with 20%–25% in the general population. HLA typing shows the above antigen in 40% of individuals with narcolepsy without cataplexy.

2. Intermittent explosive disorder 312.34:   The patient becomes irritable and explosive when criticized by outsiders for his disorder. However, there is no history of serious, purposeful assaultive acts or destruction of property.

3. Major depressive disorder: This diagnosis is supported by the patient's suicidality.

4. Antisocial personality disorder 301.7:   This will have to be explored. Mr. W. has anger outbursts against authority figures. Substance abuse is most likely excluded, but it is possible that the patient concealed it because he didn't want to answer questions in front of his family, especially his punitive and religious father.

Besides major psychiatric disorders, personality disorders can also pose an initial difficulty in their assessment. In the next chapter, we will explore how to interview patients with personality disorders.

CHAPTER TEN

DISORDER-SPECIFIC INTERVIEWING: PERSONALITY DISORDERS

1. **Emotional Withdrawal and Odd Behavior—Cluster A**
   Suspiciousness in Paranoid Personality Disorder
   Withdrawal in Schizoid Personality Disorder
   Irrationality in Schizotypal Personality Disorder
2. **Exaggerated, Dramatic Emotionality—Cluster B**
   Lying in Antisocial Personality Disorder
   Lability in Borderline Personality Disorder
   Phoniness in Histrionic Personality Disorder
   Grandiosity in Narcissistic Personality Disorder
3. **Anxious, Resistive Submissiveness—Cluster C**
   Hypersensitivity in Avoidant Personality Disorder
   Submissiveness in Dependent Personality Disorder
   Circumstantiality and Perfectionism in Obsessive-Compulsive
      Personality Disorder
4. **Personality Disorders Not Otherwise Specified**
   Controversy: Depressive Personality Disorder Versus Dysthymic Disorder
   Resentment in Passive-Aggressive (Negativistic) Personality Disorder
   Demanding Cruelty in Sadistic Personality Disorder
   Sacrifice and Self-Destruction in Self-Defeating Personality Disorder

SUMMARY

Chapter 10 describes how to establish rapport, select your interviewing techniques, and modify your mental status examination to diagnose patients with personality disorder.

423

▲ ▲ ▲ ▲ ▲

It is worse to be sick in soul than in body, for those afflicted in body only suffer, but those afflicted in soul both
suffer and do ill.

—Plutarch, *Moralia:* Affections of soul and body, sec. 501
E. about A.D. 95

▼ ▼ ▼ ▼ ▼

Psychologists, social workers, and psychiatrists are intrigued by personality disorders. Yet they cannot agree which personality disorders have validity nor how to assess them.

For the assessment, clinicians and researchers alike vacillate between a
dimensional approach—as for instance used in the Minnesota Multiphasic
Personality Inventory (MMPI)—and a categorical approach—as used in
DSM-IV-TR. Yet DSM-IV-TR does not present mutually exclusive personality
types but allows a conglomerate. DSM-IV-TR also allows you to use criteria
across several personality disorders and assign a personality disorder not
otherwise specified (NOS).

To give you an effective approach to deal with the 10 personality disorders in DSM-IV-TR, we offer Table 10–1. It lists 30 DSM-IV-TR criteria characteristic of 10 personality disorders of DSM-IV-TR. For the first eight criteria
the opposites (listed in parentheses) are also used. *Plus* (+) and *minus* (–)
signs indicate whether a particular criterion (+) or its opposite, respectively
(–), applies to a given personality disorder. A *blank* indicates that under
usual circumstances this criterion is not required.

The first eight criteria characterize personality disorders of more than
one cluster. They are useful to decide whether a patient has a personality
disorder or not. Criteria 9–13 are shared by personality disorders belonging
to Cluster A. Criteria 14–26 are specific for personality disorders in Cluster
B, and criteria 27–30 for Cluster C.

The 30 criteria in Table 10–1 allow you to arrive at a personality profile.
If this profile is consistent with one particular personality disorder, assign
that diagnosis.

If the profile satisfies criteria for two or more personality disorders,
make those diagnoses. If the profile fulfills some criteria of one or several
personality disorders without satisfying all the criteria for any one single
personality disorder, make the diagnosis of personality disorder NOS on

Table 10–1. DSM-IV-TR criteria for 10 personality disorders

DSM-IV-TR criteria	Cluster A			Cluster B				Cluster C		
	Schiz-oid	Para-noid	Schizo-typal	His-trionic	Narcis-sistic	Border-line	Anti-social	Depen-dent	Avoi-dant	Obsessive-compulsive
1. Isolated (attention seeking)	+	+	+	–	–	–	–	–	+	
2. Emotionally cold (exaggerated)	+	+	+	–	+	+	+			+
3. Hypersensitive (indifferent) to criticism, praise	–	+	+		+				+	
4. Self-centered (submissive)				+	+		+	–		+
5. Grandiose (low self-esteem)					+	+		–	–	
6. Dependent				+		+		+	–	
7. Exploiting (altruistic)					+		+			
8. Pleasure-seeking (ignoring it)	–									–
9. Suspicious		+	+							
10. Ideas of reference		+	+							
11. Magical thinking			+							
12. Illusions			+							
13. Odd speech			+							
14. Suicidal gestures				+		+				
15. Labile affect				+		+	+			
16. Impulsive				+		+	+			

(continued)

Table 10–1. DSM-IV-TR criteria for 10 personality disorders *(continued)*

	Cluster A			Cluster B				Cluster C		
DSM-IV-TR criteria	**Schizoid**	**Paranoid**	**Schizotypal**	**Histrionic**	**Narcissistic**	**Borderline**	**Antisocial**	**Dependent**	**Avoidant**	**Obsessive-compulsive**
17. Temper tantrums						+	+			
18. Nongenuine				+						
19. Feels entitled (undeserving)					+					
20. Fantasy of success					+					
21. Unstable relations						+				
22. Disturbed identity						+				
23. Empty, bored						+				
24. Law-breaking							+			
25. Lying							+			
26. Stealing							+			
27. Acceptance-craving									+	
28. Preoccupied with details										+
29. Indecisive										+
30. Workaholic										+

Note. + = present. – = opposite criterion (given in parentheses) present.

Axis II. Clinicians may also assign a personality disorder NOS for personality disorders that are not represented by a set of criteria in DSM-IV-TR. Examples are passive-aggressive (negativistic) and depressive personality disorders.

Each of the 10 personality disorders listed in DSM-IV-TR poses specific obstacles to interviewing. For instance, a patient with dependent personality disorder may endorse symptoms that, in fact, he has not experienced but feels compelled to admit to in order to please the interviewer. In contrast, a patient with antisocial personality disorder may falsify his past and deny problems to impress the interviewer.

It is the interviewer's task to spot such deceptive behavior and trace its origin (Othmer and Othmer 2002). Such a pursuit often leads right to the core of personality pathology. Since patients with a personality disorder have no or only limited insight into their disorder, and therefore cannot report their pathology in terms of symptoms, the observation of the patient's behavior during the interview becomes an important tool for the diagnosis of personality disorders.

To facilitate this process we have highlighted the pathological behavior of each of the 10 personality disorders and 3 personality disorders NOS that most likely emerge during and interfere with the diagnostic interview. Personality changes due to a general medical condition and their eight subtypes have to be ruled out. In addition, DSM-IV-TR allows us also to code a personality change due to any type of dementia. This code is, however, made on Axis I. DSM-III-R (American Psychiatric Association 1987) and DSM-IV (American Psychiatric Association 1994) included a personality change as a criterion in their definition of dementia, and therefore you could not code personality change when due to dementia.

1. EMOTIONAL WITHDRAWAL AND ODD BEHAVIOR—CLUSTER A

Three personality disorders are in Cluster A: paranoid, schizoid, and schizotypal. The mental status of a patient belonging to Cluster A is characterized by emotional withdrawal, lack of warmth, and odd or eccentric behavior. Throughout the interview he lacks spontaneity, appears cold and sometimes sarcastic, and seems even to hide his feelings from you. Regardless of your technique, and the type of question you ask, the patient has a tendency to answer with "yes" and "no." It is difficult to induce him to talk spontaneously and the interview does not flow. You seldom get the feeling that you are truly in touch with him and have established rapport.

The interviewing process differs according to the type of personality disorder, but in all cases you will experience a lack of rapport. If you analyze the reason for this deficit, you will find the patient's coldness is the culprit. Make it the point of departure for your interview. Explore whether the patient showed these characteristics throughout his life, resulting in social isolation. After exclusion of the Axis I disorders such as schizophrenia and delusional disorder, you have narrowed down your diagnostic options to a personality disorder.

Suspiciousness in Paranoid Personality Disorder

Rapport: Rapport with a patient who has paranoid personality disorder is hampered by his pervasive perception that everybody, absolutely everybody, will harm or exploit him. He screens all questions for hidden meaning and conspiratorial content. He questions your trustworthiness; your friendliness, which he may assume is fake, a cleverly disguised attempt to take advantage of his weaknesses; your limit setting, assuming a strategy of revenge; and your offer to help him, seeing it as a Trojan horse. You cannot win because he has exposed you. He is nobody's fool because he is nobody's friend.

Genuine openness on your part may persuade him to temporarily trust you with some of his problems. If you openly tell him how suspicious you find him, he may be impressed by your frankness, or he may interpret your statements as hostile, critical, or insulting. He may decide to cooperate with you, but may, at any moment, feel betrayed and disappointed, and lash out at you with a hostile counterattack.

Technique: Interviewing the patient with paranoid personality disorder is a delicate operation. As he assumes all your questions to have a hidden, and threatening meaning, he will scrutinize them:

> "Why do you ask that?"

But he resents being scrutinized himself. Smooth transitions work best. Any abruptness will be experienced as an unjustified switch in topic and may lead to anger, counterattack, or abrupt termination of the interview. He will confront you but not tolerate confrontation himself.

Mental status: The mental status of a patient with paranoid personality disorder is overshadowed by hypervigilance and suspiciousness. His attire may be meticulous so as not to give anybody reason for criticism, or show some neglect if he is depressed. He may then express that he is not interested in pleasing anybody. His speech is usually fluent and goal-directed. But the content of these goals is characteristic of his disorder: checking out your intentions, expressing that he looks through your maneuvers, and voicing his displeasure about your secret plans. His affect vacillates between anxiousness and overt hostility. Memory and orientation are intact, but his judgment is impaired by his suspiciousness. He may acknowledge his suspiciousness but staunchly defend it as justified and not accept it as a part of a personality disorder. Only short-lived hallucinations and delusions may occur under stress.

Diagnosis: The patient does not present any difficulty other than having to interview him with great caution in order not to trigger his suspiciousness and hostility. Since his hostility is so pervasive, it emerges early on. To establish a diagnosis of paranoid personality disorder, exclude persecutory delusions and any type of hallucinations; this eliminates schizophrenia, paranoid type, and brief psychotic disorder. The dementias or psychotic disorders due to a general medical condition; substance abuse; depression; and bipolar, mixed states, may be associated with suspiciousness and ideas of reference, however this suspiciousness rarely remains on a nondelusional level. The latter is also time-limited, and shows a circumscribed beginning and is associated with other symptoms of a specific disorder.

If social withdrawal, aloofness, and coldness emerge during the interview, and if the patient expresses some odd and superstitious ideas, explore the differential diagnosis of the personality disorder of Cluster A. Notice that the border between delusional disorder (Axis I) and paranoid personality disorder (Axis II) is fluid. While the patient with delusional disorder sees his behavior as the best response to a danger he perceives as real, the patient with paranoid personality disorder, who has an awareness of his increased suspiciousness, usually tries to keep it to himself but finds reasons to justify it. Here is a more severe case:

I: Hi, would you like to come in?
P: What do you mean—like to come in?
I: Didn't you want to talk to me?
P: Who gave you that idea?
I: Well, you made an appointment, didn't you?
P: Are you holding this against me? Maybe I shouldn't have.
I: Since you are here, why don't you sit down.

P: You think you've got me already. OK. Let's get on with it. I will sit down, but
     don't think that I will submit to your tricks. I have had some experience with
     psychiatrists. They are basically all the same. They trick and outmaneuver
     you—at least that's what they try to do, but not with me.
I: You don't seem to like or trust me.
P: Besides the Washington politicians, I have not found anyone I trust as little as a
     psychiatrist.

Withdrawal in Schizoid Personality Disorder

Rapport: Rapport with the patient with schizoid personality disorder is
hampered by his pervasive emotional withdrawal. There is no affective response at the start of the interview, and none at the end. If you express empathy—it leaves him cold. He may talk about his depressive feelings, but you
don't feel his suffering. Since emotional warmth is missing, you cannot judge
whether the problems he talks about are central to him. You cannot appreciate whether he likes, trusts, and respects, or resents you. It does not help
when you ask him about it, because he does not know; and if he knows, it
does not matter, because he does not care. He is indifferent. Rapport is a state
where the patient is willing to reveal and discuss his symptoms, problems,
and innermost feelings. Since the schizoid personality does not appear to
have those feelings, you never get the impression of having rapport.

Technique: You notice from the beginning that the patient only answers
with "yes" and "no," or with very short, seemingly absent-minded replies.
You may misinterpret this poverty of words as sensitivity and become cautious not to hurt his feelings, but this would be an incorrect assumption.
Any strategy seems to fail. No matter whether you invite him to talk about
any topic of his choice, or try to push him with highly structured questions,
the flow of information remains restricted. You will detect that his limited
verbal and emotional expression is not due to self-protection, but to mental
and emotional emptiness. Therefore, you can start and end where you
want—abruptly—it does not matter.

Mental status: It is characterized by edgy body movements, lack of facial
expressions, and frozen and clumsy gestures. His speech is goal-directed
but lacks detailed elaboration. The tone of voice rarely ever changes, not
even when he talks about the most intimate or traumatic events in his life.
Neither the death of his mother nor the loss of a friend seems to affect him.
This lack of responsiveness underscores his main impairment: affective
withdrawal.

The more intelligent patient with this personality disorder sometimes complains about his lack of interest and motivation. He may even name this state "depression," but he usually does not report associated sadness, guilt, or anguish.

A patient with schizoid personality disorder rarely hallucinates or displays delusional thinking except under stress; he may have some ideas of reference and a feeling that others don't care for him, but if they did, it would burden rather than please him. His memory is usually intact. He sees himself as less animated than others but does not consider this lack of interest a disturbance. His judgment concerning future plans is usually adequate; he rarely overestimates his potential unless he develops a schizophreniform disorder. Only if he is threatened with losing his job or spouse (male patients with schizoid personality disorder rarely marry) will he possibly consult a therapist. Then he usually reports vegetative symptoms and depressed mood for which he seeks treatment.

Diagnosis: A patient with schizoid personality disorder usually comes to your attention when he develops a clinical disorder (Axis I) such as substance abuse, depression, or a schizophreniform disorder, or struggles with psychosocial stressors (Axis IV).

The combination of a clinical disorder with schizoid personality disorder is a source of confusion. A concomitant depression, for instance, may present in a younger person as a simple schizophrenia because of severe blunting of affect and severe social isolation. Fleeting hallucinations, due to substance abuse such as LSD, may make you consider incipient schizophrenia. The accuracy of your diagnosis will however be assured if you routinely include in your differential the combination of an Axis I disorder with an Axis II personality disorder.

Usually, it is not so much the chief complaint of the schizoid personality, but the observed mental status that will tip you off. With your suspicion aroused, scrutinize the patient's social history. His life history is marred by loneliness, isolation, and desertion, which seem to be more significant to you than to him.

The schizoid personality's behavior pattern and interactions seem to correspond to the symptomatology of patients with negative symptoms of schizophrenia: the same lack of initiative, blunted affect, poverty of gestures, and verbal productions are seen. However, these patients are not hallucinating, they do not harbor delusions or show a formal thought disorder, and their reality testing is intact.

The following segment illustrates rapport and mental status with Mr. Forster, a patient with schizoid personality disorder.

I: Mr. Forster, can you tell me what kind of problems made you come to our clinic?
P: My work.
I: Would you tell me about the problems that you have at work?
P: No interest.
I: It must feel bad to work all day without being really interested.
P: Hmm.
I: What kind of work do you do? Tell me more about it!
P: Lab work.
I: What kind of laboratory do you work at?
P: Animal.
I: Please tell me what you do in your lab?
P: Setting up experiments.
I: For how long have you had a problem with not being interested?
P: From the start.
I: How long have you been working at your present job in that laboratory?
P: Some years.
I: Has your interest always been that low?
P: No.
I: When did this problem start?
P: Lately.
I: Can you give me a more accurate time frame?
P: Maybe spring of this year.
I: How have you been feeling lately?
P: Not so good.
I: I'm sorry to hear that you have not been feeling so good. What seems to give you the most trouble? Is it the type of work? Or other people at work? Can you give me some idea?
P: I'm feeling bad.
I: Can you pinpoint this?
P: Not really.
I: How are things at work? What is it about your work that makes it so uninteresting?
P: It's slow.
I: Are you getting your work done in time?
P: Barely.
I: Does anyone complain, push you, or threaten you?
P: No.
I: Or does anybody ask you to do more work?
P: There isn't that much to do.

No matter how hard you try, no matter how emphatic you are, whether you ask short, elaborate, open- or closed-ended questions, his responses are monotonous and short. He does not elaborate. Any affective tone is missing. To establish a differential list you will have to review a laundry list of symptoms using structured questions that permit yes and no answers. Such an interview will frustrate you but not the patient, who will return for the next appointment and will be as monotonous and uninspired as the first time around.

Irrationality in Schizotypal Personality Disorder

Rapport: When you try to establish rapport with a patient with schizotypal personality disorder, you will be amazed by his unusual formulations, surprising statements, and peculiar ideas. Rapport is hampered as long as the patient feels that you cannot appreciate his experiences.

Empathy for his feelings and thoughts can lure him out of his reserve. When you indicate that you don't reject him, and that you understand his perceptions and feelings, his confidence in you will grow and he will open up to you the sanctuary of his secret, autistic world. He will share with you his insights, personal references, sensitivities, and an individualized awareness that transcend reality. Unlike your efforts with the patient with schizoid personality disorder, you can shape rapport with the schizotypal patient.

Technique: The patient answers all types of questions if you have established rapport. You frequently have to ask him to specify his impressions and give you examples. In this clarification process you detect that he sees relationships among events and people that are not obvious to you. You can follow the direction of thinking without being fully able to appreciate its elements. Any empathic and interested approach to listening together with continuation techniques usually suffice to make the patient explain his experiences. In contrast, doubting questioning and expressions of rejection of his views or confrontation with his reality cause the patient to recoil.

A bright patient with schizotypal personality disorder often desires to find out whether you have experiences similar to his. For him it is not enough that you are interested in his views; he hungers to communicate on the same wavelength. To handle this situation is more a question of rapport than a problem of how to formulate questions most effectively.

Mental status: The mental status shows several characteristic features. The patient's attire may be somewhat peculiar; he may carry a talisman around his neck. He may use words with an unusual meaning, or in an unusual context. His sense of humor may strike you as bizarre, and his thoughts may be hard to follow. He will make an effort to communicate his thoughts and feelings to you, provided he trusts you and believes it would be worthwhile talking with you.

The patient's thought content is indeed remarkable. It may show paranoid ideation, suspiciousness, ideas of reference, and magical thinking. He may claim to have access to a fourth dimension, to have out-of-body experiences, extrasensory perception (ESP), telepathy, and premonitions. The peculiarities in formulation and thought content give you the impression that the patient is odd, strange, eccentric, and superstitious. His affect changes with the thought content. He may appear aloof and cold when you involve him in topics of your choosing, but become lively and even intense in his affect when he talks about his telepathic experiences and his convictions. As with the two other personality disorders of Cluster A, the patient with schizotypal personality disorder may experience very brief psychotic episodes under stress.

His orientation, memory, and information processing are intact and his speech is coherent. However, his judgment is influenced by thoughts situated outside the realm of verifiable reality. He has partial insight; he knows that others consider him odd, strange, and sometimes hard to understand. But he sees them as unable to look beyond a simplistic reality and not as critics of his poor reality testing.

Diagnosis: The patient's oddities remind you of a schizophrenic patient with positive symptoms. Yet, when you hunt for delusions or hallucinations, you sometimes find very short-lived episodes in stressful situations. His thinking is reminiscent of a thought disorder, with overvalued ideas and ideas of reference. Scrutiny of the patient's past will reveal that even as a teenager he was considered odd and strange. Such chronicity alerts you to the presence of a personality disorder of Cluster A.

The lack of predominantly paranoid ideas differentiates the schizotypal patient from the paranoid patient, preoccupation with the occult and the supernatural from the patient with schizoid personality disorder.

The following interview with Mr. Kevin P. illustrates some of the characteristics of schizotypal personality disorder:

1. I: Where shall we begin?
   P: I may as well start with them, the character disorders.
2. I: Tell me about them!
   P: I think the people who give you the most trouble—that's who they are.

3. I: It sounds as if some people bother you a lot.
   P: You see, it all depends. I hate the character disorders who are cruel and who hurt you. You can feel their aggressive thoughts, but I quit my job so they can't get at me anymore.
4. I: It must feel awful to be harassed by those people.
   P: I just have to stay away from them.
5. I: Did they try to harm or persecute you?
   P: It's their thoughtlessness that hurts you.
6. I: Have they ever tried to follow you, observe your house, tap your phone, bug your bedroom, or living room?
   P: No, but I'm surprised that you ask. Are you in tune with them?

Mr. P. uses formulations such as "who are cruel and who hurt you" rather than "who are cruel and who hurt me." Such formulations declare his experiences as generally true. This interpretation is supported by his direct question (A. 6):

"Are you in tune with them?"

The interviewer evades a direct answer and emphasizes that he wants to understand Mr. P.'s feelings.

7. I: I want to understand how they bother you, how they get to you.
   P: The way they look at you, the way they don't talk to you.
8. I: Have you ever heard them even when they were far away?
   P: No, not really.
9. I: Have you heard any voices ever?
   P: My own thoughts, I think them in words. I imagine how they would sound if I were to speak them out loud. There is the quality of sound in thoughts. Thoughts go beyond people. They interconnect and survive.
10. I: Do you have access to those interconnecting thoughts? Are you familiar with ESP?
   P: I can sense them, I can sense the hostile thoughts of the character disorders.
11. I: Tell me about these character disorders! Who are they?
   P: Those people who impose on your thoughts—you meet them everywhere. These thoughtless, callous mental morons.
12. I: Do you think they are like a fraternity? Sticking together and conspiring against you?
   P: No, they are not like a conspiracy—more here and there you know, just like people you meet and don't like. I don't think they are organized. It's more like a mind game.

After he found the interviewer receptive, Mr. P. communicates freely about his perceptions. The interviewer's attitude toward the patient's odd views is similar to the position taken toward hallucinations and delusions (see Chapter 4); he takes the position as if interviewing an astronaut who has visited a remote planet. What the patient reports was certainly his experience even though not immediately verifiable by the listener.

2. EXAGGERATED, DRAMATIC EMOTIONALITY— CLUSTER B

The four personality disorders in Cluster B are the antisocial, borderline, histrionic, and narcissistic personality. The mental status of a patient belonging to Cluster B impresses you by the erratic, exaggerated, dramatic, and seemingly nongenuine emotional display with colorful affect. Most of the time the patient is not aware of her affectation or inappropriateness. Her speech is usually fluent but often vague and evasive. Frequently, she gets caught in contradictions. She intends to impress you by her behavior rather than by the revelation of her problems or suffering.

Superficially, this type of patient is easy to interview. Open-ended questions usually lead to lengthy, emotionally colorful answers decorated with similes and metaphors. You have to ask her to specify, to narrow down; you have to curb the flow and steer her direction. Usually she is not irritated by accentuated or abrupt transitions but is easily hurt and angered by interpretations.

However, because of her superficially exaggerated emotionality, and her desire to impress you, it is difficult to establish rapport during the interview. You do not feel she is leveling with you. She may threaten, complain, beg, flirt, or tease. It is difficult for you (and for her) to get in touch with her true feelings, which seem hidden behind the emotional display. The mental status and the type of rapport alert you to a personality disorder of Cluster B.

Lying in Antisocial Personality Disorder

Patients with antisocial personality (sociopaths) rarely consult a mental health professional for behavior problems. Instead, they come to see you for alcohol detoxification, to get a certificate as excuse from work, to obtain stimulants or sedative hypnotics (drugs with street value), or to avoid prison after committing a crime by claiming a mental disorder. The male-to-female ratio is 3:1.

Rapport: Rapport with such a patient is a problem. It is easy to talk to him as long as you play along, but he will criticize you and be angry when you resist his manipulations. It is difficult to direct him to focus on deficits such as his lack of emotional control and his unwillingness to act responsibly, or to consider the negative consequences of his behavior. This lack of sincerity and genuineness prevents rapport. If he perceives you as an authority figure, he will protest against you clandestinely or even openly.

It has been said that the person with antisocial personality disorder lacks a sense of suffering. He is usually not remorseful about his lying, stealing, angry outbursts, or hurting others, but he can be made aware of the fact that nothing is going right for him and that he is ruining his life. You can establish rapport and review the patient's difficulties free of lies and distortions when you show him empathy for the consequences of his behavior and his failures:

> "I agree that you've had a fair share of trouble. Maybe we can find a way to prevent it in the future by finding out where things go wrong."

When he feels that the interviewer is an ally who does not scold, judge, or punish him, but supports his constructive goals and shows understanding for his inability to obey rules and regulations—he may occasionally start to form a therapeutic alliance and become cooperative, dependent, trustful, and willing to level with the therapist. Then it is temporarily possible to discuss as part of his disorder his need to impress, his inability to postpone gratification, his lack of temper control and dependability, and his tendency to lie, steal, and cheat. However, it is rare for the sociopathic patient to sincerely attempt to change his behavior.

Technique: His outfit (see below: Mental Status) may be the starting point for a conversation. Ask the patient to discuss his opposition to comply with social rules. Although the patient may seek help for his drinking, substance abuse, or depression, his mental status may serve as an opener.

The patient with antisocial personality likes attention. He may use bragging and lies to get attention. He glows in the limelight. His attention span is often short, rewards are strived for without delay. You can make him talk if you encourage him to boast, as in:

> "You are quite a salesman."
> "What a con-artist you must be."
> "You seem to be able to put anything across to people."
> "Were you quite a fighter?"

Such comments will stimulate him to display his accomplishments. The tendency of the person with antisocial personality disorder to lie and cheat will distort his stories. If he talks freely, avoid a judgmental or accusatory tone so as not to lose his cooperation. Do not approve of his crimes. Accept his boasting but explore the negative consequences of his deeds at the same time.

If the patient is uncooperative, not willing to answer questions, or if he adopts a complaining or hostile posture, withdraw your attention, display indifference, and initiate the termination of the interview:

> "You don't seem to be in the mood to discuss your problems now. Maybe we would hit it off better some other time."

Be vague about "some other time," maybe several days "down the road." Given the fact that patients with antisocial personality have short attention spans, he may quickly change his attitude.

A similar tactic is to offer the assistance of someone lower in rank:

> "Maybe you would like to talk to the medical student (or the aide)—she can tell me later what's troubling you."

If the patient is interviewed in front of staff, offer to release the staff so that you can talk to him alone. Usually, the loss of audience is painful for him, and he may quickly become cooperative.

If an inpatient with antisocial personality disorder and affective disorder becomes homicidal or suicidal but is unwilling to cooperate with the assessment or treatment plan, set limits, forcefully, and right away:

> "I want you to write a letter to the hospital administration right now, so that I can start commitment procedures against you."

Mental status: Antisocial patients from lower socioeconomic classes usually try to make a quick impression through their appearance and behavior. The male patient may try to look very masculine. The female may try to appear seductive and feminine. Alternatively, both may wear an outfit that is neglectful and sloppy, showing contempt or lack of interest in social rules.

Motor behavior, speech, and mood of sociopathic patients reveal some common characteristics, depending on whether they want to appear cool and relaxed, sexy or masculine, or display an "I don't care" attitude.

Speech may reveal stiltedness, boisterousness, or—in males—a certain hoarseness trying to appear smart and impressive with foul language or words he does not quite understand. His statements are rarely clear, detailed, and informative but instead exaggerated, vague, and contradictory, which suggests lying.

His mood may be irritable, depressed, or elated. He may portray a special emotional state such as modesty, which you will soon recognize as being merely a pretense to get you on his side and have his way with you. Usually, he shows a lack of emotional control when caught lying or when asked to follow rules.

The insight of the person with antisocial personality disorder may be limited. He may have a tendency to blame the environment for his failure. However, when you do have rapport with him, he may admit that he screwed up his life with self-destructive behavior. Judgment is often poor as well. On a superficial basis he may be able to read social expectations accurately, but he is rarely able to accept expectations as justified and is therefore unable to comply with them. A person with antisocial personality disorder also lacks remorse, which allows him to use unethical shortcuts in the pursuit of his goals.

Diagnosis: The diagnostic process is simple when you suspect antisocial personality disorder. All it takes is establishing rapport and collecting a list of teenage and early adulthood infractions against social standards and laws with questions such as:

> "Did you have disciplinary problems in school? In the service? Did you have problems with the law? At work?"

> Here is an interview with Mr. Brewster B., a 26-year-old, white male, who was brought to a Veterans Administration hospital by two friends. They had found him with a shotgun in his hand aimed at his mouth filled with water. He was pulling the trigger. Because the safety was on, the gun did not go off and they wrestled the weapon away from him.

1. I: I heard from the admitting resident what you were up to. You must have really meant business.
   P: You are damn right. They meant well, but I wish these assholes would have let me do it.
2. I: Why do you want to shoot yourself?
   P: My best friend got shot in one of the street fights that we had in L. He was just buried 2 days ago. I felt real bad.
3. I: You felt real bad?
   P: I let him down. I was a real ass. I betrayed him.
4. I: In what way did you betray him?
   P: I screwed his old lady. Can you imagine? My best friend . . . and I take his old lady to bed. He trusted me all the way. That's the jackass I am.
5. I: You are really down on yourself.
   P: You aren't kidding. Jesus, what a smart ass [cursing at the doctor].

6. I: Okay, let's get on with it.
   P: Listen, doc, I'm tired of talking to you. You can shove it.
7. I: Okay. You can talk to the resident. I'll be back on Monday.
   P: Screw you.
8. I: Well, I can't help you if you don't talk to me.
   P: Listen, doc, I didn't want to be here in the first place. Just let me out of this damn joint.
9. I: No way. You tried to shoot yourself. We have to evaluate you.
   P: I want to sign out.
10. I: You can write a letter to the chief of staff requesting your release, but I can tell you what will happen.
    P: What's that?
11. I: We'll have to commit you. In the staff's opinion you are a danger to yourself. You may suffer from a depression and I agree with them. So, I'll see you on Monday. I hope you will feel better by then.
    P: Damn, doc, I don't want to sit here the whole weekend just waiting until you come back. Let's get it over with.
12. I: Okay.
    P: What do you want to know?
13. I: I really don't want to know anything.
    P: What kind of shit are you pulling on me?
14. I: I really want to understand how you get yourself in that mess. What made you so upset?
    P: Well, I messed up my whole fucking life. I just can't lick it. I can't get myself to do anything useful.
15. I: You're not working?
    P: Nope. Well, I'm service connected. I got a medical discharge. They told me that I have schizophrenia.
16. I: How did this come about?
    P: I was on this ship. I was always on the shit list. They made me scrub the deck. I tripped, I fell down the steps, must have bumped my head. I passed out. After that I told them that I had these bursting headaches. I could not concentrate. They would not let me go. So I got drunk and ran my jeep into a light post. Then they sent me to a psychiatrist. I told him that I hear the voice of my dead grandfather and that he tells me to kill myself. That got me some action. The shrink said that I have schizophrenia and that I have no business in the service. So I'm 26 years old and I already have a nice pension.
17. I: Can you live off it?
    P: I suppose I could. If I take an apartment in the ghetto, and live off fast food.
18. I: How do you live?
    P: Do you have to know all that?
19. I: I don't have any feeling for what's really bugging you.
    P: Well, I live with a motorcycle gang. They're the only friends I've got.
20. I: You mean you stay with them all the time?
    P: Yeah. We're hanging around in a trailer park.
21. I: Really?
    P: That's all confidential, isn't it?

22. I: It's confidential.
    P: We go out and get our kicks.
23. I: How's that?
    P: We stalk shopping centers. We wait till everybody is gone and then we move in. We grab the manager—he is usually the last to leave. We make him turn over the cash. But first we let him beg. We let him go down on his knees and we pull a pistol on him, We play some Russian roulette with him—click—click [laughs].
24. I: You seem like one of those tough guys.
    P: You better believe it. That's the only thing that gives me a kick, to see a guy piss in his pants and beg us. We tell him that if he plays his cards right, we may let him off. Then we let him pay for his life, take his cash, kick him in the ass, and run off.
25. I: Aren't you afraid that you might get caught?
    P: Oh shit. We put a scare in him. We tell him if he opens his fucking mouth, some of us will be back. We tell him we know where he lives. We won't get just him. We will blow off his whole shitty family. He understands. The police are busy dishing out speeding tickets to car pooling mothers—they ain't doing anything. They go where it's easy.
26. I: Is that how you always got your kicks?
    P: What do you mean?
27. I: What did you do in school?
    P: Well, my father was a colonel in the army and my mother was a rehabilitation officer [laughs]. They kicked the shit out of me.
28. I: Did you get in any trouble at school?
    P: No. We lived on base. We moved around a lot.
29. I: Were you a good fighter in school?
    P: Well, I could take and give a good lick.
30. I: You could?
    P: Yes.
31. I: Did you ever do it?
    P: I kicked the assistant baseball coach and gave him one with my bat. He woke up in the hospital.
32. I: What did the school do?
    P: Not much. They suspended me, but my dad got me back in. Then we moved to another base.
33. I: Ever had a problem like this again?
    P: One of the kids was a real smart aleck. I straightened him out. I knocked his teeth out. That taught him something.
34. I: Did you get in trouble for that?
    P: His dad tried to start something, but my dad put on his uniform and went over to his house. He told him to tell his son not to provoke people and that he had told me that I should take care of myself if somebody crosses me. So I did. The teachers wanted me out, but my dad straightened them out.
35. I: How are you getting along with your dad now?

P: He doesn't want to have anything to do with me anymore. I got in some kind of trouble and I finally ran away. I enlisted with the Marines. I lied about my birthday. They shipped me right over to Nam.

36. I: How did you get along in the service?

P: I had a great time in Saigon. We had pot and speed and heroin—everything. And you would screw the hell out of those little girls. We got hold of some stuff from the navy and sold it. No problem. We always had money. But coming back was the pits.

37. I: What did you try to do here?

P: I tried to work as a trucker. I got in an argument. I tried to work as a scuba diver, but everything bores me.

38. I: And now?

P: And now I've had it.

39. I: Did you really want to pull that trigger?

P: I felt like it, but I put them on. I knew that the safety was on. But it put the scare in them.

40. I: So you really wanted them to get you here?

P: I guess, I must have.

41. I: So you really wanted to do something about your problems?

P: I guess.

42. I: I see.

P: I'm messing up my life. I can't go on like this. I have nothing to look forward to. I can't just live for the kicks. I have to grow up.

43. I: Does that mean you want to get more out of life?

P: Yeah.

44. I: Let's talk about it. Will you level with me?

P: We'll see.

45. I: Okay. Let's see. I want to know about the voices.

P: Oh shit, I pulled one over on this clown.

46. I: You did?

P: I know enough psychology to give young Freud his hour's worth. I made it up. I just wanted to get out of there. This shrink couldn't tell a shit.

47. I: Okay.

P: What do you think is wrong with me?

48. I: Well, I think you don't care about rules, you don't care about lying, you don't care about cheating. You live on impulse. If you get angry you just get mad.

At the beginning, Mr. B. appears angry but cooperative. Showing him empathy seems to work. However, he starts to test the interviewer's ability to control the situation in A. 5. When the interviewer sets firm limits (Q. 7, 9–11), Mr. B. cooperates again. The interviewer expresses interest in him and in the way he gets himself into difficulties (Q. 14). The patient becomes willing to discuss his problems—at times even sincerely. He finally levels, gives up his boisterous display of anger, and tells his recent distress starting with A. 14.

Lability in Borderline Personality Disorder

Rapport: The patient with borderline personality disorder presents special resistance to rapport by the instability in her mood, goals, and in relating to the interviewer. She may show intense emotions, then unexpectedly switch her tone. She seems to trust and like you and tell you that you are the best doctor she has ever met. Then she will reverse her judgment when she feels lack of support and understanding.

You may handle rapport with a patient with borderline personality by focusing in an empathic manner on her instability. Attempt to separate it as a pathological part that needs to be explored for the patient's benefit. However, since the lability in feelings, judgment, and goals also affects her relationship to you, it is difficult to maintain her instability as the focus of the interview. To neutralize the negative influence on rapport, you may have to come back to it many times. When you thus demonstrate that you recognize the instability, the patient may be more willing to open up to you, thus furthering rapport.

Technique: It is difficult to keep the patient on a subject. You have to direct her, encourage her pursuit of a topic with remarks of support, and curb her diversions. She may tell you about her goals and then renege on what she just told you. She may talk enthusiastically about a new relationship just to devalue it, moments later, when some unpleasant experience in this relationship comes up.

Confront her with her contradictions but express that you understand the nature of her ambivalent feelings—what appears good and right at one time may seem the opposite at another.

The patient with borderline personality disorder usually talks in a more genuine way if you ask open-ended questions and help her to stick with a subject by curbing, rather than trying to get precise answers with closed-ended, pointed questions.

Mental status: The overriding feature in mental status is the intense but labile affect. It varies from euphoric to depressed, from appreciative to angry and critical. The affect shows a close relationship to both the content of the patient's story and the way she experiences you, the interviewer. The labile affect is paralleled by the description of a labile mood, which you can abstract from the patient's reports about life events.

The excessive intensity of affect and mood is impressive. Unlike histrionic personality disorder in which the affect appears more intensely expressed than felt, the patient with borderline personality disorder genuinely experiences an intense affect and mood. The flair of phoniness is missing. Investigators have found that the patient with borderline personality disorder shows a strong relationship to the patient with bipolar disorder and may be a variant. Mood and affect in bipolar disorder again are intense by nature but not by the patient's intent.

The lability in emotions persists also in the patient's social attitude. Intense ambivalence to close friends leads to contradictory reports about their characteristics: they are either overidealized or devaluated. Since a patient with borderline personality has no distance from her intense feelings, she has no insight into the source of her difficulties.

Diagnosis: The diagnostic process is fueled by the patient's report of a string of intense interpersonal conflicts, possibly suicidal or self-mutilating behavior, and by your mental status observations. All you have to do is collect the pieces that complete the set of DSM-IV-TR criteria. Unless you disrupt your interview by critical, rejecting remarks, you will have no problems with the diagnosis.

> This is an interview with Ms. Janet M., a 29-year-old, white female demonstrating this instability.

1. I: What brought you here today?
   P: They sent me up here from the emergency room. I had taken too much Parnate and too much cold medication. They gave me an infusion, because my blood pressure went so high.
2. I: What made you take so much medication?
   P: I had an argument with my boyfriend—I wanted to teach that bastard a lesson.
3. I: How would it teach him a lesson, if you end up in the emergency room?
   P: I really don't like your questions. They're really dumb, reminds me of my boyfriend.
4. I: So you must have felt really desperate.
   P: [sarcastically] Mustn't I? Why else would I take an overdose?
5. I: Can you tell me a little bit about what brought on that argument with your boyfriend?
   P: Oh, just his stupidity.
6. I: How is that?
   P: It really tears me to pieces. But he can be so nice at other times. We bought a house real cheap and fixed it up together to live there . . . [after a pause] I really think I should call him. He probably wonders what's going on.
7. I: You just told me that you have these bad arguments with him and that you were ready to teach him a lesson.
   P: Maybe it's all my fault and I shouldn't have been so impulsive.

8. I: Are you impulsive often?
   P: He brings out the worst in me. But I still love him a lot.
9. I: It seems difficult for you to sort out these feelings.
   P: You hit it right on the spot. [sarcastically] You must really be a pretty good psychiatrist.

A suicidal gesture or suicide attempt in a young female suggests border-line personality disorder to be included in the differential. This diagnostic impression is substantiated for Ms. M. when the reason for her suicide attempt is not depressed mood and delusional guilt but anger and revenge (A. 2).

Despite the evidence of a borderline personality diagnosis, the interviewer makes a mistake in technique in Q. 3. Rather than being supportive and understanding and telling her:

"This fellow must have really hurt you that you were pushed so far as to overdose,"

she asks a rational and critical question—and Ms. M. lashes out in response. When the interviewer tries to correct her mistake (A. 4) by expressing her empathy, Ms. M. remains sarcastic.

When the interviewer restrains herself from supportive statements and focuses on the facts instead, Ms. M. provides them freely. While she reconstructs her last argument with her boyfriend that led to the overdose, surprisingly, she changes her feelings about the event. The expression of her anger seemed to have freed her positive feelings about her boyfriend, and she shows a bout of guilt (A. 7). When the interviewer pursues her insight and makes an implicit interpretation that it seems difficult for her to sort out her feelings, she abandons the insight track. She rejects the interviewer's interpretation with sarcasm, demonstrating her defensiveness against facing a core symptom of her personality disorder.

Phoniness in Histrionic Personality Disorder

In a clinical setting, histrionic personality disorder is more frequently diagnosed in females than in males. Structured assessments show a 1:1 sex ratio.

Rapport: When you attempt to establish rapport, you deal with exaggerated emotionality and lack of depth. Together with frequent contradictions in her story, she gives you the impression that she lacks sincerity; she appears "phony." Because of this feature, the patient may be disliked and disrespected.

With a male interviewer the female histrionic patient likes to flirt, to impress him with stories of sexual adventures, and to display her physical attributes seductively. With female interviewers, she may initiate rivalry or a power contest. Since the histrionic patient seems to be more interested in approval and admiration than in a professional relationship, rapport is hampered.

Technique: You have to overcome the patient's vagueness and dramatic exaggerations to obtain specific information for a diagnosis. Unstructured, open-ended questions may not work, because the patient becomes sidetracked and gets lost in reproducing stories in which she was adored or victimized. Therefore, settle on a main theme, like a marriage problem, a conflict at work, or a fight with her children, and keep her focused on this theme with curbing and specification. Get concrete examples. Even then you may not get a clear picture because the patient contradicts herself. Confrontation with her contradictions often results in anger and a loss of rapport. To get her to reflect on her behavior, you have to express understanding and encouragement. Use phrases like:

"You seem to be a sensitive person."
"You seem to feel that other people can't appreciate what you went through."

When the patient expresses that she feels understood by you, you may ask her:

"How do you think your husband would report the same event?"

By comparing his and her perception you may help her to develop a better understanding of her conflicts and give her some insight. Such insight, however, is usually short-lived.

You can sometimes help her to develop insight into her behavior by asking emphatic questions. When you side with her, the patient may be encouraged to admit at times some of her deficiencies. As soon as she feels that your support, understanding, and empathy are slipping away, she will return to dramatization. A histrionic female patient has often experienced rejection that she does not understand. She tries to overcome it by exaggerating her pain and this tactic often earns her contempt rather than empathy.

Another approach is to address the exaggerated dramatic behavior from the patient's point of view, such as:

"It seems to me that you have a hard time making people understand what you are going through. You tell them about your problems and they just don't seem to care. I think we should try to understand why this happens."

If pursued, the patient may complain about being rejected and ridiculed even by her family. She may admit that she wants to be loved, praised, and admired. Those admissions bring you closer to her true feelings and allow you to overcome her strategy.

The next step is to induce the patient to tell you the reasons why she is criticized. This may lead to a confession of her weaknesses. At this point, you have temporarily helped the patient to overcome her phoniness—at least for the moment.

Mental status: The mental status of a histrionic patient is dominated by a display of emotionality: vivid facial expressions, dramatic gestures, and a highly modulated voice. However, she can be interrupted and redirected to a different topic, which she will take up in the same dramatic fashion. Her distractibility differs from mania, since there is no push of speech or flight of ideas (see Glossary). The constant drama gives you the impression that she does not really experience any intense feelings. Her strong show of emotions is for your benefit, not a catharsis for her. In spite of excessive facial expressions and abundant gesturing, she appears uninvolved in her story. The term *la belle indifférence* has been coined for this internal emotional distance.

Diagnosis: As for most personality disorders, it is the patient's mental status that will alert you. When you suspect a histrionic personality disorder, invite the patient to tell you how she is getting along with people close to her. Since the histrionic patient usually has conflicts, for example, with parents, children, or spouses, she will report lifelong conflicts with them. She often divides her relatives into "the good and the bad guys." Besides the exaggeration typical of the patient with histrionic personality, you will also often encounter passive-aggressive features and intense ambivalent feelings typical for the patient with borderline personality disorder.

This is an interview with Ms. Jane R., a middle-aged, white, married female who has chronic marital conflicts.

1. I: What kind of problems brought you here?
   P: Before we begin let me tell you something. I understand that you wanted me to be seen by some other doctor in the clinic, but I wanted the best. That's why I insisted on seeing you.

2. I: Thank you. But what makes you say I'm the best?
   P: Well, you are the director of the clinic, aren't you? And Dr. T., who referred me here, said you specialize in sleep problems.
3. I: Tell me about your sleep problems.
   P: Oh, it's terrible. There are whole nights when I can't sleep at all. I toss and turn, and I get up in the morning without having closed my eyes for even a second.
4. I: This happens only some nights?
   P: It happens when I have these terrible, terrible fights with my husband. He just tears me to pieces [rolls her eyes dramatically upward].
5. I: Does he or anybody else notice what you are going through?
   P: They don't have the foggiest idea [shakes head vigorously]. I can scream and yell and they still don't understand [shrugs shoulders].
6. I: When you have these fights, is your mood affected?
   P: I get these devastating depressions [looking up to the ceiling] and I have to cry the whole time.
7. I: What are these fights about?
   P: I'm not sure. Just anything. We have not had sex for the last 4 months. I can't understand how a man can be so cruel and hateful.
8. I: I have a hard time understanding what your fights with your husband are all about.
   P: He criticizes me and puts me down. He has left me more than 30 times in the last few years.
9. I: Maybe you can give me an example?
   P: Well, he comes back from his trips and rips me all apart.
10. I: So his criticism is the main part of your problems?
    P: I suffer so terribly much. A nice man like you probably cannot understand how a man can be as mean as my husband.
11. I: Maybe I should have a chance to talk to both of you.
    P: I'd rather not do that. He tells his side of the story in such a way that it fools everyone.
12. I: What do you think he would say?
    P: Just the same old thing, that I'm a bad housekeeper, that I haven't done anything, that I'm just sitting on my fanny while he has to do all the work. He'll just carry on like that.
13. I: So he talks about your shortcomings. Does he ever ask you how you feel and why you are having trouble getting things done?
    P: He has no understanding whatsoever. It's like he's made of wood and he looks so cold. I'm getting tired easily and when I rest and watch television, the time is gone and I can't get things done.
14. I: I see. Do you think then that he has a point?
    P: Are you taking his side? I thought I'm your patient, I'm the one who's suffering. I thought you understood that.
15. I: Okay. Let's start to talk about your problems and talk with him later.
    P: Well, when you talk to him you will not believe how nasty and mean he can be.
16. I: At this point do you see a future for your marriage?
    P: I still love him, I enjoy the closeness when we have sex.

17. I: Well, as you said, that has not happened for a long time.
  P: Oh, it was just last Friday. And some hours later he was tearing me apart.
18. I: I thought you had not been intimate with him for quite some time.
  P: Why do you use whatever I say against me? Can't you understand? I meant the time before last time.

Even though Ms. R. talks freely, it is difficult to get precise information. At first, she does not describe the circumstances of the fights with her husband, nor does she agree to have him interviewed. She expresses her suffering in an exaggerated way but she is reluctant to furnish the facts. She wants the interviewer to feel sorry for her; the mere fact that she suffers should be reason enough for the interviewer to side with her.

Her vagueness is temporarily overcome when the interviewer asks her to project what the husband would report about her. But when he tries to explore whether the husband's statements are to some extent justified, she protests. She prefers to indulge in suffering rather than to analyze her underlying problems.

When the interviewer explores whether she considers a divorce, her dependency needs surface. She has a hard time fending for herself. She starts to emphasize her husband's positive features. Thus, it appears that the patient is more interested in complaining about her problems than solving them.

Grandiosity in Narcissistic Personality Disorder

Throughout the interview, the patient with narcissistic personality gives you the feeling that you are there to endorse his self-promoted importance. As long as you play along, you will be idolized as a wonderful interviewer. However, if you support his grandiose self-perception, you will not help him to test his grandiosity against the reality of everyday life. Yet, helping the patient recognize his limits shatters his self-inflated ego.

To you the grandiosity is in glaring contrast with reality, but the patient has no insight to tell the difference between his healthy, critical self and his pathological tendencies. Alliance between you and the patient's healthy part is not possible. His lack of insight prevents rapport.

Here is an interview with Henry, a child psychiatrist at an eastern pediatric department:

1. I: Hello, Henry.
  P: Before you say anything, let me give you the background of my visit. I am here to discuss with you, as a smart and knowledgeable insider, some of the

problems that I have dealing with incompetent diagnostic morons. One should call them medical technicians; they have no grasp of the essence of the problems they deal with. We have a long-standing conflict that is now coming to a head. Even after I published my book, they doubt my expertise in the field. I have to make a decision whether I should quit this clinic that supports those morons or try to get them fired.

2. I: What does Dr. L. [the clinic director] think about it?

   P: I have been over that one with her several times. I have pushed her toward an ultimatum, I had her crying, but she is incapable of taking the necessary actions.

3. I: Who are the doctors that you have a conflict with?

   P: Several pediatricians at my clinic. They have no clinical savvy whatsoever. Their judgment with regard to the trustworthiness of molested children is just horrendously impaired.

4. I: How's that?

   P: As a forensic child and adolescent psychiatrist, I have the experience that allows me to decide whether or not a child is lying. But all they are concerned about is the evidence: did the child have a conduct disorder, or did he abuse drugs? Intuition, recognition of defenses, and understanding of the family dynamics escape them completely.

5. I: Well, Henry, I'm not up on the field, maybe you can tell me on what kind of criteria you base a child's trustworthiness.

   P: That's so obvious. I'm surprised that you ask such a question. Haven't you read my book? I did send you a copy. Do you really expect me to teach you the basics here?

6. I: Well, since one of your discussions with your colleagues centers around trustworthiness of witnesses, I would like to know how you approach the question.

   P: Let me tell you what. I'll give you six criteria: experience, experience, experience, knowledge, understanding, and judgment. How does that strike you? I guess that does not sit well with your obsessiveness.

7. I: Come on, Henry. You can do better than that.

   P: You have really lost your clinical touch since you have been away from psychoanalysis. Your neurology training has gotten the better of you. I guess there is no sense in talking to you any longer!

8. I: Okay, Henry, I think I'm not helping you. It seems the pediatricians really do not grasp your contributions.

   P.   Now we're getting somewhere.

9. I: I'd like to know why you think they misunderstand you!

   P: I told you! It's their intellectual flat-footedness!

10. I: Okay, if that's right, is there anything you could do to improve matters?

    P: Listen, don't put it on me! Who do you think I am? You know I have dealt with all kinds of people who were not the smartest, but at least they had intuition, and esprit. You don't really expect me to get down to their level and worry about what pediatricians think!

11. I: Well, it depends on your goals.

    P: What do you mean? I am not on trial here. You always point at me, thanks anyway—thanks, but no thanks!

12. I: Come on Henry, we have been friends, I want to help you to find out what's going wrong! Do you want to show them how ignorant they are, or do you want to get your diagnostic reasoning across?

    P: Bull . . . I'm not enjoying this conversation. Let's forget it.

13. I: Well, Henry, you seem to feel insulted and misunderstood.

    P: The hell, I do. They think because they are pediatricians, they have one up on me. And you seem to be on their side too, just because they think they are real doctors just like you seem to think. Maybe you did the right thing by going into neurology. Next time around I would do the same [his eyes fill with tears]. You don't believe how much I have suffered in this department. By the way, do you know Rick D., the surgeon? We have the same little nursing student in the works. She really is a cute ass. Are you still giving talks?

14. I: A few of them. Why do you ask?

    P: If you know anyone who needs a speaker, I would be willing . . . you can recommend me.

This interview shows how a patient with narcissistic personality disorder tries to maintain his self-importance in light of an adverse reality. The interviewer's attempts to make Henry review his behavior are overrun. When the interviewer expresses empathy for his repercussions (due to his grandiose distortion), the patient collapses briefly but attempts to regain his posture by bragging about his amorous success.

As with other personality disorders, an empathic addressing of the narcissistic goal such as:

"You only feel worthwhile when you convince yourself and others that you are tops,"

or empathy for the consequences of the narcissistic behavior such as:

"I see you are hurting. Let's find out how you get hurt and how we can stop it,"

may only temporarily enable the patient to consider his narcissistic behavior as the cause of his problems. Usually, each insight is followed by a grandiose repair of his shattered image.

3. ANXIOUS, RESISTIVE SUBMISSIVENESS— CLUSTER C

Three personality disorders fall into Cluster C: the avoidant, the dependent, and the obsessive-compulsive personality disorder. The mental status of a patient in Cluster C is dominated by an anxious, tense, and dysphoric affect. She worries whether you accept her. Her speech appears overcontrolled, and she weighs each word to avoid mistakes. Cluster C personality disorder patients have more insight into their behavior than patients in Clusters A and B—anxiety produces self-awareness and self-consciousness.

Rapport develops along a specific pattern. The patient watches you closely to find out what you think of her. If she finds you supportive, receptive, nurturing, and nondemanding, she strives to overcome her anxiety by paying reverence to your authority. She may flatter you, ask your advice, laud you as an expert, and tell you what she thinks you want to hear. She clings to you, and expects you to take charge. Rapport becomes lopsided.

One of the personality disorders of Cluster C is more difficult to interview: the obsessive-compulsive personality. As the interview with her progresses, you may find it was only a token reverence that the patient paid you. After you respond with empathy and act protective of her, her internal resentment creeps up. Gestures and remarks slip out that indicate reluctance to cooperate. She may ask probing questions and let you know your inadequacies. She feels that you were not really worthwhile or powerful enough to justify her initial anxiety; she may resent her submissiveness and may shut you out. Special techniques will be discussed for the interview with the obsessive-compulsive personality disorder patient.

Hypersensitivity in Avoidant Personality Disorder

Rapport: In a patient with avoidant personality disorder anxious guardedness and reticence can be approached with reassurance and empathy. Avoid confrontation that she may interpret as criticism. Instead, express empathic understanding for her suffering, which may encourage her to share her past tortures and her present anticipatory fears. If the patient feels that you understand her sensitivity and are protective of her, she will trust you and cooperate with you. The result is rapport. After she feels accepted and safe, the character of the interview may change dramatically. She may become explicitly detailed, may give you examples of social insults she has endured, and report to you the reliving and resuffering of her traumata.

Technique: After you have established rapport, the patient is easy to interview. She feels relieved when she can describe her social fears of being criticized and rejected because she feels your empathy. She may experience these fears of being embarrassed as silly and express this. However, if you identify with this position, she may feel ridiculed and criticized and may withdraw again.

Mental status: The avoidant personality initially shows withdrawal and this feature dominates her mental status. She is monosyllabic, vague, and circumstantial. Initially she may appear suspicious and paranoid, or anxious and phobic, but void of clear-cut symptoms of DSM-IV-TR clinical disorders. After she feels comfortable with you and develops trust, she may reveal her sensitivity to being misunderstood and her tendency to be easily hurt by criticism or disapproval. She may then discuss her fear of rejection and inappropriate behavior.

Diagnosis: The patient's anxiousness and restricted affect at the beginning of the interview usually attract the interviewer's attention—early clues. If she opens up, the diagnostic interview follows the standard phases (see Chapter 7).

> Ms. Donna K., a 27-year-old, white, single female, had never been in treatment. When she entered the office, she sat down and put her hands in her lap, and then hung her head down glumly. She refused to have coffee by shaking her head and mumbling no. She appeared unusually tense. The interviewer decided—since small talk seemed to make her more uncomfortable—to ask for her chief complaint.

1. I: Maybe you can tell me what kind of problems bring you here . . . [pause]. What would you like to talk about?
   P: [silent, looking down at her hands with a tense expression on her face, then looking back at the interviewer]
2. I: How do you think I can help you?
   P: I don't know.
3. I: Maybe you can tell me what's bothering you.
   P: [looks down and shakes her head] People, I guess.
4. I: [silent, looking at her]
   P: [getting tenser and still looking down at her lap]
5. I: [in a soft, soothing voice] People? What is it about people?
   P: I can't really tell.
6. I: You seem to be scared of people.
   P: [nods]
7. I: What makes you scared of them?
   P: I don't know. I feel like they are closing in on me.
8. I: You feel they are out to harm you?
   P: No, not really out to harm me. They are so loud and pushy; they shut me up.
9. I: I understand. You feel that they can run over you any time; they close in on you and crush you . . . [remains silent] . . . Is this close to how you feel?
   P: Pretty close.

10. I: Is there anyone in particular?
    P: My father's brother. He comes in, pushes me aside, laughs at me. I hear it all
         the time: "Come on Donna, come off it, Donna, that's crazy, Donna, you're
         so impractical, Donna, damn, get your shit together, Donna, and put your
         foot down." [shakes her whole body] I can't stand it. I would like to hide in
         my room.
11. I: You must go through a lot.
    P: [sighs] Yeah . . . yeah, really. [for the first time looks at the interviewer and
         establishes eye contact]
12. I: How long has this bothered you?
    P: As far back as I can think. My past is full of hurts.
13. I: School must have been hell for you.
    P: Oh, it was. I remember when I had written a poem and the teacher made me
         read it to the class.
14. I: What happened?
    P: I did not want to do it. I was ashamed of having written a poem.
15. I: Did the teacher understand and help you out?
    P: She told me I could stay in my seat and read it there—it was awful.
16. I: What was awful?
    P: When I started to read, the kids in the front yelled: "Read louder, we can't
         hear you!" I started to swallow—finally, the teacher took the poem and read
         it. The whole class laughed. I swore that I would never write a poem again.
17. I: You have thin skin. Everything seems to get right through to you.
    P: I have no skin at all. I seem to be much too sensitive.
18. I: That makes it hard for you to speak up.
    P: I'll die before I open my mouth in front of a whole bunch of people again.

It takes the interviewer eight questions to piece together Ms. K.'s chief
complaint. Rapport is established with Q. 9 and 11; Q. 9 expresses cognitive
understanding and Q. 11 empathy. In Q. 9 the interviewer summarizes what
was learned. He focuses then on the person Ms. K. most dreads. For the first
time the patient gives a somewhat longer and emotionally laden account of
a person she fears and hates at the same time. The interviewer expresses
empathic understanding in Q. 11. The patient relaxes and the interviewer
is now able to follow the standard interview and get the patient's history
(Q. 12–18).

The overlap between avoidant personality disorder and social phobia,
generalized type, is substantial (American Psychiatric Association 2000, p. 720).

Submissiveness in Dependent Personality Disorder

Rapport: It is easy to establish rapport with a patient with a dependent
personality; after she loses her initial anxiety, she puts her trust in you. As

long as you give support and show empathy for her indecisiveness and failures, the interview flows easily.

However, if you try to explore the background of the patient's submissiveness, she becomes uncomfortable and tries to persuade you not to be too harsh on her. If you pursue exploring her dependency, and if you do this from your own, rather than from the patient's point of view, she will show you how much she suffers. If you don't soothe the pain, the patient may change therapists to find a more sympathetic ear.

Technique: Interviewing the patient with dependent personality disorder is easy. She cooperates and tries to meet your expectations. She answers questions to the point. She clarifies her answers on demand, so you can easily steer the direction of the interview. She tolerates accentuated and abrupt transitions, and allows you to probe very personal feelings. What she cannot tolerate is confrontation with and interpretations of her dependency.

Mental status: The mental status is colored by the associated disorders that bring her into therapy in the first place. The overriding features, however, are her dependency, submissiveness, anxiousness, and her need to please you. She tries to give you answers that she thinks you will like. Her affect strikes you often as anxious and depressed with some obsessive features.

The thought content mirrors themes of low self-esteem, desertion, and anxiety about doing the wrong thing. The patient with dependent personality disorder is oriented to her surroundings and has good memory but fails to appreciate the degree of her lack of initiative and its effect on her life. Her judgment is hampered by her dependency.

Diagnosis: Several features of the interview tell you that you are dealing with a patient with a dependent personality. From the very beginning the patient elevates you to a superior position.

Her social history shows that she always seemed to share quarters with a person who took charge of her life. The combination of these features rather than any one alone will suggest to you that the patient has a dependent personality disorder. After you have included this diagnosis in your differential, show, first, that the pattern of dependency is lifelong, and second, that her dependency can be separated from the symptoms of a disabling clinical disorder, or from justifiable responses to such a disorder.

Ms. Susan C., a white, divorced female in her late 30s has been attending a psychiatric outpatient clinic regularly for many years. During the first interview with a new psychiatrist, she demonstrates some characteristic features of the dependent personality.

1. I: I'm taking over for Dr. V. I understand that you have been coming to this clinic for quite some time.
   P: Oh yes, at least the last 15 years.
2. I: What seems to be the problem?
   P: [pauses] I don't know how to answer that question. Maybe you can tell me what's going on.
3. I: Hmm. Maybe you can help me by telling me what you've been struggling with lately.
   P: I really need your guidance. You can probably sort it all out. That's why I am coming here. I need your help and advice.
4. I: You have a hard time to get along?
   P: Yes, since my husband deserted and divorced me, people have been taking advantage of me, says Dr. V. I'd been better off if my husband hadn't divorced me. But he always said I cling to him too much. And so he left me, and I had done everything for him.
5. I: It seems you still miss him.
   P: I still see him once in a while. He's married again. They have three children. It gives me a pain in the chest when I see them and how happy they are, and I'm so miserable. Maybe you can help me.
6. I: Are you living alone now?
   P: No, I moved back in with my mother. She never liked my husband. Now I'm not dating at all. I don't even go out. I don't want to hurt my mother.
7. I: Have you ever thought of marrying again?
   P: My mother wouldn't like it. It would be like deserting her a second time. Sometimes I think it would be nice to find a man who would love me and would like to take care of me. Maybe an older man.
8. I: Why don't you want to find a man your own age?
   P: They are so demanding; they want you like a partner and not as a wife. I'm pretty traditional when it comes to marriage. I think the husband should be a gentleman and show you love and care for you.
9. I: Being a partner in a marriage seems to be tough for you.
   P: I think with real love men will be understanding. I feel that you understand.
10. I: It sounds to me that you have to find out how much you have to be on your own, how much responsibility to take.
    P: You sound like Dr. R. He did not seem to like me. He was not like Dr. V., who was always on my side.
11. I: I feel I have touched on something very painful for you.
    P: [silent]
12. I: I think it may be helpful for you if we can discuss it.
    P: My mother criticizes me all the time . . . but I don't make enough money to live by myself [her eyes fill with tears]. I'm really trapped. Please don't criticize me, I can't take it, I want you to help me.

Most long-term patients have a chronic disorder—one of the Axis I disorders that is, such as schizophrenia; rapid cycling, nonresponding bipolar disorder; or nonresponsive major depressive disorder. If such a disorder is missing, yet the patient visits the clinic over many years, a personality disorder of Cluster C is likely, especially dependent personality.

This may surprise the reader since by definition all personality disorders are chronic. However, not all result in long-term therapy as the Cluster C disorders do. Therefore, a patient who is psychologically minded, with deep, nonresolving dependency needs, is a prime candidate for long-term psychotherapy. The interview with Ms. C. bears it out.

From the beginning of the interview Ms. C. attempts to put the interviewer in charge (A. 2, 3). He does not confront her with this tendency but assesses her life circumstances instead. She describes a situation typical of the dependent personality.

In Q. 10 the interviewer attempts to address her ability/inability to rely on her resources. Ms. C. misunderstands this exploration as an implicit criticism and responds with tears and a plea to not be criticized. This response shows how stressful it is for her to be confronted with her pathological dependency in the first interview. Instead, explore the patient's view of her dependency and then make her gradually aware of the consequences of her behavior. Chances are that, in spite of your therapeutic skills, you may not be able to make the patient self-sufficient.

Circumstantiality and Perfectionism in Obsessive-Compulsive Personality Disorder

Rapport: The obsessive patient is fixated on details. Therefore, in the interview you will be involved in a struggle about words, issues, and who is in charge without being able to develop an atmosphere of cooperation and understanding.

If you show empathy you will have a problem. He is proud that he doesn't have any feelings, that he is objective. Therefore, he is perturbed when you express empathy for his suffering and rejects it as irrelevant. Not his suffering but his problems are important; however, they are unsolvable. This struggle may prevent you from establishing the split between the healthy and the diseased part of his personality.

You may overcome this struggle by continually trying to get and keep the patient in touch with his anger. This may work as long as he believes that you feel his anger is justified. But if you attempt to make the anger the object of the interview, he will defend or deny it. He will put forth more obstructive obsessive thinking, actively preventing a split between the healthy and the sick part of his personality. To form an alliance is difficult, and the interview often consists of aborted attempts, struggles, and frustrations.

Technique: Your position as interviewer is precarious because the patient's ambivalence is hard to overcome. He doubts your assurances. Your open-ended questions lead to confusion. He wants more circumscribed questions, but if you comply he interprets them as too narrow.

Mental status: The mental status of the patient with obsessive-compulsive personality is overshadowed by one difficulty—making decisions. This shows in his ambivalence and the way he keeps you in limbo when answering questions. Should he open up to you, or would he be misunderstood? He may decide not to open up, but will wonder, is that right? Should he spend his money on seeing you and then risk not getting a true reading of his problems? How can he get your best opinion if he holds back? Are you really the right person to talk to? Probably not. He has to find out from you what's wrong. He should ask the questions; you should provide the answers. Who is in charge? Him? Or should you be in charge, since you are supposed to be the expert?

The obsessive-compulsive patient perceives himself as being neutral, a quite distorted view. You sense a low-grade, chronic anger that can flare up into tenacious, persistent, bothersome questioning that cannot be satisfied by any answer. His anger will become overt when his obsessive expectations are not met, when he feels shortchanged in interviewing time, overcharged for his visit, or not rewarded with useful answers to his questions.

Diagnosis: The mental status gives the patient's diagnosis away; no secret here. The problem is to get the details of the associated disorders, if any. If such a patient presents at a clinic, obsessive-compulsive disorder itself, depression, phobic disorder, and sometimes delusional disorder occur as comorbid conditions.

> Here is an example of an obsessive-compulsive personality found in Mr. Wynn G., a 35-year-old scientist:

1. I: How can I help you?
   P: I'm concerned about a letter I wrote to my coauthor. She did not take it well at all.
2. I: What was the letter about?
   P: I don't know whether I should discuss this here. You may know her.

3. I: Are you concerned that something may leak out?

P: Obviously ... But maybe I can tell you if you can assure me of complete confidentiality.

4. I: How can I help you if you can't talk about it?

P: Maybe the content of the letter is not the problem, but her reaction.

5. I: What is it about her reaction that concerns you?

P: I'm just thinking that you can't really understand her reaction if you don't know about the letter.

6. I: Let's look at the whole package.

P: You are pushing me. Maybe I should think more about what I should tell you.

7. I: Alright.

P: If I break off now, you couldn't really charge me for that short a visit, because it isn't me who can't guarantee confidentiality.

8. I: I'm sorry, this hour was reserved for you, I will charge you for my time.

P: You really have a way with words. OK, if you charge me anyway, I may as well use the time. My coauthor agreed with one of the harshest critics who reviewed our paper. This really incensed me, because she's not really an expert in the area.

9. I: So you became angry.

P: Not angry. I am very rarely distracted by my feelings. I consider them irrational. What I basically did is ask her to change the paper according to her criticism.

10. I: Could she do it if she is not an expert in the area?

P: I cannot understand how someone can criticize work if they can't change it. Then she shouldn't have criticized it in the first place.

11. I: But wasn't her intention ...

P: I don't really care about intentions, I'm looking at facts. The facts are that she criticized the paper without being able to improve it. It's as simple as that.

12. I: But don't you miss the point, when you look at the facts without including the intentions?

P: I don't think you have any appreciation for the facts. You are unable to see the facts. You have a hang-up on the emotional side. You are obviously biased.

13. I: My statements seem to make you angry.

P: I'm not an emotional person. I just want to get the facts straight. But you won't let me do that.

The interviewer demonstrates a struggle that frequently evolves with a patient suffering from obsessive-compulsive personality disorder. Since he questions everything that he does and that you propose by considering the opposite, no resolution is forthcoming. However, the patient with obsessive-compulsive personality disorder has a specific sensitivity that allows you to channel the interview—he wants to be considered logical. He cannot stand to give up something for nothing. He is stingy with emotion, time, money, and control and does not want to lose out to anyone. Therefore he continues with the interview when he hears that he may get charged anyway if he breaks it off. Thus the interviewer can motivate him to complete the interview even though it appears that the interviewer is not in charge when indeed he is. Progress will not be straightforward but will move three steps ahead and two steps back.

4. PERSONALITY DISORDER NOT OTHERWISE SPECIFIED

Two personality disorders are classified NOS in DSM-IV-TR: depressive personality disorder and passive-aggressive (negativistic) personality disorder. Both are considered disorders that need further study. Since you are likely to encounter these disorders when you interview patients, we have included them here.

Controversy: Depressive Personality Disorder Versus Dysthymic Disorder

In DSM-IV and DSM-IV-TR, depressive personality disorder has been proposed as a criteria set for further study. A controversy arises from the difficulty in differentiating depressive personality disorder and dysthymic disorder. For instance, criterion A for dysthymic disorder is similar to criterion A1 of depressive personality disorder. Criterion B4 of dysthymic disorder resembles criterion A2 of depressive personality disorder. Criterion B6 of dysthymic disorder expresses a similar outlook for the future as that reflected in criterion A6 of depressive personality disorder.

The difference seems to be the area emphasized. Dysthymic disorder emphasizes vegetative symptoms such as disturbances in appetite, sleep, and energy (B1–B3), whereas depressive personality disorder emphasizes negative attitudes, such as being critical and derogatory toward self and critical and judgmental toward others, as well as having feelings of brooding and being prone to guilt.

Semantically we can draw such a distinction indeed. Empirical studies are needed, however, to investigate whether there exists a distinctive group of patients with a negative attitude who are relatively free of appetite and sleep disturbances and who show an adequate level of energy; or, vice versa, whether there are patients who fulfill criteria for dysthymic disorder but lack guilt feelings, worrying, and a critical, judgmental attitude toward themselves and others.

It appears that the more chronically nonsuicidal depressed patients are diagnosed with depressive personality disorder when they assertively display their negative attitude, but when they lack assertiveness they may be diagnosed with dysthymic disorder. Nevertheless, the exclusion criterion B for depressive personality disorder does not allow the diagnosis of depressive personality disorder if dysthymic disorder could better account for the observed depressive psychopathology.

In your interview for your final diagnosis, you may focus on the vegetative complex that would support the diagnosis of dysthymic disorder, whereas its absence in the presence of lifelong, critical judgment against self and others, combined with worrying, guilt, and remorsefulness, would tilt your diagnosis toward depressive personality disorder after major depressive disorder has been excluded.

Resentment in Passive-Aggressive (Negativistic) Personality Disorder

Rapport: Like the patient with dependent personality disorder, the patient with passive-aggressive personality disorder establishes and maintains rapport as long as you agree with him and take his side. When you challenge his view, you trigger his anger. He is especially sensitive to demands put on him; he resists them with tardiness, sulking, evasiveness, arguments, and occasionally open anger.

If you address his resentment toward demands, he becomes guarded, monosyllabic, and often hostile. If you fail to appreciate this sensitivity to demands, or even sympathize with the demanding person, you lose rapport. You regain it only if you return to the patient's point of view.

Technique: Slowly and carefully explore the patient's deep aversion to demands. The skillful interviewer expresses that she understands the patient's needs for leniency but points out at the same time that if he leaves expectations unfulfilled, it may cause disappointment and resentment in others. She knows that if she temporarily sympathizes with the patient's resentment about demands, the patient may cooperate and allow her to explore his personality disorder and its comorbidity (see below: Diagnosis).

Mental status: During the interview the patient may not show much psychopathology. His affect appears to be well adjusted and pleasant except when he starts to talk about situations where he was asked to perform.

Then he shows signs of resentment, irritability, or anger. If you fail to identify these trigger situations, you may miss his underlying personality disorder.

Diagnosis: A patient with passive-aggressive personality disorder rarely consults you for problems related to his disorder. His associated Axis I disorders bring him to see you, such as alcoholism, mood disorder, or an anxiety disorder.

His story becomes transparent when he talks about social disappointments, interpersonal conflicts, and bad breaks. Typically, the patient does not openly oppose demands but accepts commitments and makes promises even when he knows he will not keep them. He says "yes" but acts "no." This characteristic leads to disappointments and rejection by colleagues, friends, and family members. And the patient complains bitterly about being rejected without understanding how he sets it off.

If you hit upon the "say yes/act no" attitude, explore whether it is limited to certain people, situations, or certain life periods when the patient was depressed. If this attitude tints all relationships lifelong, your patient has passive-aggressive personality disorder.

> Mr. Andy O. is a 34-year-old businessman with a family history of bipolar disorder, but without a psychiatric history of his own.

1. I: How can I help you?
   P: I just have to talk to somebody about the things that happened to me at work.
2. I: OK, Andy.
   P: It will probably upset you as much as me.
3. I: You must have gone through some rough times.
   P: Have I ever . . . boy, if I could tell you. This friend of mine accepted a job down here and when I talked to him he asked me if I wouldn't like to join him.
4. I: So you did?
   P: Well, I did because I trusted him. So I went to work with him, and I thought we'd have a good time, because the guy seemed to be a lot of fun.
5. I: Was he?
   P: Let me tell you—the first thing he did was start with staff meetings in the morning—did I ever resent them. That was his sneaky way of forcing us to be on time.
6. I: Was there a problem with that?
   P: A problem? We were friends and he knew I had good ideas, but they don't necessarily come at 8 o'clock in the morning.
7. I: Well . . .
   P: When I came late, when I had car trouble, or when I had to run an errand, he didn't say anything, but I could feel that he didn't like it.

8. I: Was he ever late himself?

P: Are you kidding? That guy is a workaholic. He was there in the morning and he stayed late in the evening. If I'd known that he was such a slave driver, I would not have come here in the first place. But I got back at him when I had that accident. I don't know whether he believed me, but I brought the splinter from my foot with me back to work to show it.

9. I: Did your friend see it?

P: I showed it to some colleagues when he was passing by in the hall.

10. I: Did he see it?

P: You know what that bastard said? "If you don't believe Andy's story today, he'll bring a bigger splinter in tomorrow!" Boy, was I miffed.

11. I: So you expected him to treat you more as a friend than as an employee.

P: That's exactly right. What's the use of working for a friend, if you have to slave along anyway?

12. I: So he should have given you some privileges and leeway.

P: Isn't that obvious? You don't suppose that I should run like clockwork for that guy.

13. I: Well, you said he's at work at 8 o'clock.

P: Listen, I think I made a mistake talking to you about it. You seem to be just like him. I want you to know there is more to life than work, work, work.

14. I: Let's go back, Andy, and explore some more of your feelings about your friend's demands.

P: Listen, my friend, I have to explore nothing with you any more. I'm here of my own free will. I resent your domineering attitude.

15. I: I'm sorry. I must have missed the point completely. I failed to see how your friend's pettiness has cost him your friendship and devotion.

P: [sarcastic] What a sudden turn in your view.

16. I: [ignoring the sarcasm] You're right, I failed to see things from your vantage point. Your friend knew you before you went to work for him—he should have told you what to expect.

P: That's right. I would never have worked for him if he'd told me that it's worse to work for a friend than for just any other employer.

The patient makes the underlying assumption that everybody who works for a friend can expect privileges such as being tardy, taking it easy, and extra time off. When the interviewer addresses these expectations indirectly (Q. 8), Mr. O. avoids a response such as:

"You are right, he sets a good example, why shouldn't I do the same?"

but instead criticizes the friend as a workaholic. Mr. O. responds with anger when his friend humors him for missing work because of a splinter in his foot (A. 10).

When the interviewer confronts Mr. O. with his expectation of receiving privileges, he becomes hostile. His response shows that he is more interested in mustering support for his position—if he indeed discusses his conflict—rather than facing his distorted expectation.

To stay engaged in the interview with a patient suffering from passive-aggressive personality disorder, explore *his* point of view. Use *his* angle to look at his conflicts. The interviewer started this in Q. 15. Over many future sessions, the patient would have to become aware of his perspective and learn to detect why that perspective causes friction and resentment with others. For instance, Andy has to experience how colleagues resent the privilege that he demands by his overt behavior. He has to experience that granting him these privileges would be an unfair practice that erodes morale at the workplace. To apply these techniques exceeds the scope of a diagnostic interview. For the purpose of the diagnostic interview, you only need to be able to identify the patient's perspective and use it in the interview.

Two other personality disorders NOS were proposed in DSM-III-R: sadistic personality disorder and self-defeating personality disorder. They are not included among the DSM-IV-TR personality disorders NOS. Nevertheless, when you encounter them in your practice, you still have to classify them as NOS.

Demanding Cruelty in Sadistic Personality Disorder

What are the characteristics of the patient with sadistic personality disorder? The physical and mental cruelty and lack of empathy that such a patient shows for his victims will impress you each time you encounter one. He is quite capable of finding victims—usually he chooses somebody under his control, such as a child, wife, student, employee, or elderly person. If his rank does not assure him superiority, he will pick on somebody physically weaker.

He finds pleasure in dominating, torturing, and inflicting pain on his victim. Not only is he interested in the dominance and the ensuing increase in self-esteem, but in the pain that he can unnecessarily and deliberately cause.

Means that can enhance both dominance over and torture of others have a magic fascination for him. Therefore, he likes weapons, the martial arts, and professions that allow him to use them.

A patient with sadistic personality disorder does not seek treatment to have his sadism diffused. Sometimes, you may encounter sadistic features in patients who suffer from other problems such as persecutory delusions or alcohol or substance abuse, and you diagnose the sadistic personality disorder as a comorbid condition. Usually, however, you meet him through his victim.

When you interview such a person, he may attempt to intimidate, bluff, and make you, too, suffer. He will use his ways to impose his will upon you.

> The following interview takes place between a psychiatrist and the husband (H) of a patient who demands his wife's release from the hospital. Mr. Mambrino is a pale, 5'8", thin man with dark, slightly disheveled hair. He sits stiffly and straight up on a chair with his fists pressed against the armrests, white knuckles protruding. Out of narrowed eyes he stares piercingly at the interviewer without blinking.

1. I: Hi, Mr. Mambrino. I'm Dr. O., the attending physician here. Our nurse, Mrs. J., just called me and told me that you would like to talk to me.

   H: [stands up, walks toward the interviewer and positions himself in front of him, with legs spread and with a low, pressed voice] You got that right. I want to sign out Irene [his wife]. She just took off from home and the next thing I know is that the social worker calls me and tells me that she has checked into this hospital here.

2. I: Hmm . . .

   H: And she tells me that Irene doesn't even want to talk to me.

3. I: [frowns] I don't understand . . . [with a puzzled look on his face] and you want to check her out?

   H: [with suppressed excitement in his voice] You can't hold her here.

4. I: [stretching out his right hand nearly touching Mr. Mambrino's chest] Wait a moment . . . What did the social worker tell you?

   H: She told me that Irene has checked in here and that Irene wanted her to let me know that she's here, but that she doesn't want to talk to me.

5. I: Hmm . . .

   H: She didn't even want to come to the phone when I called back.

6. I: [shrugging] Well . . .

   H: [protruding his chin] Well . . . what?

7. I: [shrugging some more and leaning slightly backwards] Seems like your wife has made her wishes clear.

   H: [steps forward half a foot] I don't believe that. That's a bunch of crap. She wouldn't dare do that! It's the social worker who put her up to that. I know those bitches. They put their noses into everything.

8. I: [raises his eyebrows] You say your wife wouldn't dare? [puzzled] I don't understand.

   H: [with emphasis] She wouldn't! She knows better than that! We have a kind of old-fashioned marriage. She knows what I expect from her. But you liberals wouldn't understand that.

9. I: [with a very low voice] Maybe you're right I don't understand.

H: [loud but less pressed] In our marriage my wife is the wife and I'm the man. She wouldn't go against me.

10. I: [leaning his head to the side with a thin slightly provoking smile] What makes you so convinced?

H: [with open anger in his voice] Listen, I don't owe you any explanation [condescending] but I'll tell you anyway.

11. I: [turns his back to the husband, walks to a chair, and sits down, stretching out his feet and looking the husband straight in the face but not saying anything]

H: When we got married my wife was quite immature. Whenever we had an argument she was on the phone to tell her mother. I put a stop to that shit.

12. I: [with mild interest] How did you do that?

H: [walking toward the interviewer and standing in front of him] I guess you don't believe me. Let me tell you what. I'll give you an example.

13. I: [interrupting] Why don't you sit down?

H: [insecure, looking around the waiting room, and finally taking a seat but sitting stiffly and bent forward] Okay, I told my wife not to call her mother anymore. The next thing I know she's writing her a letter. That was it for me.

14. I: What do you mean "That was it"?

H: I grabbed that bitch by the neck and gave her a good shake and then . . .

15. I: And then what?

H: And then I let her eat her words.

16. I: [raises his eyebrows] What do you mean?

H: I let her read the letter to me aloud and I just looked at her. When she was through, I told her: "Eat it!" She looked at me and knew that I meant it. I had her tear up the letter in pieces and eat it.

17. I: That is what you did? What did you expect to get out of that?

H: Exactly what I got. She quit doing that crap. And now she has the rules down pat.

18. I: Hmm.

H: Let me tell you a joke that my father used to tell. He was from Italy, the old country, you know.

19. I: Alright, go ahead if you have to. Why don't you sit down!

P: [Mr. Mambrino takes a seat but sits just on its edge]

There was a newly wed guy and after a few months of marriage he met his friend and his friend asked him:

"How's it going with your marriage?"

"Bad," the newly wed guy said. "My wife is doing as she pleases and I feel like a clown. She talks about me to her family and friends and makes fun of me."

The friend laughed and said: "You forgot to rip the cat apart."

When the newly wed guy said that he didn't get it, his friend said: "You see when I got married, I came home, grabbed the cat by its legs and ripped it apart. The cat was my bride's pet. She understood who's the master."

"Well," the newly wed guy said, "my wife has a cat too."

A few days later, the newly wed guy met his friend again. The friend was surprised because the newly wed guy had a black eye and wore a bandage around his neck.

"What happened?" he asked him.

"Well, I followed your advice. I came home, I grabbed the cat and killed it. My wife took a big wooden spoon, hit me in the face, and took the kettle with boiling water and threw it at me."

The friend laughed and couldn't stop laughing. "You fool, now it's too late. You should have killed the cat on your wedding night."

I never forgot that story. It stuck with me. And I thought when I get married I make sure that I wear the pants. And I do.

20. I: So . . . that kind of kids' stuff impresses you?

H: Okay, let's just stop beating around the bush. I will take my wife home, and I mean now.

21. I: But Mr. Mambrino, I don't understand you. You just heard from the social worker that your wife doesn't even want to talk to you. Why do you think she wants to go home with you now?

H: Listen, buddy, I tell you what. I want her to tell me that to my face, and then we'll see.

22. I: Your wife doesn't want to see you. Mr. Mambrino, you just heard that your wife doesn't want to talk to you face to face. Is that so hard to understand?

H: That's enough of that [he jumps up from his chair]. I consider this a case of kidnapping. If my wife is not down here in 2 minutes, you will hear from my lawyers.

23. I: [remains seated] Mr. Mambrino, that is just fine. If I can be of any help, here is the telephone.

H: Your kind really gets to me. I want to tell you something in confidence. I've been a hit man for the Mafia. It doesn't mean a thing to me to blow anyone away.

24. I: Mr. Mambrino, I realize you are angry. There is no reason for threats. You can't tear apart any cat here. I would prefer you sit down and answer a few questions about your wife. I believe you have some concern for her, even though you have a hell of a way of expressing it.

H: [stares at the interviewer; after a few seconds] Ha . . . let's see what you can come up with.

25. I: That all depends how much you can tell me to make me understand what's going on between you and your wife. You already gave me a little taste of it.

H: Damned, that was exactly what I was afraid of.

26. I: I guess you're right. If you did not get mad about all this, nothing on earth would have gotten you here to talk to us. So since you're here, we may as well make use of it.

H: Holy cow . . . I don't believe this . . . but let's get on with it.

This encounter shows some of the key features of sadistic personality disorder as described above. The interviewer uses a set of strategies that seem to work for this man.

First, whenever Mr. Mambrino makes an implied threat, the interviewer tells him that he does not understand, to force Mr. Mambrino to spell out the threat. That gives Mr. Mambrino the message that he cannot intimidate the interviewer "indirectly." That way, Mr. Mambrino is placed in a position comparable to a flasher who gets deflated when his intended victim asks him:

"Is that all you've got? Why do you show it off?"

Second, when the patient with sadistic personality disorder spells out his threats, the interviewer shows no emotion, especially not disgust, horror, or intimidation. Instead, he indicates his lack of understanding for the patient's fascination with violence. He shows him a neutral, unimpressed, "professional" side.

Third, the interviewer does not give way to the threat nor does he try to make a counterthreat. Instead, he confronts Mr. Mambrino with his aggression and tells him that nothing can be accomplished with it.

Fourth, he sidesteps the affront and focuses on a legitimate topic of conversation, namely the husband as the informant for the patient's psychiatric problems.

Sacrifice and Self-Destruction in Self-Defeating Personality Disorder

You encounter a patient with self-defeating personality disorder (once called masochistic personality disorder) under one of two sets of circumstances:

1. The patient has a clinical disorder. At the beginning of the treatment you often notice some social problems that you think can be interpreted as resulting from the major psychiatric disorder. Typical problems are related to work and to relational problems in the family. Since the patient often suffers either from a major depressive or anxiety disorder, you see her problem as the consequence of her coping deficit or her guilt feelings. However, you notice during treatment that many of the relational problems persist and that new problems surface that the patient had hidden from you previously. Thus, your view of the patient's disorder can change dramatically during treatment; increasingly, you notice that her coping deficits are due to her personality disorder.

2. A patient consults you with symptoms that superficially fit criteria for adjustment disorder with depressed, or anxious mood, or mixed emotional features, or with withdrawal or disturbance of conduct. However, at closer examination you detect that similar adjustment reactions under similar circumstances have occurred before. You notice that her prob-

lems are less specific to stress than to a coping deficit. The patient seems to arrange some of the failures, reminding you of Freud's notion that some patients seem to have a compulsion to repeat their mistakes. Behind the adjustment problem, the self-defeating personality disorder emerges.

Under both sets of circumstances the characteristics that the patient displays are the same. She sacrifices her own interests for others. She gives up her pleasure and her professional opportunities in favor of somebody else's. Her sacrifice is often not solicited, and therefore a bother to others and not appreciated, which can cause rejection. Typically, she misinterprets the reason for this rejection. She believes that she has not given enough and thus she increases contempt rather than ameliorates rejection. Dysphoric feelings and hopelessness result.

If you explore her needs and confront her with her denial of those needs, she will indicate that they are egotistical and that it is repulsive to her to pursue those needs. She seems to consider it a sin to even talk about them. If you point out how her self-denial contributes to her misery, she may reject you as materialistic and nonunderstanding, and lose interest in you.

You will find this pattern more often in physically, sexually, or psychologically abused females, and in passive men who often serve loyally in underpaid, dependent positions (Spitzer et al. 1989; Kass et al. 1989).

This is an interview with Ms. Marion T., a 38-year-old, white, separated female. She has been hospitalized and was treated with fluoxetine (Prozac); all vegetative symptoms of her major depressive disorder had improved. She could concentrate better in recreational therapy, signs of psychomotor retardation were gone and she denied depressed mood, but she still stayed by herself in her room lying on her bed. When the interviewer enters her room, she is in bed. She has a thin smile on her lips. When he walks up to her, she sinks back into her bed. She looks several years older than her stated age.

1. I: [with a soft voice] Ms. T., you have been with us here for a while; you sleep well now, you eat well, you seem to get around the hospital fine, but you look like you carry a big cross. You seem sad most of the time.

  P: Yes, I'm here in the hospital when I should be at home taking care of my kids [patient has eleven children].

2. I: Well, I'm concerned because you stay so much by yourself; that's why I thought you should stay a little while longer.

  P: But I really feel better.

3. I: That's what they say in the staff meetings, and also the recreational and the occupational therapist say that you're doing so much better.

P: I am, at least for the last week or so.

4. I: [surprised and slightly irritated] Why didn't you tell me? I talked to you every day . . .

P: I thought you would tell me when I'm ready.

5. I: [puzzled] Hmm, you said you felt overpowered by all your problems.

P: [sitting up] Yeah, but I wasn't depressed anymore.

6. I: [with doubt] But you isolated yourself and stayed in bed and . . . you're still back here in your room.

P: Because I don't want to bother others with my problems, they have enough to worry about themselves, Really, I think I should be with my kids now.

7. I: Who takes care of them now?

P: My sister and her husband. But that's not right. They shouldn't be doing that just for me. I'm really letting them down so much . . . [tears well up in her eyes].

8. I: Ms. T., you were pretty depressed. I think it's best for all of you that the family helps out.

P: [shakes her head] No, I have to go back to work to make some money for food and the rent.

9. I: What about your husband?

P: He left.

10. I: He left? . . . Why didn't you ever tell me about it?

P: I was ashamed . . . but we are still married . . .

11. I: I'm sorry to hear he left . . . How long ago did he leave?

P: Nearly a year now.

12. I: What happened?

P: Well, I guess it became too much for him.

13. I: What do you mean?

P: Well, when he came home there were always the children, always a lot of commotion, they were all over the place, I guess he just couldn't take it.

14. I: [surprised] Couldn't take it?

P: You know, he had a lot of pressure at his job and he couldn't get along with his foreman anyway and then he came home and there was some more pressure.

15. I: But they are his kids, aren't they?

P: Well—yeah, of course, we had a good marriage and it lasted for 15 years; but then when I was pregnant with John, he just couldn't take it anymore.

16. I: Couldn't take it?

P: He had the problem before; and once in a while when it got too much for him, he would just stay out.

17. I: Stay out?

P: With a lady friend of his or just with the guys from work.

18. I: How did you handle that?

P: Well, he told me there is no discipline with the kids, they are all over the place. He said it was my fault that I couldn't control them any better.

19. I: But what about him? Couldn't he help out?
    P: Well, he was at work and not around much.
20. I: And what about you?
    P: I worked too most of the time, because we couldn't pay the bills on one paycheck; but he didn't like it. He liked me to be home when he came back at night from his job.
21. I: Hmm.
    P: We argued a lot and there was a lot of fighting.
22. I: [surprised] Fighting? You never mentioned that before.
    P: I guess I felt guilty.
23. I: What were the fights about?
    P: Oh, about anything, but often about me working.
24. I: You working?
    P: Yeah . . . He said I rub it in . . . When we went bowling, I let everybody know that I had to work. It made him mad and he started fighting.
25. I: Physically?
    P: Physically and mentally. When he was drinking, he could get pretty upset.
26. I: He was drinking? That's news.
    P: Well, I'm sorry, I didn't know you and I didn't want to tattle on him.
27. I: Hmm.
    P: I must have angered him a lot.
28. I: Angered him?
    P: Yeah, he got pretty mad. I got him so angry one time that he hit me in the face and broke my nose.
29. I: Hmm.
    P: Another time he hit me in the eye and my retina came off. That's when I lost my job, because I couldn't see well enough any more to put the chips in the holes and do the soldering.
30. I: Ms. T., it sounds like you took a lot of abuse.
    P: But it was my fault, he told me. I brought it on.
31. I: What did your kids say when there was so much fighting?
    P: They got mad at him and then he got mad at me, because he said I put them up to it. So I tried to hide it from them because he's still their father and I don't want them to be caught between us.
32. I: Where is your husband now?
    P: He's around somewhere.
33. I: Does he not pay child support?
    P: He's supposed to, but he don't.
34. I: Don't you want to take him to court?
    P: No, he was my husband, and I don't believe in suing him. And I don't want to do it because of the kids . . . so I'm stuck.
35. I: Stuck? But he let you down . . . Can't you get any other kind of child support?
    P: If I apply for that, those agencies will go after him and I don't want that to happen.
36. I: But Ms. T., your husband ran away and let you hold the bag.
    P: I have to get through it. There is no need to talk about it. I just have to.

37. I: Do your older children help out?
    P: They really want to be with their high school friends, you know, go out with them and have a good time—I just have to get through with it by myself. I'm trapped, I just have to do it. There's no way out. I have to get through it.
38. I: Are you living alone with your children now?
    P: Well, kind of . . . There is a friend of mine who stays with me most of the time.
39. I: Oh, I see. Does he help out?
    P: Well, George has enough problems of his own. He's a veteran, he got injured in Vietnam, they had to amputate his foot, and he still has pain in the foot even though it's off. It really got to him mentally. He just got out of the state hospital; they said he had schizophrenia.
40. I: How do you feel about that?
    P: I feel bad about it because I'm Catholic and I think it's a sin. Because as a Catholic I'm not really divorced.
41. I: That's not what I meant. I mean how you feel about George.
    P: I feel sorry for him, because he's not able to work and he has only the V.A. pension.
42. I: So you took on an additional burden . . .
    P: I can't help him as much as I should because since I lost my job at the plant because of my bad vision, I have to work as a waitress and that doesn't pay enough to really help him out.
43. I: It appears to me that you have a hard time thinking about yourself and your own needs.
    P: I don't think one should just think about oneself. I can't just feel sorry for myself. And it wouldn't help anyway.
44. I: We should try to find out why you can't think about yourself . . .
    P: I'm not that kind of a person.

It is easy to get apparent rapport with the patient. And that is the first difficulty. She seems to open up and is ready to talk about her failures in spite of all of her efforts. That is where the interviewer can get trapped. It might escape him—as in Ms. T.'s case—that the patient carefully edits what she reports so that she appears as a victim.

Another difficulty arises when you attempt to discuss her problems and make her recognize her behavior as self-defeating. If the interviewer focuses on the underlying self-sacrificing behavior, the patient feels criticized without being able to see its pathological nature.

Self-defeating personality disorder is one of the few conditions in which expression of empathy does not work because it devalues the patient's self-sacrifice as a symptom. The patient still suffers from the nagging feeling of not investing enough. If you suggest that she is overburdened, you threaten her identity, which she cannot comprehend as pathological. If you suggest to her that she denies her needs and forgoes assertiveness to gain love and protection through sacrifice, she will be appalled by your misunderstanding of her motives. Since the patient cannot be helped without gaining insight into her behavioral traits, her personality disorder defeats effective help.

EPILOGUE

▲ ▲ ▲ ▲ ▲

Shall I tell you what knowledge is? It is to know both what one knows and what one does not know.

—Confucius, 551–479 B.C.

▼ ▼ ▼ ▼ ▼

GLOSSARY

This glossary defines those terms in the text that are not found in the DSM-IV-TR Glossary. It also expands on a few DSM-IV-TR definitions.

abreaction   Discharge of emotional tension by recalling or acting out a painful experience that had been repressed (see *catharsis*).

acalculia   Inability to do arithmetic operations, seen in parietal lobe lesions; acalculia is a type of aphasia.

activity level   The ability to make decisions, to initiate and complete actions, and feel satisfied. A variety of brain areas participate in this complex mastery: the reticular activating system contributes alertness; the limbic system regulates emotional tone and motivation; the dominant hemisphere provides various parts of memory and language functions; the frontal lobe directs control and executive functions.

agraphia   Loss of ability to communicate in writing, usually attributed to cerebral disorders and often affecting the receptive or expressive language areas.

akathisia   A condition marked by motor restlessness, ranging from anxiety to inability to lie or sit quietly or to sleep, as seen in toxic reactions to neuroleptics. It is associated with pacing, foot tapping, and walking on the spot.

amnesia

> **amnestic states**   A state of memory disturbance manifested as the inability to learn new information or to recall previously learned information.
>
> **anterograde**   Refers to forgetting of events that follow a brain insult. The patient cannot store permanently new memory traces. He is unable to recall what you have discussed with him a few minutes ago. If you repeat the same joke several times during the interview, the patient will repeatedly laugh at the punch line.

chronic, Alzheimer type   Depends on the degree of cortical involvement; patients suffer first recent and immediate memory loss; later they lose their remote memory. Relatives usually do not understand memory disturbances. They may quote as "good memory" the recollection of events in the patient's childhood.

chronic, amnestic state, Korsakoff type   Occurs when recent memory is disturbed, but immediate and remote memory are intact. Korsakoff patients may be able to lay down new memory traces, but are unable to retrieve them spontaneously. They can, however, recognize some of the material that they were exposed to.

impaired retrieval   Occurs in normal forgetting and in retrograde amnesia.

psychogenic   The patient claims inability to recall certain events or claims complete loss of memory. In spite of his claimed disability, he finds his way around, is able to learn new material, and take care of himself. Inconsistencies in his memory failure can often be detected. Hypnosis and sodium Amytal interview may lead to recovery. This type of memory disturbance is a pseudo-neurological symptom that occurs in somatization and conversion disorder and in dissociative identity disorder. Psychogenic amnesia has to be distinguished from simulation.

retrograde   The patient has forgotten events prior to a brain insult. Psychiatrists encounter that state, for instance in patients treated with electroconvulsive therapy.

simulated   The patient with antisocial personality disorder or factitious disorder may simulate amnesia to win compensation. This patient knows that he is simulating. He is usually suspicious and hostile when he feels that you as interviewer make attempts to retrieve the lost memory. Hypnosis and sodium Amytal are not helpful in this situation.

anniversary reaction   Symptoms or disturbed behavior that occur on an anniversary of a significant experience in the patient's life (often a loss).

apraxia   1) Inability to perform purposeful movements without sensory or motor impairment or 2) Inability to properly use objects.

attention   This is the ability to focus on one subject or activity. It requires the interaction of the ascending reticular activating system that regulates alertness, the frontal lobes that regulate voluntary focusing, and the limbic system that adds emotional value to the focus of attention.

body type (Kretschmer 1925; Sheldon and Stevens 1942)

> **dysplastic** Obese with abundance of fat tissue on the torso and the limbs.
>
> **ectomorphic** Predominance of the structures developed from the ectodermal layer of the embryo: slender, thin, with relatively long limbs—thought to be associated with schizophrenia.
>
> **endomorphic** Predominance of the structures developed from the endodermal layers, *pyknic type*—(fat body with protrusion of the abdomen)—thought to be associated with bipolar disorder.
>
> **mesomorphic** Predominance of the structures derived from the mesoderm, athletic body build.

catharsis A technique of freeing the mind by having a person recall a traumatic event or experience. This technique was used by Freud initially in his psychotherapy. Catharsis is a method used to bring about *abreaction*.

coma Loss of consciousness and responsiveness to outside stimuli.

concentration The ability to maintain attention to outside stimuli as well as to mental operations such as puzzle solving and calculations. The ascending reticular activating system that regulates alertness, the frontal lobes that regulate voluntary focusing, and the limbic system that adds emotional value participate in this function.

congruency of hallucinations and delusions Refers to the relationship between the content of hallucinations or delusions and the patient's prevailing mood. For example, if the mood is depressed, voices that belittle the patient, accuse, or scold him are congruent with his mood; so are delusions of chronic illness, destruction, unforgivable sin, and eternal guilt. In contrast, command hallucinations or ideas of thought insertion, of being controlled by outside forces, or of living by somebody else's will do not reflect a depressive mood—they are mood incongruent.

Related to congruency of mood is the phase relationship between presence of hallucinations or delusions and abnormal mood. If hallucinations and delusions only occur when the mood is clearly disturbed, then they are in phase; otherwise, they are out of phase.

consciousness   A state of subjective awareness and appropriate responsiveness to external stimuli. It is controlled by the ascending activating system, which originates in the reticular formation of the brain stem and extends to the cortex via the diffuse or nonspecific thalamic projection system. A lack of alertness points to involvement of subcortical centers. Isolated cortical damage does not lead to loss of alertness (for details, see Strub and Black 1993).

delusion   (compare DSM-IV-TR glossary) A fixed false belief firmly held despite obvious contradictive evidence. This belief is not ordinarily shared by others. Empirical evidence or logical arguments cannot change the patient's conviction. These ideas do not withstand reality testing. Fixed false ideas are also called *apophanous phenomena,* a term introduced by Conrad.

congruency   see *congruency.*

primary (apophany)   Experiences not deducted from other events. They take three forms: delusional mood, delusional perception, and sudden delusional (autochthonous) ideas. Delusional mood refers to the patient's feeling that he is in danger, or persecuted, or that something is brewing at work, that people are talking about him and avoid talking to him.

Delusional perception is based on a real perception to which the patient assigns a new meaning: a patient gets up during group therapy and explains that suddenly he understands communication among people. He explains that he saw a girl at a party putting her hands on her waist, spreading her index and middle finger thus forming an inversed letter "V". This meant that she wanted to make love to him. He also explained other signs: touching an earlobe means she does not want to get involved. He explained that suddenly he understands this language and can respond to it.

The primary delusional (autochthonous) idea refers to the sudden occurrence of a fully formed delusion. A patient claimed that he was looking at his fingernails and detected white spots in them. All of a sudden he understood that he was supposed to enter the race for mayor and that he should choose his sister-in-law for adviser.

Distinguish a delusional idea from delusional misinterpretations in which the perception may have a logical place within the delusional system. For instance, a patient talks to her ex-husband on the phone and hears a cracking noise in the line. She concludes that he must be making a recording to prove that she is an unfit mother.

secondary Arise from other morbid experiences, for instance, from disturbed mood or hallucinations: a patient hallucinated that she hears the voices of her family over a long distance. They tell her that she looks like an ape. She concludes that her family wants her to be an animal, so her husband can be free and can control her. In this example, the delusion is secondary to the auditory hallucination.

dysgeusia Impairment or perversion of the sense of taste. Patients with depression often report that meat has a strawlike, repugnant taste.

dyslexia A condition in a person with normal vision and normal intelligence who is unable to interpret written language.

ego-dystonic Denotes any thought content or impulse that the person experiences as not his own and not under his voluntary control and repugnant to or inconsistent with his conception of himself (its opposite is *ego-syntonic*).

ego-syntonic Denotes ideas or impulses that are acceptable to and compatible with an individual's self-perception. The person experiences them as his own and under his control.

euphoria Morbid or abnormal state of physical and emotional well-being.

euthymia Joyfulness or mental tranquility.

excitement A paroxysmal increase in motor activity. It may occur in the same disorders that are associated with stupor, namely schizophrenia, catatonic and paranoid types, and mood disorders.

manic The patient displays hostile or euphoric affect; shows flight of ideas and increase of goal-oriented and expressive movements.

paranoid Patients with schizophrenia, paranoid type may experience an increase in intensity of phonemes (hallucinations of conversing voices) and react with increased psychomotor activity.

folie à deux   Occurrence of a similar disturbance, often a delusion, in two closely associated persons occurring at the same time.

fright   Extreme sudden fear.

Gerstmann syndrome   Joseph Gerstmann (1888–1969), American neurologist, described a symptom complex: it consists of finger agnosia, right-left disorientation, acalculia, and agraphia. Additional features may be present: constructive apraxia, word-finding difficulties, disturbed ability to read, impaired color perception, absence of optokinetic nystagmus, and disturbance of equilibrium.

Gjessing's periodic catatonia   Gjessing has shown in systematically controlled investigations that motor functions, ideation, and perception in periodic catatonia are closely correlated with changing levels of positive or negative nitrogen balance. Stuporous or excited catatonic states change periodically in these patients but can be arrested by continuous administration of thyroxine (Gjessing 1946, 1953a, 1953b; Gjessing and Gjessing 1961).

hallucination   (compare DSM-IV-TR glossary) A sensory perception without an exterior stimulus occurring during wakefulness. A hallucination is different from a dream, which also contains perceptions without exterior stimuli but occurs during sleep. Hallucinations can affect all senses. There are auditory, visual, olfactory, gustatory, haptic (tactile), and vestibular hallucinations. Even hallucinations of pain may occur. The most common type of hallucination in a psychiatric population is auditory, followed by visual and haptic hallucinations. Hallucinations may occur in a subjective rather than in an objective space, such as voices may be heard in one's mind rather than outside the head. This is seen in both schizophrenia and mood disorders.

> **auditory**   Such hallucinations are also called *phonemes*. Patients with functional psychosis report three types of phonemes: 1) voices that give the patient orders (command hallucinations), which he may follow or resist; 2) voices that comment on, criticize, or praise the patient's actions and repeat his thoughts; or 3) thoughts that become audible (the technical term is a German word, *Gedankenlautwerden,* which can best be translated as *thought echo*). These three types of phonemes, listed by Kurt Schneider (1959) as so-called first-rank symptoms, were thought to be pathognomonic for schizophrenia. However, the specificity of

these hallucinations has not been verified by clinical studies. Manic patients also experience first-rank symptoms.

complexity Hallucinations vary from simple to complex. Examples of simple hallucinations are noises, light flashes, or sudden unpleasant smells or tastes (elementary hallucinations). They often occur in delirium or dementia, less often in schizophrenia. They may precede seizures, especially temporal lobe seizures, and migraine headache attacks (classic). Hallucinations can be *complex and organized,* such as music, intelligible voices and conversations, or dramatic scenes.

congruency see *congruency*

dysmegalopsia The objects in visual hallucinations may occupy more space and appear larger *(macropsia)* or smaller *(micropsia)* than in reality. Both experiences are called *dysmegalopsia.*

gustatory Hallucinations of taste are often reported by schizophrenic patients with persecutory delusions whose food tastes drugged to them, as if somebody slipped something into it (see *dysgeusia).*

haptic Perceptions of touch. They are more common in cognitive disorders. An example is the sensation that insects are crawling over the patient's skin as reported in delirium tremens due to alcohol and sedative withdrawal. This sensation may occur isolated from a visual perception and is then called *formication.*

hypnagogic Visual and auditory hallucinations that are associated with sleep-onset rapid eye movement (REM) periods. Dreamlike phenomena occur prior to sleep. These experiences are reported by patients with narcolepsy.

hypnopompic Occurs at the end of sleep (see *hypnagogic).* They are associated with REM sleep but persist after cessation of dream sleep.

mood congruency see *congruency*

olfactory Hallucinations of smell can precede seizures, especially temporal lobe seizures; they are described as elementary hallucinations of short duration, usually of unpleasant quality, like burned rubber, and they may not always be followed by a grand mal seizure. Patients with persecutory delusions suffering from either schizophrenia or cognitive disorders may report a strange smell such as of gas penetrating the house. Some patients report that they emit a foul-smelling body odor originating from their sexual organs. This may occur as a monosymptomatic hallucination. These monosymptomatic, chronic, olfactory hallucinations are often resistant to treatment with phenothiazines, tricyclics, sedatives, MAO inhibitors, carbamazepine, phenytoin, ECT, and combinations thereof. Some may respond to those neuroleptics that are also calcium channel blockers, such as pimozide (Orap).

pain   Schizophrenic patients report hallucinations of pain, such as some force tearing flesh off their bones. They also report the sensation that an animal such as a snake is eating them alive from inside their bodies. Distinguish this hallucination from a delusion. The sensation of actual pain is absent in the latter.

space and time distribution   Hallucinations may occur outside the usual sensory space. A patient may see a person exactly behind him where he normally could not see him, or the patient can hear two people conversing over hundreds of miles (without telephones). These hallucinations have been called *extracampine.*

vestibular   Visual images affected by vestibular stimulation, often seen in alcoholic hallucinations. "Under vestibular irritation, these images show changes such as occur when the subject is submitted to passive rotating movements" (Campbell 1981).

visual   These hallucinations may occur isolated or combined with auditory ones. They are more frequently encountered in acute cognitive disorders in combination with clouding of consciousness. A special form is the vision of small crawling animals (insects, mice, or rats), either seen on the floor, or on the patient's skin. This perception seems to be common in delirium due to withdrawal from sedative hypnotics or alcohol.

insight   Refers to the patient's knowledge that the symptoms of his disorder are abnormal and morbid; for instance, a patient has insight when he realizes that his hallucinations or delusions are incompatible with reality and therefore a product of an illness. He has no insight when he assigns reality to them and claims, for instance, that only he has the ability to perceive them because of his special powers.

irritability   Hypersensitivity and hyperreactivity to outside stimuli.

lability of affect   Extreme changes in affect—within minutes—occurring spontaneously or triggered by change in thought content, frequently seen in patients with cognitive or bipolar disorders.

mannerism   A peculiar modification or exaggeration in movements, speech, writing, or dressing.

memory   The ability to recall past events, experiences, facts, and impressions. It is usually subdivided.

> **immediate or short-term**   Recall of events from the last few seconds.

> **recent**   Recall of events from the last few months and days up to the last few minutes.

> **remote**   Recall of impressions from childhood and years ago. These three types of memory correspond to different brain functions needed to reproduce them: the language cortex is essential for immediate recall, limbic structures for recent memory, and the association cortex for remote memory.

mental status   Cross-sectional aspect of psychological and higher cortical functioning, as opposed to the patient's history, which reflects the longitudinal view of his psychiatric problems. The time frame of the mental status examination is the duration of the interview, whereas that of the psychiatric history is the patient's life. The history reflects the experiences reported by the patient and significant others, the mental status includes the patient's current symptoms and the objective signs and behaviors observed by the interviewer. The patient's history reflects the recurrent and stable features of mental functioning, the mental status the ever-changing here and now. Often, interviewers include phenomena such as hallucinations and delusions in their mental status examination, even if they do not occur during the interview but were present during the previous 24 hours.

mood   The feeling of pleasure or displeasure by which a person experiences himself, the outside world, and his reactions to both. Distinguish mood from affect. Affect is the external manifestation of emotion observable by you. Mood is the subjectively experienced background emotion that is not written on face and body but that you have to ask for.

> **reactivity**   Refers to mood changes due to external events, such as a depressed mood that normalizes in response to favorable experiences.

movements

athetotic Slow, coarse, and wormlike writhing, involuntary movements of the extremities; they are more pronounced in the distal than in the proximal part of a limb.

choreic or choreatic Rapid, abrupt jerking, involuntary movements that resemble parts of expressive and reactive movements.

expressive They project the patient's emotions in facial expressions, gestures, and posture.

goal-directed Necessary to accomplish all physical tasks and purposeful actions.

grooming see *spontaneous*

myoclonic Sudden muscular contractions restricted to one area of the body.

reactive They occur in response to unexpected tactile, visual, or auditory stimuli. The responder startles and flinches, and automatically turns his head toward the stimulus.

spontaneous (or grooming) They include nose and hand rubbing, ear lobe pulling, mouth covering, throat clearing, blinking, swallowing, foot tapping, pacing, nail biting, finger picking, grimacing, and stereotyped movements.

stereotyped They are carried out in a uniform way. They may resemble goal-directed or expressive movements; for instance, grimacing is a stereotyped movement of the facial muscles.

mutism Absence of speech.

akinetic The patient is mute and immobile but his eyes follow people around and can be diverted by sound. A painful stimulus sometimes evokes a reflex or weak movements but no manifestation of pain or emotion. Akinetic mutism is presumably due to incomplete interruption of the reticular activating system.

myoclonus see *movements, myoclonic*

omega sign Eyebrows drawn together with medial ends raised obliquely producing vertical and horizontal furrows on the mid-forehead. This sign is thought to indicate the presence of depression.

orientation   Refers to the patient's ability to identify himself (orientation to person), to know where he is (county, state, city, address, hospital, room number—orientation to place), and to know the time (year, month, date, and time of day—orientation to time).

paraphasia or paraphrasia   Disorder characterized by incoherent speech.

perplexity   A sign observed most commonly in cognitive disorders but sometimes also in mood and anxiety disorders. The patient shows disturbance in grasping a situation, in association, memory, attention, and will.

phonemes   see *hallucinations, auditory*

posture   Maintenance of muscle tone against gravity.

   catalepsy   The patient maintains an abnormal posture for minutes or hours. To diagnose waxy flexibility or catalepsy the patient has to be instructed to resume a resting position after his limbs have been passively moved, but he fails to do so.

   posturing   The patient holds his body in a strange position.

   waxy flexibility   The patient offers some plastic resistance to movements imposed by the examiner, and maintains the final posture for some time.

pseudohallucination   The term has several meanings. Hallucinations may be perceived in a subjective rather than in an objective space: "It is a voice in my mind," rather than "I hear the voice like I hear your voice." The patient may deny that his perception has the same quality as a real perception. He may feel that he has control over it, can make it appear and disappear, or he has insight and can identify it as a hallucination.

pseudoseizure   A clinical event that resembles a grand mal seizure but lacks essential components of it, such as electroencephalic changes, and has clinical features incompatible with a grand mal seizure, such as being induced or stopped by a simple command or a hypnotic suggestion. Such patients often claim they can hear and see what is going on in their environment but they cannot respond. Self-injuries from a fall, tongue biting, and incontinence are extremely rare.

simulation   Pretense of having a disease, or a symptom.

speech   The mechanical forming of words by the muscular apparatus of the mouth, tongue, diaphragm, and vocal cords, and by the central directing and organizing functions of the speech centers in the dominant hemisphere of the brain.

> **concept of words**   The way words are used. If words are used correctly in the conventional manner and with the right level of abstraction.
>
> **flow**   The continuity of verbal production.
>
> **mumbled**   Hesitant speech with low intensity, poor articulation, and unnatural pauses and slowing (Huntington's chorea).
>
> **neologism**   A newly coined meaningless word.
>
> **paraphasic**   Speech in which the patient substitutes the correct word with a wrong word. This wrong word may be invented; for example, "I write a letter with my cryston" (neologistic paraphasia). The wrong word may be correct semantically but not logically; for example, "I write a letter with my car" (semantic paraphasia). The wrong word may show the substitution of only one otherwise correct letter; for example, "I write a letter with my nen" (literal paraphasia).
>
> **pressure of speech**   The patient has the urge to continue talking; he cannot be interrupted.
>
> **push of speech**   No pauses exist among words and sentences. Words are incomplete and flow into each other and a great deal is said in a short period of time. The patient can be interrupted, if not combined with pressure of speech.
>
> **retarded**   Slow, with many pauses.
>
> **scanning**   Vowels and sounding consonants (m, n) are stretched. Speech is slow with sliding cadence (multiple sclerosis).
>
> **staccato**   The opposite of scanning speech—consists of words that are clipped and abruptly presented (psychomotor epilepsy).

stressor   A stressor is a stimulus that taxes the patient's ability to respond. Be aware of the circularity: a stressor is what causes an intense reaction; an intense reaction identifies a stressor. A stressor may be related to a psychiatric disorder in six different ways: 1) time marker, 2) magnifier, 3) consequence, 4) pathological thought content, 5) trigger, or 6) cause of a dysfunction.

time marker   The patient considers a life event as the "cause" of his disorder, but reveals that the event merely occurred at the same time, often after the onset of the disorder.

magnifier   The stressor is part of the patient's routine life but suddenly he is unable to deal with it. The stressor reveals and magnifies the patient's dysfunction. For instance, a patient who could previously take over the responsibilities of a vacationing colleague cannot do so when depressed. He may blame the increased work load as the cause of his depression, rather than the depression as a cause for his inability to cope.

consequence   Divorce or job loss reported as the precipitating event of a mental disorder are in fact its result. Analysis of the sequence of events reveals, for instance, that the disorder preceded the event. The irritability, social withdrawal, and decreased sex drive associated with depression did result in marital discord or divorce rather than the divorce resulting in depression.

pathological thought content   During a depressive episode some patients who experience guilt feelings screen their past for reasons to feel bad. Sometimes these reasons are quite delusional in character. For instance:

"When I was 5 years old, I stole a stamp. Now people found out and I have to suffer the consequences. That makes me depressed."

Others may talk about recent bad news that pulls them down. Recognize these reasons as a secondary filling, that is, the fitting of a content to the pessimistic outlook typical for depression.

trigger   A stressor may be a trigger of a psychiatric disorder if the patient has a predisposition for the psychiatric disorder. Such a stressor may be a disabling medical disorder, personal loss, or job loss. Females may also report the onset of a depressive episode after a biological and psychological stressor such as childbirth (postpartum depression) or after the onset of menopause (involutional depression). However, the literature is controversial with respect to such a trigger function of a stressor.

cause According to DSM-IV-TR, two types of disorders are caused by stressors: posttraumatic stress disorder and adjustment disorder. Posttraumatic stress disorder requires extraordinary stressors like earthquakes, floods, war, rape, or atrocities. An adjustment disorder may be caused by a more common stressor such as physical illness, job loss, or loss of support. If you encounter such a stressor, examine the patient's response. For symptoms and signs of both disorders, see DSM-IV-TR.

It is unknown what makes these stressors pathogenic for some people but not for others. It is also not clear what makes them more noxious at one but not at another time. Before you accept a stressor as sufficient cause of an adjustment disorder, exclude alternate possibilities.

stupor

1. Level of alertness: the patient appears unconscious and responds to pain only with some defensive movements or utterances. This is usually due to interruption of the impulses from the reticular activating system of the pons and midbrain to the cortex.
2. Special psychiatric condition: psychogenic stupor occurs as a fright reaction. The patient appears motionless and mute, but is alert without incontinence of urine or feces. Hypnosis or sodium Amytal will interrupt this state.
3. In stupor due to a medical condition, such as akinetic mutism, space-occupying lesions of the third ventricle, the thalamus, or the midbrain can be found. These patients appear alert, react slightly to pain, but are unable to talk or follow commands. Patients usually have complete amnesia for this state if they recover. Some stuporous states are associated with repeated bursts of discharges in the EEG similar to grand mal seizures, or spike and wave charges. In Gjessing's periodic catatonia, slow waves in the EEG have been described.

   catatonic The patient is mute, has increased muscle tension especially in the anterior neck muscles, masseters, and the muscles around the mouth, giving rise to the so-called snout spasm. The patient does not respond to painful stimuli or anesthesia, is incontinent of urine, and may show catalepsy. The patient is usually alert. Sodium Amytal injections may break the muteness, as does ECT.

   depressive The patient may appear confused, perplexed, and bewildered. There is usually no obstruction, opposition, catalepsy, or increase in muscle tension. The patient is alert, but appears depressed. There is no incontinence of urine or feces; response to emotional stimuli is present. Most stuporous patients should have an EEG and lumbar puncture to rule out medical causes.

suggestibility A condition in which a person responds readily to suggestions or opinions of others to the point of uncritical acceptance.

tardive dyskinesia A neuroleptic-induced, often irreversible movement disorder. It presents with mouth smacking, rotating tongue movements, and flapping finger movements, and can progressively involve the trunk and limbs.

thinking

> **abstract** The ability to use symbols such as "dog" and to generalize to a class of symbols such as "a dog is a four-legged barking animal."

> **concrete** The inability to abstract.

> **thought blocking** Sudden involuntary cessation in the train of thought.

torpor Abnormal inactivity, dormancy, numbness, apathy.

transference The unconscious shifting of an affect and behavior pattern from one person to another; especially the transfer of the patient's emotion originally directed toward parental figures to the therapist as a result of unconscious identification.

tremor Rapid alternation of contraction of antagonistic muscle groups of the eyelids, tongue, lips, head, upper trunk, extremities, and hands. Tremors can be classified by their frequency, amplitude, regularity, and relationship to volitional movements. The latter criterion is customarily used in most descriptions.

> **action** Occurs when the limb is voluntarily maintained in a certain position. It disappears when the limb is relaxed. Normal people have very fine action tremor. It is 6 counts per second in children, and 10 counts per second in adults.

> **hepatic flapping** A special form of an action tremor. It is best demonstrated when the patient's hands are held in front of the body and sharply dorsiflexed, with the fingers maximally spread apart. Periodically, the

hands will fall due to gravity. Voluntary attempts to bring them back into position leads to bursts of rapid, arrhythmic flexion and extension movements (asterixis).

intention   A tremor that occurs with movements. It often increases near the end of the completion of the movement. If a patient is asked to touch the examiner's finger, the patient's finger may oscillate more and more the closer it comes to the goal.

static or resting   Occurs when a limb is in repose. It shows 3–7 beats per second and is suppressed temporarily with voluntary movements. Therefore it does not interfere much with voluntary motor acts such as writing.

Verhältnisblödsinn   Discordance between ambition and comprehension, between desire and capabilities. Many patients with Verhältnisblödsinn continuously start new businesses, persuade others with false arguments to invest money into their ventures, and then lose financial control, fail everywhere, and involve others in their downfall. Some patients obtain large grants or scholarships to presumably develop artistic talents that they don't have. The intelligence of patients with Verhältnisblödsinn suffices for a modest social level; however, such patients maneuver themselves into positions that they can't fill. Many of these patients have confused thinking (translated from Bleuler 1972, p. 585).

vigilance   The ability to sustain attention to an outward stimulus over some arbitrary time period.

waxy flexibility   Often seen in catalepsy, permitting the limbs to be molded into unusual positions in which they persist.

word salad   Continuous, senseless word fluency without pauses and with incorrect nouns. Consecutive words are not linked by meaning. Word salad is frequently an indication of damage of Wernicke's speech center in the dominant temporal lobe.

The Executive Interview (EXIT) and the Qualitative Evaluation of Dementia (QED)

The disturbance of executive control functions is an important diagnostic criterion of dementia as defined in DSM-IV-TR (American Psychiatric Association 2000). Royall et al. (1992) developed an instrument, called the Executive Interview (EXIT), to measure these functions at the bedside. They also developed a rating scale, the Qualitative Evaluation of Dementia (QED; Royall et al. 1993), which separates dementia into two clinical types—the cortical type, which is characterized by disinhibition, and the subcortical type, which is characterized by apathy. Although it remains to be seen whether these represent homogeneous subtypes, they provide the clinician with an operational procedure to assess and describe qualitative differences in cognition and behavior.

The Executive Interview (EXIT)

Patient's name: _____

Date: _____

Age: _____

Sex: _____

Diagnosis: _____

Education level in years: _____

TOTAL TEST SCORE: _____

Global Testing Observations

During the interview, record signs and behaviors that indicate a disturbance of executive functions. Seven types of pathological behaviors can be observed:

1. Perseveration
2. Imitation behavior
3. Intrusion
4. Frontal release signs
5. Lack of spontaneity/prompting needed
6. Disinhibited behavior
7. Utilization behavior

Source. From Royall DR, Mahurin RK, Gray KF: "Bedside Assessment of Executive Cognitive Impairment: The Executive Interview." *Journal of the American Geriatrics Society* 40:1221–1226, 1992. Used with permission. Edited, adapted, supplemented, and reformatted for this book by Ekkehard and Sieglinde C. Othmer. We thank Drs. Royall et al. for granting us permission for use of this instrument here.

Notice that each of the 25 test items of the EXIT may reflect one or more pathological behaviors. We give short definitions of the seven types as they apply to the EXIT and examples for each below. (I = interviewer; P = patient)

1. Perseveration. Patient responds with a requested behavior but repeats it over and over, inappropriately.

Examples
  Test Item 1:
    P: 1A, 1A, 1A.
    or, P: 1A, 1B, 1C.
    or, P: 1A, 2A, 3A.
  Test Item 2:
    P: America, America, America.
  Test Item 3:
    P copies one of the test examples or one of his/her own pictures over and over.

2. Imitation behavior. Patient repeats the interviewer's words (echolalia) or behaviors (echopraxia) rather than responding to them.

Examples
  Test Item 1:
    I: 1A, 2B, 3—?
    P: 1A, 2B, 3—?
  Test Item 2:
    P: People, pot, plan.
  Test Item 3:
    Patient copies both test figures.
  Test Items 16, 20, 25:
    Pathological response.

3. Intrusion. Inappropriately, patient includes items of a previous task in his/her response.

Examples
  Test Item 2:
    Watch for intrusion from the local environment.
    P: America, axe, bird, chirping, nest . . .

Test Item 3:
   The patient starts one or two figures but then begins to draw related fig-
   ures, such as cross, box, window, house, tree, car.
Test Items 6 and 7:
   Pathological responses.

4.   Frontal release signs.   These are reflexes that occur in patients with
frontal lobe damage. Two of these frontal release signs, the grasp reflex and
the snout reflex, are tested in test Items 10 and 13, respectively.

Examples
Test Item 10:
   Pathological response. Note when the patient's grasp is so firm that you
   can draw him/her out of the chair.
Test Item 13:
   Pathological response. Note if the patient, in addition to a snout reflex,
   shows puckering even before tapping (suck reflex).

5.   Lack of spontaneity.   The interviewer has to encourage the patient
again and again to respond to the tasks. The patient responds with a long
latency time. He/she gives only one response when a series of responses is
requested.

Examples
Test Item 1:
   P: 1
   I: And what letter?
   P: A.
   I: What comes next?
   P: 2.
   Patient answers correctly but needs prompting to go on.
Test Item 5:
   Pathological response.
Test Item 22:
   P: December *[and looks at the interviewer]*
   I: Keep going!
   P: November *[then stops again]*

6.   Disinhibited behavior.   The patient responds as requested but ignores
limiting test specifications.

Examples

Test Item 1:
   The patient continues after the stop signal has been given, such as saying, "6F, 7G, 8H."

Test Item 2:
   P: America, America *[starts singing "God shed his grace on thee, and
   bound thy good with brotherhood from sea to shining sea."]*

Test Item 4:
   Pathological response.

Test Item 25:
   P: *[Touches interviewer's wrist]* "Wrist."

7. Utilization behavior. The patient substitutes the logical or the requested response with a response that reflects a social habit or frequent
usage.

Examples

Test Item 3:
   P looks at the sheet and signs his/her name.

Test Item 11:
   P: You are welcome.

Test Item 24:
   Pathological response.

Materials Needed for the EXIT

- Stopwatch
- Three test cards with test Items 5 (cat chasing bird), 7 (brown), and 23
  (four fish and shell)
- Two recording sheets for test Items 2 (word fluency) and 3 (design fluency)

Test instructions	0	1	2	Score
1. NUMBER-LETTER TASK I: I'd like you to say some numbers and letters for me like this: "1A, 2B, 3"—What would come next? P: C. I: Now you try it, starting with the number 1. Keep going until I say stop. P: 1A, 2B, 3C, 4D, 5E . . . . I: Stop.	No errors	Needs prompting	Does not complete task	
2. WORD FLUENCY I: I'm going to give you a letter. You have ONE MINUTE to name as many words as you can think of that begin with that letter. For example, with the letter *P* you could say "people," "pot," "plan," and so on. The letter is *A*. Go! *[Start stopwatch, record P's words on Recording Sheet 1 for word fluency (see p. 504) and stop after 1 minute.]*	10 or more words	5–9 words	Fewer than 5 words	
3. DESIGN FLUENCY *[Draw two pictures on Recording Sheet 2 (see p. 505).]* I: Look at these pictures. Each is made with only four lines. I'm going to give you ONE MINUTE to draw as many different designs as you can. They each must be different and be drawn with four lines. Now, go! *[Hand P Recording Sheet 2, on which you drew the two designs. Then start the stopwatch and stop after 1 minute. Correct figures can contain curves.]*	10 or more unique drawings, no copies of examples	5–9 unique drawings	Fewer than 5 unique drawings	

	No errors	One or more errors	Continues one or more sentences
4. **ANOMALOUS SENTENCE REPETITION** I: Listen very carefully and repeat these sentences exactly: 1) I pledge allegiance to those flags. 2) Mary fed a little lamb. 3) A stitch in time saves lives. 4) Tinkle, tinkle little star. 5) A B C D U F G.	No errors	One or more errors	Continues one or more sentences (e.g., "Mary had a little lamb whose fleece was white as snow.")
5. **THEMATIC PERCEPTION** [*Show P the picture of the cat chasing the bird.*] I: Tell me what is happening in the picture.	Tells spontaneous story (story = setting, three characters, action)	Tells story with one prompt ("anything else?")	Fails to tell story despite prompt
6. **MEMORY/DISTRACTION TASK** I: Remember these three words: book, tree, house. [*Have P repeat words until they are registered.*] Remember them. I'll ask you to repeat them later. Now, spell *cat* for me. . . . Good. Now, spell it backward. OK. Tell me those three words we learned.	Names all three words correctly without *cat* [*I may prompt, "Anything else?"*]	Other responses (describe)	Names *cat* as one of the three words (intrusion)
7. **INTERFERENCE TASK** [*Show the card with the word* brown *and sweep index finger over all letters.*] I: What color are these letters?	Black	P: Brown [*Repeat question once*]; P: Black.	P: Brown [*Prompt*]; P: Brown (intrusion)
8. **AUTOMATIC BEHAVIOR I** I: Please, hold your hands forward, palms down. Relax while I check your reflexes. [*Rotate P's arms one at a time at the elbow as if to check for cogwheeling. Gauge P's active participation/anticipation of the rotation.*]	Remains passive	Equivocal	Actively copies the circular motion

Note. I = interviewer; P = patient.

Test instructions	0	1	2	Score
9. AUTOMATIC BEHAVIOR II I: Please, hold your hands out palms up. Just relax. [*Push down on P's hands—gently at first, becoming more forceful. Gauge P's active participation in the response.*]	No resistance, remains passive	Equivocal	Active resistance or compliance	
10. GRASP REFLEX I: Please hold your hands out with open palms down. Just relax. [*Lightly and simultaneously stroke both palms of P's hands from roots to fingertips with both of your hands palms up, fingers gently curved upward. Look for grasping/gripping actions in P's fingers.*]	Absent	Equivocal	Present	
11. SOCIAL HABIT [*Fixate on P's eyes. Silently count to 3 while maintaining P's gaze. Then say:*] I: Thank you.	Replies with a question (e.g., "Thank you for what?")	Other responses (describe)	P: You're welcome.	
12. MOTOR IMPERSISTENCE I: Stick out your tongue and say "aah" until I say stop . . . Go! [*Count to 3 silently. P must sustain a constant tone, not "ab . . . ab . . . ab . . ."*]	Completes task spontaneously	Completes task with I modeling task for patient	Fails task despite modeling by I	
13. SNOUT REFLEX I: Just relax. [*Slowly bring your index finger toward P's lips, pausing momentarily 2 inches away. Then place finger vertically across lips, touching lips, and tap the finger lightly with the other hand so that the crossed finger touches P's upper lip. Observe lips for puckering before and after the tapping.*]	Not present	Equivocal	Present	

14. **FINGER-NOSE-FINGER TASK** [Hold up your index finger.]

I: Touch my finger. [Leaving your finger in place, say:]

I: Now touch your nose.

Complies, using same hand	Other response (describe)	Complies, using other hand while continuing to touch examiner's finger

15. **GO/NO-GO TASK**

I: Now when I touch my nose, you raise your finger like this. [Raise your index finger (F).] When I raise my finger, you touch your nose like this. [Touch your nose (N) with index finger.]

I: Please, repeat my instructions. [Begin task. Leave finger in place while awaiting P's response. Circle P's response. Left column shows P's correct responses.]

Interviewer	Patient	
F	N	F
N	F	N
F	N	F
F	N	F
N	F	N

Performs sequence correctly, e.g., N-F-N-F	Correct, requires prompting/repeat of instructions	Fails sequence despite prompting/repeat of instructions

16. **ECHOPRAXIA I**

I: Now listen carefully. I want you to do exactly what I say. Ready? Touch your ear! [Touch your nose and keep finger there.]

Touches his/her ear	Other response (describe). [Look for midposition stance]	Touches his/her nose

Note. I = interviewer; P = patient.

Test instructions	0	1	2	Score
17. LURIA HAND SEQUENCE I I: Can you do this? *[In the air, make a single hammering-like movement with your arm, the hand forming a fist. Then repeat the arm motion with an open palm, making a cutting motion. Alternate between hammering and cutting hand motions. Stop movement. P may use either arm.]*	Four cycles without error after I stops	Four cycles with additional verbal prompt ("Keep going") or modeling	Unsuccessful despite prompting/modeling *[Watch for mid-position stances.]*	
18. LURIA HAND SEQUENCE II I: Can you do this? *[Model three hand movements on your knee or table surface: 1) slapping with palm, 2) hammering with fist, 3) cutting with edge of opened hand.]* I: Now follow me. *[Repeat the sequence of three movements.]* I: Keep doing this until I say stop. *[Stop, let P repeat three cycles, then ask P to stop.]*	Three cycles without error after I stops	Three cycles with additional verbal prompt ("Keep going") or modeling	Unsuccessful	
19. GRIP TASK *[With both hands, form a pistol (e.g., a fist with stretched index finger and erected thumb). Point both index fingers toward each other in front of yourself, leaving a 1-inch space between the index fingers.]* I: Squeeze my fingers.	Grips fingers	Other response (describe)	Pulls I's hands together	
20. ECHOPRAXIA II *[Suddenly and without warning, slap your hands together.]*	Does not imitate I	Hesitates, uncertain	Imitates slap	

21. COMPLEX COMMAND TASK I: Put your left hand on top of your head and close your eyes. . . . That was good. *[Remain aloof; quickly begin next task.]*	Stops when next task begins	Equivocal—holds posture during part of next task	Maintains posture throughout completion of next task—has to be told to cease
22. SERIAL ORDER REVERSAL TASK I: Please recite the months of the year. *[Disregard P's errors.]* I: Now, start with January and recite them backward! *[Ask P to stop after September if correctly recited.]*	Recites January, December November, October, September . . . . I: Stop!	Correct response but with prompting	Unsuccessful despite prompting
23. COUNTING TASK *[Show P the fish picture.]* *Tap each item in a clockwise direction.]* I: Please count the fish in this picture out loud.	Four	Fewer than four	More than four
24. UTILIZATION BEHAVIOR *[Hold a pen near its point and dramatically present it to the patient asking:]* I: What is this called?	P: Pen	Reaches, hesitates	Takes the pen from I
25. IMITATION BEHAVIOR (ECHOPRAXIA III) *[Hold your wrist up, flex it up and down, and point to it.]* I: What is this called?	P: Wrist	Other response (describe)	Flexes wrist up and down

SCORE

TOTAL SCORE

Note. I = interviewer; P = patient.

EXIT Recording Sheet 1 for Test Item 2: Word Fluency

Write down all words that P gives you within 1 minute.

1. _____

2. _____

3. _____

4. _____

5. _____

6. _____

7. _____

8. _____

9. _____

10. _____

EXIT Recording Sheet 2 for Test Item 3: Design Fluency

Draw two pictures using only four lines for each.

EXIT Scores and Activity of Daily Living (ADL)

EXIT scores	ADL
0–10	Independent, normal, unsupervised living of control subjects (normal 11-year-old and older)
11–12	Equivocal
13–17	Living with minimal supervision in apartments, using parking space and kitchen appropriately (normal 8- to 10-year-old)
18–23	Group home, residential care, no driving, not institutionalized, common dining, no independent shopping or cooking (normal grade schooler)
24–32	Skilled nursing facility, institutionalized, nurses, charts, fed on the unit, rehabilitation activity (normal preschooler)
33–50	Dementia of the Alzheimer's type, special care units

Test card for Item 5

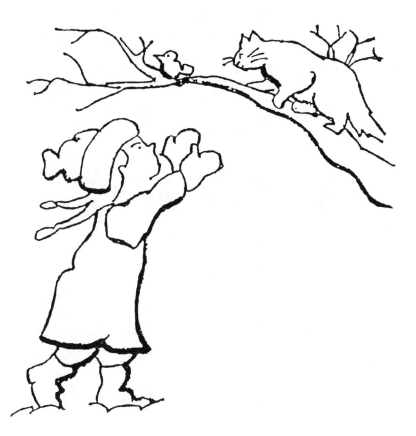

Test card for Item 7

brown

Test card for Item 23

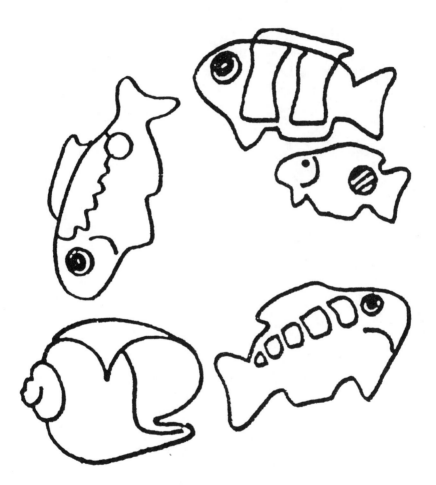

Qualitative Evaluation of Dementia (QED)

The Qualitative Evaluation of Dementia (QED) is an instrument designed to operationalize, standardize, and quantify the clinical concepts of cortical and subcortical dementia. The classical example of a predominantly cortical dementia is dementia of the Alzheimer's type; examples of predominantly subcortical dementias include vascular dementia and dementia due to major depressive disorder. This subtyping of dementia overlaps and parallels the subtyping of irreversible and reversible dementia, active and passive dementia, and disinhibited and apathetic dementia.

The QED discriminated patients with probable dementia of the Alzheimer's type (n = 17) from 1) those with no dementia as defined by criteria of the National Institute of Neurological and Communicative Disorders and Stroke (NINCDS) and the Alzheimer Disease and Related Disorders Association (n = 22), and 2) dementia patients without evidence of aphasia, agnosia, constructional apraxia, or memory deficits who did not improve with prompting (n = 46) (Royall et al. 1993). In another study, the QED distinguished 29 subjects with dementia due to major depressive disorder from 35 subjects with either dementia due to probable Alzheimer's disease (n = 22) or frontal lobe–type dementia (n = 13). The latter two cortical dementias could not be discriminated (Royall et al. 1994).

Source. Reprinted from Royall DR, Mahurin RK, Cornell J, et al.: "Bedside Assessment of Dementia Type Using the Qualitative Evaluation of Dementia." *Neuropsychiatry, Neuropsychology, and Behavioral Neurology* 6:235–244, 1993. Used with permission. We thank Drs. Royall et al. for granting us permission to reproduce this instrument here.

Directions

For each domain, first determine if an abnormality exists. If not, rate **NORMAL = 1.** If deficit is present, you **MUST** choose between the available alternatives. If insufficient information is available, rate as 1.

Domain	Clinical features			Score
	0	1	2	
Interview	Not spontaneous Short replies Little elaboration	Normal	Spontaneous and/or tangential. May be pressured	
Interview	Led to interview Little participation Prompting needed	Normal	Disinhibited Socially adroit but inappropriate	
Memory	Recalls 1–2 of 3 words spontaneously aided by prompting	Normal	Unable to recall 3 words after distraction. Not aided by prompts	
Orientation	Disoriented to time only	Normal	Disoriented to location or person	
Language	Word finding or mild comprehension deficits only	Normal	Paraphasias Poor comprehension Fluent or nonfluent aphasia, vague or empty speech	
Speech	Dysarthric Hypophonic	Normal	Perseverative, flat, effortful, or mumbling	
Frontal release	Gegenhalten or motor soft signs but no snout or grasp	Normal	Snout or grasp present	
Judgment	Worried, complains, ruminates Says "I don't know" or "I can't"	Normal concern	Little insight Denies deficits Confabulates	

TOTAL PAGE 1

Domain	Clinical features			Score
	0	**1**	**2**	
Constructions (See Mini-Mental State Exam [Folstein et al. 1975])	Recognizable but distorted by flattening or omissions	Normal	Unrecognizable Disorganized	
Praxis	Rarely initiates self-care/household chores, but does well if prompted	Normal	Tries to participate in self-care/household chores, but uses tools/appliances inappropriately	
Motor/gait	Shuffling Dyskinetic "Apractic" Prominent tremor	Normal	Spastic Hemiparetic or ataxic	
Mood	Depressed Apathetic Cries without provocation	Normal	Can be outgoing, even euphoric at times Sings, claps, can be prone to catastrophic reactions	
Behavior	Sits around Needs prompting or encouragement	Normal	Into trouble Habit driven Environmentally dependent Resists change Wanders	
Personal care	Cares for himself/herself, but disheveled, inattentive to details or appearance	Normal	Requires personal assistance in dressing, bathing, or toileting	
Community affairs	Rarely asks to leave house, room, unit	Normal	Goes out but needs constant supervision at home or in public Easily lost, anxious, or confused	

TOTAL PAGE 2

QED TOTAL

A QED score of 0 indicates pure subcortical dementia characterized by apathy, and a score of 30 indicates pure cortical dementia characterized by disinhibition. A score of 15 indicates normal function.

BIBLIOGRAPHY

Adler A: Problems of Neurosis. New York, Harper & Row, 1964

Akiskal HS, Webb WL (eds): Psychiatric Diagnosis: Exploration of Biological Predictors. New York, SP Medical & Scientific Books, 1978

American Psychiatric Association: Diagnostic and Statistical Manual of Mental Disorders, 2nd Edition. Washington, DC, American Psychiatric Association 1968

American Psychiatric Association: Diagnostic and Statistical Manual of Mental Disorders, 3rd Edition. Washington, DC, American Psychiatric Association, 1980

American Psychiatric Association: Draft, DSM-III-R in development (10/5/85). Washington, DC, American Psychiatric Association, 1985

American Psychiatric Association: Diagnostic and Statistical Manual of Mental Disorders, 3rd Edition, Revised. Washington, DC, American Psychiatric Association, 1987

American Psychiatric Association: DSM-IV Draft Criteria (3/1/93). Washington, DC, American Psychiatric Association, 1993

American Psychiatric Association: Diagnostic and Statistical Manual of Mental Disorders, 4th Edition. Washington, DC, American Psychiatric Association, 1994

American Psychiatric Association: Diagnostic and Statistical Manual of Mental Disorders, 4th Edition, Text Revision. Washington, DC, American Psychiatric Association, 2000

Arnold WN: Vincent van Gogh: Chemicals, Crises, and Creativity. Boston, MA, Birkhäuser, 1992

Baker AB, Joynt RJ (eds): Clinical Neurology, Revised Edition, Vols. 1 & 2. Philadelphia, PA, Harper & Row, 1985

Bandler R, Grinder J: Frogs into princes, in Neurolinguistic Programming. Edited by Stevens, JO. Moab, UT, Real People Press, 1979

Barrett J, Hurst MW, Discola C, et al: Prevalence of depression over a 12-month period in a nonpatient population. Arch Gen Psychiatry 35: 741–744, 1978

Ben-Yishay Y, Diller L, Gerstman L, et al: The relationship between impersistence, intellectual function and outcome of rehabilitation in patients with left hemiplegia. Neurology 18:852–861, 1968

Berne E: Transactional Analysis in Psychotherapy. New York, Grove Press, 1961

Berne E: Games People Play. New York, Grove Press, 1964

Black DW, Noyes R, Phohl B, et al: Personality disorder in obsessive-compulsive volunteers, well comparison subjects, and their first-degree relatives. Am J Psychiatry 150:1226–1232, 1993

Bleuler E: Lehrbuch der Psychiatrie, 12th Edition. Revised by M. Bleuler. Berlin, Springer-Verlag, 1972

Boxer PA: Assessment of potential violence in the paranoid worker. J Occup Med 35: 127–131, 1993

Cameron N: Personality Development and Psychopathology: A Dynamic Approach. Boston, MA, Houghton Mifflin, 1963

Cameron N: Experimental analysis of schizophrenic thinking, in Language and Thought in Schizophrenia. Edited by Kasanin JS. New York, WW Norton, 1964

Cameron-Bandler L: They Lived Happily Ever After. Cupertino, CA, Meta Publications, 1978

Campbell RJ: Psychiatric Dictionary, 5th Edition. New York, Oxford University Press, 1981

Chapman J, McGhie A: Echopraxia in schizophrenia. Br J Psychiatry 110: 365–374, 1964

Cohen S, Chiles J, MacNaughton A: Weight gain associated with clozapine. Am J Psychiatry 147:503–504, 1990

Confucius: The Sayings of Confucius. Translated by Ware JR. New York, New American Library, Mentor Books, 1955

Cormier WH, Cormier LS: Interviewing Strategies for Helpers. 2nd Edition. Monterey, CA, Brooks/Cole, 1985

Corsini RJ: Current Psychotherapies. Edited by Wedding D. Itasca, IL, FE Peacock Publishers, 1984

Cox A, Hopkinson K, Rutter M: Psychiatric interviewing techniques II: naturalistic study: eliciting factual information. Br J Psychiatry 138:283–291, 1981

Cox A, Rutter M: 1985. Diagnostic appraisal and interviewing, in Child and Adolescent Psychiatry: Modern Approaches, 2nd Edition. Edited by Rutter M, Hersov, L. Oxford, England, Blackwell Scientific, 1985

Cox A, Rutter M, Holbrook D: Psychiatric interviewing techniques. A second experimental study: eliciting feelings. Br J Psychiatry 152:64–72, 1988

Critchley M: The Parietal Lobes. New York, Hafner Press, 1953

Darwin C: The Expression of the Emotions in Man and Animals (1872). With a preface by Konrad Lorenz. Chicago, IL, University of Chicago Press, 1965

DeBetz B, Sunnen G: A Primer of Clinical Hypnosis. Littleton, MA, PSG Publishing, 1985.

Dijkstra W, Van der Veen L, Van der Zouwen J: A field experience on interviewer-respondent interaction, in Research Interview: Uses and Approaches. Edited by Brenner M, Brown I, Canter D. London, Academic Press, 1985

Dobson KS (ed): Handbook of Cognitive-Behavioral Therapies. New York, Guilford, 1988

Dubois P: The psychological origin of mental disorders. New York, Funk and Wagnalls, 1913

Edward RH, Simon RP: Coma, in Clinical Neurology, Vol 2, Revised. Edited by Joynt RJ. Philadelphia, PA, JB Lippincott, 1992

Ekman P: Autonomic nervous system activity distinguishes among emotions. Science 221:1208–1210, 1983

Eppright TD, Kashani JH, Robinson BD, et al: Identity: Comorbidity of conduct disorder and personality disorders in an incarcerated juvenile population. Am J Psychiatry 150:1233–1236, 1993

Erikson E: Identity: Youth and Crisis. New York, WW Norton, 1969

Fenichel O: The Psychoanalytic Theory of Neurosis. New York, WW Norton, 1945

Fish F: Clinical Psychopathology. Bristol, England, John Wright, 1967

Folstein MF, Folstein SE, McHugh PR: Mini-mental state: a practical method for grading the cognitive state of patients for the clinician. J Psychiatr Res 12:189–198, 1975

Foulds GA: The Hierarchical Nature of Personal Illness. New York, Academic Press, 1976

Franklin J: The diagnosis of multiple personality based on subtle dissociative signs. J Nerv Ment Dis 178:4–14, 1990

Freedman AM, Kaplan HE, Sadock BJ: Comprehensive Textbook of Psychiatry, 2nd Edition, Vols. 1 & 2, Baltimore, MD, Williams & Wilkins, 1975

Freud A: The Ego and the Mechanisms of Defense. Translated by Baines C. New York, International Universities Press, 1946

Freud S: Gesammelte Werke chronologisch geordnet, Vols 1–17. London, Imago Publishing, 1952–1955

Frosch JP (ed): Current Perspectives on Personality Disorders. Washington, DC, American Psychiatric Press, 1983

Fulton M, Winokur G: A comparative study of paranoid and schizoid personality disorders. Am J Psychiatry 150:1363–1367, 1993

Gauron EF, Dickinson JK: Diagnostic decision making in psychiatry: I. Information usage. Arch Gen Psychiatry 14:225–232, 1966a

Gauron EF, Dickinson JK: Diagnostic decision making in psychiatry: II. Diagnostic styles. Arch Gen Psychiatry 14:233–237, 1966b

Gedo MM: Picasso: Art as Autobiography. Chicago, IL, University of Chicago Press, 1980

Gjessing R: II: Biological investigations in psychoses. Introductory lecture. Biological investigations in endogenous psychoses. Acta Psychiatr Neurol Scand Suppl 47:93–104, 1946

Gjessing R: Beiträge zur Somatologie der periodischen Katatonie. Mitteilung VII. Archiv für Psychiatrie und Nervenkrankheiten 191:247, 1953a

Gjessing R: Beiträge zur Somatologie der periodischen Katatonie. Mitteilung VIII. Archiv für Psychiatrie und Nervenkrankheiten 191:297, 1953b

Gjessing R, Gjessing L: Some main trends in the clinical aspects of periodic catatonia. Acta Psychiatr Scand 37:1–13, 1961

Golden CJ, Purish AD, Hammeke TA: Luria-Nebraska Neuropsychological Battery (LNNB). Los Angeles, CA, Western Psychological Services, 1991

Goldstein K: Methodological approach to the study of schizophrenic thought disorder, in Language and Thought in Schizophrenia. Edited by Kasanin JS, New York, WW Norton, 1964

Goodman WK, Price LH, Rasmussen SA, et al: The Yale-Brown Obsessive Compulsive Scale (Y-BOCS): Part I. Development, use, and reliability. Arch Gen Psychiatry 46:1006–1011, 1989a

Goodman WK, Price LH, Rasmussen SA, et al: The Yale-Brown Obsessive Compulsive Scale (Y-BOCS): Part II. Validity. Arch Gen Psychiatry 46:1012–1016, 1989b

Goodwin DW, Guze SB: Psychiatric Diagnosis, 4th Edition. Oxford, England, Oxford University Press, 1989

Goodwin DW, Othmer E, Halikas J, Freemon FR: Loss of short-term memory: predictor of the alcoholic "black-out." Nature 227:201–202, 1970

Greden JF, Genero N, Price HL: Agitation-increased electromyogram activity in the corrugator muscle region: a possible explanation of the "omega sign"? Am J Psychiatry 142:348–351, 1985

Griesinger W: Mental Pathology and Therapeutics (1845). Translated by Robertson CL, Rutherford J. New York, William Wood, 1882

Gunderson EK, Rahe RH (eds): Life Stress and Illness. Springfield, IL, Charles C Thomas, 1974

Gunderson JG.: Borderline Personality Disorder. Washington, DC, American Psychiatric Press, 1984

Gunderson JG, Sabo AN: The phenomenological and conceptual interface between borderline personality disorder and PTSD. Am J Psychiatry 150: 19–27, 1993

Hall RCW (ed): Psychiatric Presentations of Medical Illness. Somatopsychic Disorders. New York, Spectrum, 1980

Hamilton M: The assessment of anxiety states by rating. Br J Med Psychol 32:50–55, 1959

Hamilton M: A rating scale for depression. J Neurol Neurosurg Psychiatry 23:56–62, 1960

Health Care Financing Administration: HCFA Standard 482.61, form HCFA 1537 A, dated 4/86; Law 42 CFR, chap. IV, subchap. E, Standards and Certification. Federal Publication. Federal Register filed 10-1-1989.

Heller K, Davis J, Myers RA: The effects of interviewer style in a standardized interview. J Consult Clin Psychol 30:501–508, 1966

Helzer JE, Clayton PJ, Pambakian R, et al: Reliability of psychiatric diagnosis: II. The text/retest reliability of diagnostic classification. Arch Gen Psychiatry 34:136–141, 1977

Hersen M, Turner SM: Diagnostic Interviewing. New York, Plenum, 1985

Hill CJ: Factors influencing physician choice. Hospital and Health Services Administration 36:491–503, 1991

Hinsie LE: Concepts and Problems of Psychotherapy. New York, Columbia University Press, 1937

Holmes TH, Rahe RH: The social readjustment rating scale. J Psychosom Res 11:213–218, 1967

Hopkinson K, Cox A, Rutter M: Psychiatric interviewing techniques III. Naturalistic study: eliciting feelings. Br J Psychiatry 138:406–415, 1981

Horney K: New Ways in Psychoanalysis. New York, WW Norton, 1939

Horowitz M, Marmar C, Krupnick J, et al: Personality Styles and Brief Psychotherapy. New York, Basic Books, 1984

Isaacson RL: The limbic system, 2nd Edition. New York, Plenum, 1982

Izard C: Human Emotions. New York, Plenum, 1977

Izard C: Emotions in Personality and Psychopathology. New York, Plenum 1979

Izard CE, Ekman P, Levenson RW, et al: Autonomic nervous system activity distinguishes among emotions. Science 221:1208–1210, 1983

Jaspers K: Allgemeine Psychopathologie, 7th Edition. Translated by Hoening J, Hamilton MW. Manchester, England, Manchester University Press, 1962 (originally published 1959)

Jaspers K: General Psychopathology. Chicago, IL, University of Chicago Press, 1963

Joynt RJ (ed): Clinical Neurology, Vols 1–4, Revised Ed. Philadelphia, PA, JB Lippincott, 1992

Jung CG: Psychological Types. Princeton, NJ, Princeton University Press, 1971

Kaplan HI, Sadock BJ (eds): Comprehensive Textbook of Psychiatry/V, 5th Edition, Vols 1, 2. Baltimore, MD, Williams & Wilkins, 1989

Kasanin JS (ed): Language and Thought in Schizophrenia. New York, WW Norton, 1964

Kass F, Spitzer RL, Williams DSW, et al: Self-defeating personality disorder and DSM-III-R: development of the diagnostic criteria. Am J Psychiatry 146:1022–1026, 1989

Kent GH: E-G-Y scales. New York, Williams & Wilkins, The Psychological Corporation, 1946

Klein M: The Origins of Transference. Int J Psychoanal 33:433–438, 1952

Kleist K: Über zykloide, paranoide und epileptoide Psychosen und über die Frage der Degenerationspsychosen (On cycloid, paranoid and epileptic psychoses and on the question of degenerative psychoses). Schweiz Arch Neurol Psychiatr 23:3–37, 1928

Kluft RP: An introduction of multiple personality. Psychiatric Annals 14: 19–26, 1984

Kluft RP: The natural history of multiple personality disorder, in Childhood Antecedents of Multiple Personality. Edited by Kluft RP. Washington, DC, American Psychiatric Press, 1985, pp 197–238

Kluft RP: First-rank symptoms as a diagnostic clue to multiple personality disorder. Am J Psychiatry 144:293–298, 1987

Kluft RP, Fine CG: Clinical Perspectives on Multiple Personality Disorder. Washington, DC, American Psychiatric Press, 1993

Koenigsberg HW, Kaplan RD, Gilmore MM, et al: The relationship between syndrome and personality disorder in DSM-III: experience with 2,462 patients. Am J Psychiatry 142:207–212, 1985

Kraepelin E: Lectures on clinical psychiatry, Revised Ed. Edited by Johnstone T. New York, Hafner Press, 1968

Kretschmer E: Physique and Character: An Investigation of the Nature of Constitution and the Theory of Temperament. Translated from the second revised and enlarged edition by Sprott WJH. New York, Harcourt Brace, 1925

Leon, RL: Psychiatric Interviewing: A Primer, 2nd Edition. New York, Elsevier, 1989

Leonhard K: The Classification of Endogenous Psychoses, 5th Edition. Edited by Robins E. Translated by Berman R. Irvington, NY, Halstead Press, 1979

Lilienfeld SO, Van Valkenburg C, Larntz K, et al: The relationship of histrionic personality disorder to antisocial personality and somatization disorders. Am J Psychiatry 143:718–722, 1986

Lion JR: Personality Disorders: Diagnosis and Management (Revised for DSM-III), 2nd Edition. Baltimore, MD, Williams & Wilkins, 1981

Lovett LM, Cox A, Abou-Saley M: Teaching psychiatric interview skills to medical students. Med Educ 24:243–250, 1990

Ludwig AM: Principles of Clinical Psychiatry, 2nd Edition. New York, Free Press, 1985

Ludwig AM, Othmer E: The medical basis of psychiatry. Am J Psychiatry 134: 1087–1092, 1977

Luria AR: Higher Cortical Function in Man. New York, Basic Books, 1966

MacKinnon RA, Michels R: The Psychiatric Interview in Clinical Practice. Philadelphia, PA, WB Saunders, 1971

MacKinnon RA, Yudofsky SC: The Psychiatric Evaluation in Clinical Practice. Philadelphia, PA, JB Lippincott, 1986

McWilliams N: Understanding Character: Psychoanalytic Personality Diagnosis. New York, Guilford, 1994

Mahrer AR (ed): New Approaches to Personality Classifications. New York, Columbia University Press, 1970

Manschreck TC: Delusional (paranoid) disorders, in Comprehensive Text-book of Psychiatry, Vol 1, 5th Edition. Edited by Kaplan HI, Sadock BJ. Baltimore, MD, Williams & Wilkins, 1989

Marquis KH, Marshall J, Oskamp S: Testimony validity as a function of question form, atmosphere, and item difficulty. Journal of Applied Social Psychology 2:167–186, 1972

Masserman JH: Practice of Dynamic Psychiatry. Philadelphia, PA, WB Saunders, 1955

Mellor CS: First rank symptoms of schizophrenia. Br J Psychiatry 117:15–23, 1970

Mendel DB: On therapist-watching. Psychiatry 27:59–68, 1964

Menninger KA: A Theory of Psychoanalytical Technique. New York, Basic Books, 1958

Mesulam MM: Principles of Behavioral Neurology. Philadelphia, FA Davis, 1985

Meyer A: Psychobiology: A Science of Man. Springfield, IL, Charles C Thomas, 1957

Miller C, Swift K: The Handbook of Nonsexist Writing, 2nd Edition. New York, Harper & Row, 1988

Millon T: Disorders of Personality. DSM III: Axis II. New York, Wiley, 1981

Millon T, Klerman GL (eds): Contemporary Directions in Psychopathology: Toward the DSM-IV. New York, Guilford, 1986

Morris D: Bodywatching: A Field Guide to the Human Species. London, Grafton, 1987

Morrison JA: The First Interview. New York, Guilford, 1993

Murphy GE: Suicide in Alcoholism. New York, Oxford University Press, 1992

Othmer E, Desouza C: A rapid screening test for somatization disorder (hysteria). Am J Psychiatry 142:1146–1149, 1985

Othmer E, Othmer SC: The Clinical Interview Using DSM-IV-TR, Vol. 2: The Difficult Patient. Washington, DC, American Psychiatric Publishing, 2002

Othmer E, Penick EC, Powell BJ: The Psychiatric Diagnostic Interview: Manual. Los Angeles, CA, Western Psychological Services, 1981

Othmer E, Penick EC, Powell BJ, et al: The Psychiatric Diagnostic Interview. Revised by Penick EC. Los Angeles, CA, Western Psychological Services, 1989

Overall JE, Gorham DR: The Brief Psychiatric Rating Scale. Psychol. Rep. 10:799–812, 1962

Payne RW, Hewlett JHG: Thought disorder in psychotic patients, in Experiments in Personality, Vol 2, Psychodiagnostics and Psychodynamics. Edited by Eysenck, HJ. New York, Humanities Press, 1960

Powell BJ, Penick EC, Othmer E, et al: Prevalence of additional psychiatric syndromes among male alcoholics. J Clin Psychiatry 43:404–407, 1982

Putnam FW, Guroff JJ, Silberman EK, et al: The clinical phenomenology of multiple personality disorder: 100 recent cases. J Clin Psychol 47:285–93, 1986

Rado S: Psychoanalysis of Behavior; Collected Papers. New York, Grune & Stratton, 1956

Rank O: Will Therapy and Truth and Reality. New York, Alfred A Knopf, 1945

Reich W: Character Analysis. New York, Farrar, Straus & Young, 1949

Reitan RM, Wolfson D: The Halstead-Reitan Neuropsychological Test Battery: Theory and Clinical Interpretation. Tucson, AZ, Neuropsychology Press, 1985

Robins E: The Final Months: A Study of the Lives of 134 Persons Who Committed Suicide. New York, Oxford University Press, 1981

Rogers CR: Client-Centered Therapy. Boston, Houghton Mifflin, 1951

Rose FC, Bynum WF (eds): Historical Aspects of the Neurosciences: Festschrift for McDonald Critchley. New York, Raven, 1982

Ross ED: Disorders of higher cortical functions: diagnosis and treatment, in The Science and Practice of Clinical Medicine: Neurology, Vol 5. Edited by Rosenberg RN, Dietschy JM. New York, Grune & Stratton, 1980

Ross ED: The divided self: contrary to conventional wisdom, not all language is commanded by the brain's left side. The Sciences 22:8–12, 1982

Rosvold HE, Mirsky AF, Sarasow E, et al: A continuous performance test of brain damage. J Clin Consult Psychol 20:343–350, 1956

Royall DR, Mahurin RK, Gray KF: Bedside assessment of executive cognitive impairment: the Executive Interview. J Am Geriatr Soc 40:1221–1226, 1992

Royall DR, Mahurin RK, Cornell J, et al: Bedside assessment of dementia type using the Qualitative Evaluation of Dementia. Neuropsychiatry Neuropsychol Behav Neurol 6:235–244, 1993

Royall DR, Mahurin RK, Cornell J: Bedside assessment of frontal degeneration: distinguishing Alzheimer's disease from non-Alzheimer's cortical dementia. Exp Aging Res 20:95–103, 1994

Rutter M, Cox A: Psychiatric interviewing techniques: I. Methods and measures. Br J Psychiatry 138:273–282, 1981

Rutter M, Cox A, Egert S, et al: Psychiatric interviewing techniques: IV. Experimental study: four contrasting styles. Br J Psychiatry 138:456–465, 1981

Sandifer MG Jr: Psychiatric diagnosis: cross-national research findings. Proc Royal Soc Med 65:1–4, 1972

Sandifer MG Jr, Hordern A, Green, LM: The psychiatric interview: the impact of the first three minutes. Am J Psychiatry 126:968–973, 1970

Schneider K: Clinical Psychopathology. Translated by Hamilton, MW. New York, Grune & Stratton, 1959

Shea SC: Psychiatric Interviewing: The Art of Understanding. Philadelphia, PA, WB Saunders, 1988

Sheehan DV: The Anxiety Disease. New York, Scribner's, 1983

Sheldon WH, Stevens SS: The varieties of temperament: a psychology of constitutional differences. New York, Harper, 1942

Siegman AW, Pope B (eds): Studies in Dyadic Communication. New York, Pergamon, 1972

Simms A: Symptoms in the Mind. London, Balliere Tindall, 1988

Smith A: The serial sevens substraction test. Arch Neurol 17:78–80, 1967

Smith A: Neuropsychological testing in neurological disorders, in Advances in Neurology, Vol 7. Edited by Friedlander WJ. New York, Raven, 1975

Snaith RP, Harrop FM, Newby DA, et al: Grade scores of the Montgomery-Asberg depression and the clinical anxiety scales. Br J Psychiatry 148: 599–601, 1986

Sno HN, Linszen D: The déjà vu experience: remembrance of things past? Am J Psychiatry 147:1587–1595, 1990

Southwick SM, Yehuda R, Giller EL: Personality disorders in treatment-seeking combat veterans with posttraumatic stress disorder. Am J Psychiatry 150:1020–1023, 1993

Spitzer RL, Williams JBW, Kass F, et al: National field trial of the DSM-III-R diagnostic criteria for self-defeating personality disorder. Am J Psychiatry 146:1561–1567, 1989

Spreen O, Benton AL: Neurosensory center comprehensive examination for aphasia. Victoria, BC, Canada, Neuropsychology Laboratory, Department of Psychology, University of Victoria, 1969

Strub RL, Black FW: The Mental Status Examination in Neurology, 3rd Edition. Philadelphia, PA, FA Davis, 1993

Sullivan HS: The Psychiatric Interview. New York, WW Norton, 1954

Taylor MA: The Neuropsychiatric Mental Status Examination. New York, SP Medical & Scientific Books, 1981

Taylor MA: The Neuropsychiatric Guide to Modern Everyday Psychiatry. New York, Free Press, 1993

Taylor MA, Abrams R: The phenomenology of mania: a new look at some old patients. Arch Gen Psychiatry 29:520–522, 1973

Thaker G, Adami H, Moran M, et al: Psychiatric illness in families of subjects with schizophrenia-spectrum personality disorders: high morbidity risks for unspecified functional psychoses and schizophrenia. Am J Psychiatry 150:66–71, 1993

Truax CB, Mitchell KM: Research on certain therapist interpersonal skills in relation to process and outcome, in Handbook of Psychotherapy and Behavior Change. Edited by Bojin AE, Garfield SL. New York, Wiley, 1971

Vaillant GE: Empirical Studies of Ego Mechanisms of Defense. Washington, DC, American Psychiatric Press, 1986

Vaillant GE, Perry CJ: Personality disorders, in Comprehensive Textbook of Psychiatry, 4th Edition. Edited by Kaplan HI, Sadock BJ. Baltimore, MD, Williams & Wilkins, 1985

van Riezen H, Segal M: Comparative Evaluation of Rating Scales for Clinical Psychopharmacology. Amsterdam, Elsevier, 1988

Warnock JK: Tips on taking the psychiatry and neurology oral exam. Resident and Staff Physician May 15:121–123, 1991

Wechsler D: Wechsler Adult Intelligence Scale—Revised. San Antonio, TX, Psychological Corporation, 1981

Weinberg H, Hire WA: Abnormal Personalities: A Book of Case Readings. New York, MSS Information Corporation, 1992

Weintraub S, Mesulam MM: Mental state assessment of young and elderly adults in behavioral neurology, in Principles of Behavioral Neurology. Edited by Mesulam MM. Philadelphia, PA, FA Davis, 1985

Wender PH, Kety SS, Rosenthal D, et al: Psychiatric disorders in the biological and adoptive families of adopted individuals with affective disorders. Arch Gen Psychiatry 43:923–929, 1986

Wilbur CB: Multiple personality and child abuse. Psychiatr Clin North Am 7:3–7, 1984

Wilson IC: Rapid Approximate Intelligence Test. Am J Psychiatry 123:1289–1290, 1967

Winokur G, Crowe RR: Personality disorders, in Comprehensive Textbook of Psychiatry, Vol 2, 2nd Edition. Edited by Freedman AM, Kaplan HI, Sadock BJ. Baltimore, MD, Williams & Wilkins, 1975

Wolberg LR: The Techniques of Psychotherapy, 2nd Edition. New York, Grune & Stratton, 1967

Young GB, McGlone J: Cerebral localization, in Clinical Neurology, Vol 1, Revised Edition. Edited by Joynt RJ. Philadelphia, PA, JB Lippincott, 1992

Young RC, Biggs JT, Ziegler VE, et al: A rating scale for mania: reliability, validity and sensitivity. Br J Psychiatry 133:429–435, 1978

Zarin DA, Earls F: Diagnostic decision making in psychiatry. Am J Psychiatry 150:197–206, 1993

Zimmerman M, Pfohl B, Stangi D, et al: The validity of DSM-III Axis IV (severity of psychosocial stressors). Am J Psychiatry 142:1437–1441, 1985

Zuckerman M: Sensation seeking, in Dimensions of Personality. Edited by London H, Exner J. New York, Wiley, 1978

Zung WWK: How normal is depression? Psychosomatics 13:174–178, 1972

INDEX

Page numbers printed in **boldface** *type refer to tables or figures.*